Voluntary Servitude. Masochism And Morality

Le Soldat's *Voluntary Servitude. Masochism and Morality* presents an extraordinary analysis of masochism, the subject, death drive, and sexual discourse inspired by Freudian drive theory, philosophy, gender theory, political science, and mythology.

This book will certainly evoke the reader's curiosity, but even more than that it will encourage readers' critical reflection on the clandestine defensive formations between the psyche and reality that, in the author's view, obscure pleasure principle by corrupting the death drive and the body. Le Soldat presents an unprecedented formulation in psychoanalytic literature to date, one of incomparable significance not only for our clinical work but also for critical theoretical reflection on society and its vicissitudes. As a result of their defensive stances, we encounter 'masochistic subjects of servitude' enclosed in a world of wars, economical rivalries, regressive brutality of consumerism, religious dependency, and political mania.

Drawing on the work of Freud and Adorno, and balancing theoretical and clinical material, this is essential reading for psychoanalysts, psychotherapists, and anyone who seeks to understand the concept of voluntary servitude.

Judith Le Soldat (1947–2008) was a Swiss psychoanalyst, researcher, lecturer and author. She was born in Budapest and lived in Zurich, where she studied psychology and ran her own psychoanalytic practice from 1974. Her first monograph *Voluntary Servitude. Masochism and Morality* was published in 1989. In her second monograph (1994), she presented an exciting, completely new understanding of Oedipal conflicts (see the critical edition of the book published in 2020 under the title *Raubmord und Verrat - Robbery murder and betrayal*). She worked on a third monograph on male homosexuality, but left it unfinished. The book was published posthumously in 2018 under the title *Land of No Return*. The lectures Judith Le Soldat gave at the University of Zurich in 2006/07 were also published posthumously. They appeared as the first volume of Le Soldat's *Collected Works* in 2015 under the title *Grund zur Homosexualität* (Grounds for Homosexuality). *Grounds for Homosexuality* contains an introduction to both her theory of the Oedipal Conflicts and her theory of homosexuality and is therefore well suited as an introduction to her entire oeuvre. - Further publications by Judith Le Soldat, in German, s. www.lesoldat.ch

Voluntary Servitude. Masochism and Morality

Judith Le Soldat

Edited with a prologue by Andjela Samardzic, Vaia Tsolas and Michael Civin based on the critical edition by Monika Gsell

Introduction by Monika Gsell and Ralf Binswanger

Translated by Nils F. Schott

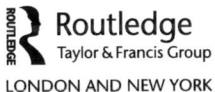
LONDON AND NEW YORK

Designed cover image: © Getty Images

First published in English 2025
by Routledge
605 Third Avenue, New York, NY 10158

and by Routledge
4 Park Square, Milton Park, Abingdon, Oxon, OX14 4RN

Routledge is an imprint of the Taylor & Francis Group, an informa business

© 2025 Frommann-Holzboog-Verlag

The right of Judith Le Soldat to be identified as author of this work; The right of Andjela Samardzic, Vaia Tsolas and Michael Civin to be identified as the authors of the editorial material has been asserted in accordance with sections 77 and 78 of the Copyright, Designs and Patents Act 1988.

Translated by Nils F. Schott

Introduction and preliminary material by Monika Gsell and Ralf Binswanger

All rights reserved. No part of this book may be reprinted or reproduced or utilised in any form or by any electronic, mechanical, or other means, now known or hereafter invented, including photocopying and recording, or in any information storage or retrieval system, without permission in writing from the publishers.

Trademark notice: Product or corporate names may be trademarks or registered trademarks and are used only for identification and explanation without intent to infringe.

Originally published in German as: Judith Le Soldat: Freiwillige Knechtschaft. Kritisch ediert, bearbeitet und kommentiert von Monika Gsell. Mit einer Einleitung von Monika Gsell und Ralf Binswanger.

© frommann-holzboog Verlag e.K. - Eckhart Holzboog 2021

Library of Congress Cataloging-in-Publication Data
Names: Le Soldat, Judith, author. | Samardzic, Andjela, 1986– editor. | Tsolas, Vaia, editor. | Civin, Michael A., editor.
Title: Voluntary servitude: masochism and morality / Judith Le Soldat; edited with a prologue by Andjela Samardzic, Vaia Tsolas and Michael Civin based on the critical edition by Monika Gsell; introduction by Monkia Gsell and Ralf Binswanger; translated by Nils F. Schott.
Other titles: Freiwillige Knechtschaft.
English Description: New York, NY: Routledge, 2025. |
Includes bibliographical references and index. |
Identifiers: LCCN 2024032309 (print) | LCCN 2024032310 (ebook) |
ISBN 9781032666235 (hardback) | ISBN 9781032666259 (paperback) |
ISBN 9781032666273 (ebook)
Subjects: LCSH: Masochism.
Classification: LCC RC553.M36 L413 2025 (print) |
LCC RC553.M36 (ebook) | DDC 616.85/835—dc23/eng/20241104
LC record available at https://lccn.loc.gov/2024032309
LC ebook record available at https://lccn.loc.gov/2024032310

ISBN: 9781032666235 (hbk)
ISBN: 9781032666259 (pbk)
ISBN: 9781032666273 (ebk)

DOI: 10.4324/9781032666273

Typeset in Optima
by codeMantra

Contents

About the editors and contributors   *viii*
Prologue   *ix*
ANDJELA SAMARDZIC, VAIA TSOLAS, AND MICHAEL CIVIN

Introduction to the Critical German Edition by Monika Gsell	1
About this volume	2
Judith Le Soldat on her masochism book–a document from the posthumous papers	5
On the two trains of thought in the masochism book MONIKA GSELL AND RALF BINSWANGER	10
On the genesis of the masochism book	47
Acknowledgments	49

I
Pulsional demand and wish fulfillment   51

1 Disentangling aggression and sexuality	53
2 The identification with the aggressor is not happening	60
3 Remarkable alliances	65
4 A "mishap" in Germany	80

5	Three lessons from an objective triumph	84
6	On the necessity of lying	90
7	The ability to remain silent and the task of theory	96
8	A disarming contradiction	103
9	From sadism to the death drive	109

II
The economy of excitation 127

1	The Drummer's dream	129
2	A female rescue phantasy	135
3	The physicist's dog	139
4	Somebody's late	143
5	The diagnostic dilemma	146
6	Two paths to masochism	151
7	Voluntary servitude	158
8	The search for the "subjective factor"	162
9	A little parapraxis	166
10	On the utilization of pulsional energy	171
11	Aggression, the difference between the sexes, and infantile neurosis	176
12	The principle of the death drive	191
13	Masturbation technique and anxiety signal	200

III
Masochistic pleasure 215

1 A contribution to decreasing tension 217

2 Pleasure and duration 226

3 The object of identification 230

4 A forgotten cultural achievement 240

5 Splendor and misery of the superego 250

6 Who's afraid of castration? 265

7 Unavoidable pain 279

*Appendix: Two unpublished prefaces from the first
version of* Voluntary Servitude 289
   Preface I: A Warning 289
   Preface II: An Explanation 289
Bibliography 291
Index 307

About the editors and contributors

Ralf Binswanger is a Psychoanalyst and Psychiatrist in private practice in Zurich. He has published on drive, sexuality, and gender, and on the psychoanalytic understanding of dreams.

Michael Civin is Co-founder and Trustee of the Pulsion Psychoanalytic Institute and co-founder and Vice-President of Rose Hill Psychological Services. He has authored many papers and book chapters and is also a psychologist and psychoanalyst in private practice in New York.

Monika Gsell is a Psychoanalyst and works in private practice in Zurich. She is the editor of Judith Le Soldat's Collected Works (in German).

Andjela Samardzic is a Psychoanalyst and Clinical Psychologist working in private practice in New York and Zurich (Switzerland) and a board member of the Pulsion Psychoanalytic Institute. She has published on many subjects including historical trauma, masochism, jouissance, and psyche-soma phenomena.

Vaia Tsolas is Co-founder, President, and Director of the Pulsion Psychoanalytic Institute, Supervising and Training Analyst at Columbia Psychoanalytic and Assistant Clinical Professor of Psychiatry at Albert Einstein College of Medicine. She is an author and editor of many psychoanalytic books.

Prologue

Andjela Samardzic, Vaia Tsolas, and Michael Civin

Yet all joy wants eternity.[1]

Our century is marked by innumerable discontents: wars, imploding democracies, ecological catastrophes, individualism versus community,[2] virtuality and avatarism versus body, and excess versus thought. These echo ethical concerns, malaises, and jouissances that demand attention.

Might we characterize Western society to have reached a capitalist impasse, where pleasure is insistently exhibited before us, where clones in the clouds configure our desires? What more could we possibly desire in a supply side economy of desire? In *The Interpretation of Dreams*, Freud notes that "nothing but a wish can set our mental apparatus working." The dream is a wish fulfillment.[3] However, in the contemporary era, we can begin to foresee a metaverse of elective, perfectionistic group avatarism in which omnipotence and omnipresence override our ideals threatening what it really means to be human. Dreaming gives sway to concrete thinking and discharges through action as one of the main solutions to drive overload.

In their most recent book, *A Psychoanalytic Exploration of the Contemporary Search for Pleasure: The Turning of the Screw,* Vaia Tsolas and Christine Anzieu-Premmereur tackle a contemporary problematic of pleasure echoed in addictions, somatizations, mechanical thinking, and disaffection to avoid pain and thought.[4] In keeping with Freud's theory of libido, contemporary pleasure structurally foregrounds a short-circuiting of the drives, a disavowal of vulnerability and limits, of passivity, of the sexual difference, of the feminine.[5]

In the new era of clicks, the cogito deteriorates into a new lalangue and a new jouissance. Freud cautioned us that the issue at hand is an economic one.[6] In keeping with Fechner's law of constancy, Freud initially formulated the pleasure principle as a homeostasis-seeking principle.[7] Consequently, in the Laplanche and Pontalis dictionary, the pleasure principle is defined as avoiding of unpleasure.[8] However, in *Beyond the Pleasure Principle*, Freud further develops the idea that an explanation is needed to explain why humans, given the pleasure principle, would repeat phenomena that result in seeking unpleasure (e.g., the *fort/da* game).[9] Earlier, for example in *Three Essays on the Theory of Sexuality,* he approached this problematic by developing the notion of the partial drives and partial drive satisfaction.[10] However, in view of the ubiquity of phenomena that stretched the limits of this explanation beyond the plausible, prominently the massive violence of World War I, he reasoned that there must be another psychical force at play. The introduction of the death drive proved to be the answer, a drive seeking death and destruction articulated in the repetition compulsion, aggression, war-like destructiveness, self-harm, etc. Lacan arrives at the concept of jouissance as the beyond, the surplus, the excess that escapes constancy and torpedoes it.[11]

In this new edition of *Freiwillige Knechtschaft: Masochismus und Moral,* Le Soldat examines pleasure and its vicissitudes, a jouissance echoed in the malaise of her time, masochism: "I observed that masochism, sadism, longing for death are topics of our time, the way, for instance, that sexuality and its suppression, hypocrisy, and defense against the drives were the issues at the turn of the century" (#7).

We feel a striking similarity three decades later, especially in how sexuality and the drives are received. A serious dedication to and examination of pulsional desires has been absent from psychoanalytic literature under the guise of obsolescence of the drives, while the hyper-focusing on "ego-driven" subjectivity, and, as an offshoot of British Object Relations theory, concretist interpersonal relations, and identities has been in vogue. Le Soldat's theory is reminiscent of Freud's metapsychology in his meticulous, archeological quest for the plague from within, the uncanny, the abject,[12] and the unconscious.

The enigma of masochism, be it sexual perversion in the taking partial-drive-pleasure in suffering (as it was initially conceived by Freud in the *Three Essays*) or be it as the guardian of life[13] in the binding the drives, has fascinated psychoanalysis and other social sciences for centuries. In the "Economic Problem of Masochism," Freud developed three forms of masochism, erotogenic, feminine, and moral masochism. Erotogenic masochism, foundational to all forms of masochism comes into play when a quantity of the death drive is not cathected to objects, but rather remains internalized and "with the help of the accompanying sexual excitation ... becomes libidinally bound there."[14] Primary erotogenic masochism, e.g., the satisfaction of the death drive the infant achieves in waiting for the reappearance of the breast. While primary erotic masochism, thus, is a function of the infant's anticipation of the part object (the breast), secondary masochism occurs when the subject withdraws a quantity of the death drive from the object and turns it toward the ego. In moral masochism, also referred to as secondary masochism, masochism has "loosened its ties with what we recognize as sexuality." While the other forms of masochism "emanate from the loved person and shall be endured at his command," in moral masochism the relationship to the object is dropped in favor of suffering *qua* suffering.[15] In feminine masochism, the "manifest content is of being gagged, bound, painfully beaten, whipped, in some way mal-treated, forced into unconditional obedience, dirtied and debased." These actions of the subject signify "being castrated, copulated with, or giving birth to a baby."[16]

Freud's focus on masochism, however, never ceased throughout his work.

According to Laplanche and Pontalis, Freud investigated the link between moral masochism and the need for punishment, unconscious sense of guilt, and negative therapeutic reactions. He had reservations, however, about the term "unconscious sense of guilt" and believed that "need for punishment" was a more appropriate term. He explained self-punishing behavior as a tension between a demanding super-ego and the ego. The term "need for punishment" highlights the driving force behind certain individuals' desire to suffer and the paradoxical satisfaction they derive from it. Freud distinguishes between individuals who exhibit excessive moral inhibition and those who engage in moral masochism. The former emphasizes the heightened sadism of the super-ego, while the latter focuses on the ego's own masochism. However, Freud argues that the sadism of the super-ego and the ego's masochism cannot be simply seen as opposing forces. In his work "Analysis Terminable and Interminable," Freud suggests that the need for punishment, as an expression of the death instinct, cannot be fully explained by the conflict between the super-ego and the ego. He proposes that other portions of the death drive may be at work in unspecified places.[17]

The Paris psychosomatic school many decades later elaborated on the enigma of masochism in the work with somatic patients. In her further elaboration of Fain's ideas, Marilia Aisenstein's work proves crucial on the consequences of incomplete primary masochism due to early traumatic situations, for the soma-psyche unity rendering the protective aspects of masochism of the binding of the drives inaccessible. In her view, the insufficient masochism fails to provide the psyche with its guardian aspect leading to the death drive surge unbound and destructive. It is an anti-traumatic defense of leaning toward discharge and behavioral solutions that make tolerating passivity difficult with an overvaluing of activity that infiltrates the ego-ideal with phallic narcissism. In consequence, what motivates the subject, therefore we might say simply, is an overly inflated phallic ego ideal instead of the protective postoedipal superego. This tyrannical ego ideal does not tolerate weaknesses and human vulnerabilities but rather seeks perfections in the black and white logic of the ideal of the inhuman. An authoritarian ego ideal is prone to seek external figures of authoritarian power to unite, identify and follow. In her article on "the destruction of thought processes," Aisenstein goes even a step further when she says that the desexualized cultural superego and the regression of the superego to the ego-ideal are insufficient to explain the pull to masochistically submit and blindly follow authoritarian destructive figures unless we see the unbound death drive energy in connection to an irreparable rift in the ego.[18]

xii   *Prologue*

Le Soldat builds on Freud's Papers on Metapsychology and Other Works (1914–1916 notion of masochism as a particular vicissitude of aggression and proposes a revision of the pulsional aggression, of the part of the sexual pair libido-aggressiveness that has particularly been prone to social amnesia, and as such particularly individually and socially virulent.[19] Freud remarks:

> I know that in sadism and masochism, we have always seen before us manifestations of the destructive instinct (directed outwards and inwards), strongly alloyed with erotism, but I can no longer understand how we can have overlooked the ubiquity of non-erotic aggressiveness and destructiveness and can have failed to give it its due place in our interpretation of life. … I remember my defensive attitude when the idea of an instinct of destruction first emerged in psychoanalytic literature and how long it took before I became receptive to it. That others should have shown, and still show, the same attitude of rejection surprises me less … The Devil would be the best way out as an excuse for God.[20]

In La Boetie's *Discourse de le servitude volontaire* (1577), echoing Aristotle, the intricate relationship between aggressiveness and social order of dominion is illuminated.

> It is unbelievable how people, once they are subjected, fall so quickly into such a deep forgetfulness of freedom that it is impossible for them to reawaken and regain it. They serve so freely and so willingly that you would say to see them that they had not lost their liberty but won their servitude.[21]

In this book, Le Soldat elucidates the phenomenon of servitude as a psychic phenomenon, a symptom that articulates aggressive vicissitudes as they become socially corrupted. In her words: "The interests of dominion require the pure gold of sexualized aggression" (#258).

In three parts, Le Soldat lays out the fundamentals of masochism, death drive, and pleasure in an unprecedentedly precise manner.

Part I: *Pulsional demand and wish fulfillment*

In her first part, the author elucidates the etiology of masochism, foregrounding a disentanglement (unbinding) of the drives of libido and aggression in favor of aggression.

Le Soldat notes that under certain internal and societal conditions, the ego becomes more "permeable" (#352) and manipulable, such that the already loose binding of libido and aggression becomes even more compromised in favor of aggression. She references Jörg Friedrich's study of post-war Germany that describes how pulsional aggressive energies found entry into the jurisprudence of the Federal Republic, resulting in the legalization of Nazi crimes.[22] The author argues that this is not a parapraxis, not a faux pas, but rather a dialectic between drives and culture, conscience, and reality.

Jacoby, in his *Social Amnesia: A Critique of Contemporary Psychology*, argues:

> This overpowering by a brutal reality ... is to be overcome, at least in thought and theory, before subjectivity can be realized ... Before the individual can exist, before it can become an individual, it must recognize to what extent it does not yet exist. It must shed the illusion of the individual before becoming one.[23]

Building on Jacoby, Le Soldat pleads for psychoanalysis with a "social place"[24] that operates as a critical theory of the subject as it initiates thinking.

Of particular note, as a point of connection with the ideas that Le Soldat presents in this part, is *Eros et Antéros*.[25] The authors argue that Thanatos does not stand in direct opposition to Eros, but rather, that position is best occupied by Anteros. Eros and Anteros are siblings (sometimes described as twins and other times as playmates). Similarly, their parents may be Poros (expediency) and Penia (poverty), Ares and Aphrodite, or Poseidon and Nerites. Eros has an insatiable hunger for his object. No barrier set between them can be strong enough to thwart his quest. The search is endless and frenzied. Anteros, "counter eros" from the Greek, is the god of requited love and, as such, divine satisfaction and satiety. For Fain and Braunschweig, the role of the death drive constitutes the radical antagonism between the two. The Nirvana of the death drive is anathema to both Eros and Anteros. For Eros, the anxiety laden, frenzied quest for the object unbinds itself from the cold calm of death, whereas Anteros, satisfied by the incorporation of the object, cannot tolerate any anxiety that might come with aggression. For Eros, there is a total triumph of object libido and annihilation of Nirvana while for Anteros there is a triumph of ego libido and a whole-cloth embracing of Nirvana. Eros discards aggression and Ateros displaces it, preferring the unchallenged satisfaction that can only come from the pleasure of being part of a group under the aegis of an authoritarian leader. "Thus, in a very interesting shift of orientation, the division between masculine and feminine is replaced by two currents of sexuality: one arising from infantile sexuality and fixed on Oedipal objects, the other distributed and refracted between hetero and homosexual group cathexes."[26]

Another argument of the book is that subtle processes of internal and external resistances, disavowals, amnesias, and thinking prohibitions are at play in resisting and obfuscating any insight that might serve to facilitate separation from the cult-like Nirvana of voluntary servitude. These processes echo fundamental individual and cultural resistances against the limit, a foundational anxiety, and aggression-free passivity inherent in limitless primary erotogenic masochism.

Part II: *The economy of excitation*

Via three clinical vignettes, Le Soldat illustrates the binding and unbinding processes of the drives with their corresponding symptoms and vicissitudes unfolding in a dynamic of servitude and disavowal of sexual difference.

1 An early aggressive inundation of the ego over time is assumed to be an important factor for masochistic development. Unbinding of aggression and libido in service of aggression leads to the waning of the drive tension associated with ambivalence, a tension that is the *sine qua non* of pleasure. The masochistic ego emerges as "uncooperative and unyielding," the superego as "vicious and full of hatred" (#81).

The fantasies about sexual differences evocative of the existential lack[27] draw aggressive fantasies causing guilt, shame, and ridicule. As a result, resistance to sexual differences leads to defensive constructions of exogenous power and submission.

As Le Soldat poignantly articulates:

> Beside the disentanglement of sexuality and aggression, a new divergence arises between *aggressive phallic wishes* that must be projected and are *idealized* in the object, and the *passive sexual wishes* bound in one's own body. The latter are the target of the remainder of aggression that cannot be projected and takes the form of *debasement and mockery (#242)*.

A further problematic of the masochistic structure, as Le Soldat argues, is masturbation. "Patients conceal their intimate actions like a secret treasure" (#232) since those are reminiscent of aggressive cathexes and subsequent pulsional anxieties.

2 Further addressed in this part is the classical association between masochism and death drive.

In usual cases, pulsional tension is formed in the ego to build structures and thus protect itself from the quanta of the pulsional energies by the id. The ego now seeks physical satisfaction as another means of fulfilling its pulsional desires.

In her abundant clinical observations, Le Soldat arrives at the conclusion that the death drive is destructive only by human projections. It represents a cessation of the life functions, precisely of the pulsional strivings in the Id.

Prologue xv

As a result of the waning pulsional demand from the id, the ego is compelled to dissolve its structures and employ aggressive hypercathexes.

Le Soldat furthermore engages with the question of pulsional temporality and argues that:

> the destruction of ego structures and the fluctuation of the pulsional pressure are everyday phenomena that are intensified and extended at the moment of biological death by the cessation of the somatic pulsional source and, second, that psychical death cannot be considered the consequence of aggressive pulsional strivings (#230).

Hence, there is no correlation between masochism and death drive. She formulates a more poignant definition of death drive in Part III.

3   Building on de La Boétie's *Discours de la servitude volontaire*, Le Soldat elucidates socio-political dynamics involved in voluntary servitude: "the majority of the pulsional energies that are not bound, not invested in the defense, unsatisfied, is ready to be socially utilized. ... In a system of dominion, the individual-psychical energy joins the means of production capital, land, and labor on equal footing" (#198).

Le Soldat building on Adorno[28] cautions against social amnesia, disavowals, and the "subjective factor" (#117) of shame and passive desires that hinder emancipation and liberation. Freud relates resistance to analytic cure to these dynamics.[29]

Part III: *Masochistic pleasure*

In this part, the author synthesizes the book's main topics, the drives, masochism, pleasure, and death drive.

Pleasure

It is the Faustian plea for eternal pleasure at the price of infinite servitude that is constitutive of masochistic pleasure. Le Soldat contends that pulsional satisfactions are possible; however, "instead of being particularly pleasurable—since they are relieved of the sense of guilt—they become rather unexciting." The masochist thus aims to synchronize somatic processes and fantasies via pain. In one of her vignettes, the analysand forms physical tension through pain stimuli that imitate the rhythmical course of a libidinal wish (#262). "In this way, the ritual completes somatically what the neurosis has torn apart psychically" (#336).

The masochistic taboo, however, often suspends this physical excitement, its instrument of pleasure. The masochistic perverse ritual is now cathected with anxiety, guilt, and shame that attenuate the already strained quality of pleasure. Psychoanalysis, as Le Soldat argues, must intervene at this impasse of the masochistic ritual. Its intervention must spur a mnemic fantasy of sexual excitation that is intertwined with the strife concerning infantile masturbation and aggression, ultimately resulting in the resolution of the oedipal crisis. She argues: "A therapy that boasts to have 'cured' masochistic symptoms was not therapy; in masochism, the perversion is an indispensable part of sexuality" (#338).

Socio-political intricacies

The author postulates the waning of Eros on the one hand and the rise of destruction and aggression on the other as a consequence of socio-political forces. She states: "The absence of ambivalence tension … that is, the loss of pleasurable equivocalness in favor of two divergent strivings, points to a socially produced disavowal, a 'forgetting'" (#435). This forgetting is echoed in the rise of belligerence, economic rivalry, obsessive consumption, political and religious obsessions, and dependencies over the past decades.

Death drive

> In keeping with Freud's theory, I see in the death drive the antagonist of the sexual drives. Yet I do not oppose libido and destructiveness to each other but conceive of aggressive and libidinous strivings as usually inseparable components of the sexual drive, which in turn is subject to the pleasure principle and the death pulsional principle simultaneously. In this way, the death "drive" is really a pulsional antagonist (#270).

The death drive rather "sets a meter or rhythm of the flow of pulsional energy" (#266) and thus generates "*a rhythmic, staccato-like course of the cathexis* in all pulsional processes" (#268). Hence, "the 'death drive' is not a dynamic drive but rather an axiom or basic law of the psyche" (#266).

Diminishing ambivalence tension in favor of sociopolitical power is thus yet another operation of the death drive, concludes the author.

Identifications

The masochistic ego introduced by Freud in *Mourning and Melancholia* identifies with the lost love object, hence it disavows the work of mourning.[30]

Le Soldat adds: "the internalization of the female phallus counts as insurance against the consequences of castration" (#282).

Masturbation, on the other hand, reignites aggressive cathexes and is thus to be sanctioned: "the taboo strikes all of autoeroticism" (#300). The authority of the superego that imposes sanctions is both strict and inadequate at the same time. Its deficiency lies in overwhelming quanta of aggressive pulsional energies that it succumbs to. This insufficiency ultimately renders "masochists all the more susceptible to external threats" (#342).

To conclude

Le Soldat argues that the masochistic problematic is that of pulsional, economic nature associated with a deficient binding of the drives, relatively diminished masturbation fantasies with insufficient sensorial and bodily pleasure, as well as with disavowal of the sexual difference as a consequence of castration threat. Like Marilia Aisenstein, Michel Fain, Beno Rosenberg, and others (see above) the author pleads to rehabilitate masochism against cultural (as well as individual) defamation.

Another argument of the book is that subtle processes of internal and external resistances, disavowals, amnesias, and thinking prohibitions are at play in resisting and obfuscating any insight that might serve to facilitate separation from the cult-like Nirvana of voluntary servitude. These processes echo fundamental individual and cultural resistances against the limit, a foundational anxiety, and aggression-free passivity inherent in limitless primary erotogenic masochism.

Marilia Aisenstein also emphasizes "the crucial importance of the need to accept passivity and of being able to find pleasure in anticipation of gratification or substitute gratifications (for instance, art, research, thought) in the face of increasing tension."[31] Accepting passivity would mean to accept the essential fluctuations of the life-death rhythm echoed in the death drive. Eros and Anteros function in a dynamically equilibrated tension, the rhythms of life and death in the perpetual anxieties of binding excitement and calm.

Like Goethe's Faust, humankind must ultimately succumb to this law of the psyche by relinquishing the imperative of endless jouissance. In *Civilization and Its Discontents*, Freud stresses that it is by a fusion (binding) of Eros and Ananke (for Fain Anteros), by the rhythm of the drives and exigencies of reality, that a civilization unfolds in "uniting separate individuals into a community bound together by libidinal ties."[32]

Notes

1 Nietzsche (1883–1885) 2006, IV.12: 264.
2 See Ottmann 1977.
3 Freud 1900, SE 5, 567.
4 Tsolas and Anzieu-Premmereur 2023.
5 See Lichtenstein 2019, Schaeffer 2018, and Aloupis 2017.
6 Freud 1895.
7 Freud 1900.
8 Laplanche and Pontalis (1967) 1973.
9 Freud 1920.
10 Freud 1905a.
11 Lacan (1959–1960) 1992.
12 Kristeva (1980) 1982.

xviii *Prologue*

13 Aisenstein 2022.
14 Freud 1924a, 163–64.
15 Freud 1924a, 167.
16 Freud 1924a, 162.
17 Freud 1937.
18 See Aisenstein 2014.
19 See Freud 1924a and Jacoby 1975.
20 Freud 1930, 119–21.
21 La Boétie (1574) 2012, 13.
22 See Friedrich (1984) 1994.
23 Jacoby 1975, 81.
24 Bernfeld (1929) 1996.
25 Braunschweig and Fain 1971.
26 Aisenstein 2018, ##.
27 Kierkegaard (1843) 1983.
28 See Adorno (1969) 2005a, 251.
29 Freud 1937.
30 Freud 1916.
31 Aisenstein 2022, 8.
32 Freud 1930, 139.

Introduction to the Critical German Edition by Monika Gsell

About this volume

This book is a translation of the fourth volume of the collected works of Judith Le Soldat, a new edition of *Freiwillige Knechtschaft: Masochismus und Moral* of 1989. The masochism book—as we will call it from here on out—was not just Le Soldat's first *published* monograph; on the level of *content*, too, it may be called her "early work." In this book, she develops a conception of masochism that is very much her own—one at odds with all previous psychoanalytic conceptions, and one that evades any alignment with Freud's well-known distinction between erogenous, feminine, and moral masochism. Le Soldat conceives of masochism as a neurosis, more precisely as a *special case of the oedipal development*.[1] It is a special case because both the initial conditions of the oedipal development and, subsequently, the conflicts, the defense formations, and the unfolding of the "masochistic" oedipal development deviate from what the classic theory leads us to expect.

Beginning with the second part of the book at the latest, however, those familiar with Le Soldat's later work will note that much of what she conceives here as a special case of the oedipal development will turn out to be the foundation and keystone of her new, general theory of the oedipal development already in the next book she published, the *Theory of Human Unhappiness* (*Theorie menschlichen Unglücks*, 1994).[2] A close reading of the volume, moreover, shows those parts of the masochism concept that did not find a place in the new Oedipus theory to merge with the special cases she conceptualizes later of the *postoedipal* stage of development, where they are further elaborated.[3]

That is why, strictly speaking, not much will be left of the concept of masochism developed in the present volume: *as a concept* of masochism, it disappears unwept and unsung or silently merges with her later work.[4]

This does not mean, though, that the masochism book has lost its significance—on the contrary: when we read this work against the background of Le Soldat's later theories, we have the impression of discovering a new archaeological layer. At first, we do not quite know how it relates to the layers we are already familiar with—until we place some "pieces" that initially seem nondescript, meaningless, or incomprehensible side by side and suddenly realize that what we have there will probably prove to be of great significance in understanding Le Soldat's work as a whole. Significant in (at least) two respects: on the one hand, the masochism book allows for tracing, with more precision than before, the genesis of Le Soldat's distinct contribution to advancing psychoanalytic theory and thereby allows both for better understanding of its content and for better situating it within the history of theory. On the other hand, the significance of the masochism book in our view is that it offers a wealth of clues for a better assessment of the structure and systematic orientation of the *unwritten* part of the theoretical edifice Le Soldat communicated only in conversation.

A detailed elaboration of our ideas about the form in which Le Soldat's later theories, both published and transmitted orally, are already prefigured in the present work must wait for a separate study. When we nonetheless present the nuclei of the later theories in the first part of our introduction, we do so for *one* reason in particular: as we will show in a number of instances, they can aid in finding our way among the imprecisions and contradictions of Le Soldat's conceptual work in the masochism book. The second part of the introduction is devoted to Le Soldat's engagement with sociopolitical issues and the question of how psychoanalysis and social theory relate to each other. These are issues that hardly ever come up in her later work.

Before we present our own reflections on the masochism book, however, we would like to let Le Soldat herself speak. Among her posthumous papers, there is a typescript of some seven pages in which the author herself lays out what the book is about, why she wrote it, and which aspects were particularly important in doing so. She must have written the document shortly before or after the book's publication, namely, for Paul Parin—as a manuscript note in the top margin of the first page tells us.[5] Here it is in full.

Notes

1 See #107 (masochism as "an autonomous form of neurosis"); #109 (analogy with hysteria); #115 (as the result of pulsional conflicts *and* a particular ego structure).
2 Republished in a critical edition, Le Soldat (1994) 2020.
3 Le Soldat's later theoretical work contains a new, general theory of oedipal development (presented in Le Soldat 1994/Le Soldat (1994) 2020; Le Soldat 2015, lectures 5–7: 117–80) as well as the conception of two different variants of a special, *postoedipal* stage of development that comes about only under certain conditions and comprises specific conflict formations. Of the two variants of this stage of development, Le Soldat elaborated only one in writing: this variant concerns a special line of development within male homosexuality (laid out in Le Soldat 2015, lectures 9–11: 209–81, and Le Soldat 2018). She did not elaborate the other variant on paper but communicated it orally in supervisions and designated it using the English term "borderline." Both variants are distinguished by a special stage of development that, as noted, takes place post-oedipally and that Le Soldat describes topographically as crossing the border from the world of the oedipal to a world beyond the oedipal. The terms Le Soldat introduced, *this side* and *beyond* the oedipal, which we take up here, refer to the distinction between these two

inner worlds or psychical states. For a comprehensive presentation of Le Soldat's theoretical work, see Fäh and Gsell 2021.
4 This also explains why Le Soldat nowhere in her later work returns to her *concept* of masochism—with a single exception: a lecture published in 1990, whose content still moves on the ground covered by the masochism book (Le Soldat 1990: "Social Masochism"). In the few passages where she later refers to the masochism *book*, she already does so from the generalized perspective. In the announcement of the work she planned but was not able to complete, which had the working title *The American Moira: Borderline, Multiple Personality* (*Die amerikanische Parze: Borderline, multiple Persönlichkeit*), too, there is no reference to the concept of masochism but instead to the other parts of her "theoretical edifice": "Following the special oedipal theory of the drives (1994) and the study on homosexuality, the investigation of the psychical symptoms that are usually summarized as borderline and multiple personality forms the third and general part of the revision of drive theory I am aiming at" (www.lesoldat.ch/über-judith-le-soldat). And even where, in her later work, she discusses sexual practices that can be classified as masochistic (BDSM, for instance), there is neither a reference to the masochism *concept* nor to the masochism *book*.
5 Paul Parin was one of Le Soldat's training analysts.

Judith Le Soldat on her masochism book–a document from the posthumous papers[1]

There are two trains of thought to the book:

1 "Masochism" is a psychosexual syndrome: a development with peculiar reactions and positions, produced by inner conflicts and constitutional factors.
2 "Masochism" is the symptom of a social force that acts on the individual: a socially conditioned and generated feeling and action of the individual.[2]

The goal of the work:

1 to localize masochism in the individual: is masochism a genuine pulsional force? An expression of a particular conflict? A kind of defense? Then: trace lines of development and name possible causes.
2 to study the social conditions that can produce masochistic symptoms in the individual.
3 most of all, however, to pace out the *intermediate realm* that links individual and society. What laws are in effect there? How is influence exerted? Which forces, which balance of forces dominate? (What does "social amnesia" (Jacoby) mean, what "social production of unconsciousness" (Erdheim); both have described phenomena but not demonstrated mechanisms, have not looked into the *gears* of the synapsis, but that is precisely what I was interested in!)

Starting point:

– I was annoyed by how thoughtlessly people (from Reik via Reich to Marcuse, Dahmer, etc., even Morgenthaler) call masochism a perversion, use it synonymously with "pleasure taken in suffering," feminine, passive, etc.
– I was annoyed by "masochism" being used as an explanatory pattern (by La Boétie, Adorno, Marcuse, etc.) when it comes to understanding how it is possible that people act against their interests and let themselves be subjugated [*geknechtet*].

DOI: 10.4324/9781032666273-3

6 *Voluntary Servitude. Masochism and Morality*

- I observed that masochism, sadism, longing for death are topics of our time, the way, for instance, that sexuality and its suppression, hypocrisy, and defense against the drives were the issues at the turn of the century.
- At the same time, it cannot be denied that at the level of the individual, the most varied masochistic symptoms crop up, as self-observation shows, as analytic work shows. Nor can it be denied that there is "something," an internal and/or external force, that drives people to submission, keeps them dependent, etc. ("Voluntary servitude" according to La Boétie's concept).
- This led me to the thesis I start from: while psychoanalysis studies the sexual libido in every respect and has made it accessible to general consciousness, aggression as a pulsional force has largely remained unexplored. It has not succeeded in establishing itself in people's minds as a "drive." While we have learned to understand the symptoms of sexuality, we are at a loss, helpless in confronting the expressions of sadism. This "preferential treatment" is no coincidence. A social force concrete interests of dominion[3] prevent the recognition of the mechanisms and paths of aggression because they want to keep their manipulation for themselves.
- There is thus a prohibition on thought imposed on the aggression drive in order to reserve use of this drive for those who have dominion, and the current symptoms are to be interpreted as a return of the repressed. (That aggression does not yield to dominion either but takes its own paths is what the first chapter is about.)[4]

From this annoyance emerged:

1 a psychoanalytic concept of masochism
2 a sociological theory of voluntary servitude
3 a theory of the connection between psychology and social theory
4 on the path to (1), (2), and (3), a series of "clarifications":

e.g. of the death drive (yes, but completely differently), of the concept "identification with the aggressor" ([which] is much more complicated than one would think since psychologically, the aggressor is always the subject itself, sociologically objectively always the instrument of the interest of dominion, subjectively, however, the individual itself), yet above all the theorems of ambivalence, pulsional fusion, pulsional defusion, etc.

Conclusion

Individual-psychological masochism—as a special solution of the oedipal conflict—and socially induced masochism result in seemingly identical symptoms, but they are entirely different as to their origin, development, balance of forces, and function, which is immediately apparent when we try to influence them analytically.

concerning (1) [a psychoanalytic concept of masochism]:

I have traced Freud's train of thought as he wavered between originary sadism and genuine masochism and finally reached the opposite conception from what he started with (that was the content of my 1986 article in *Psyche*).

I demonstrate that Freud's theoretical development on this point can be understood only if we read it as a defense against the—initially captured—insight that aggression is a genuine pulsional force.

That is the starting point of my study. Via three exemplary cases from [my] practice, I demonstrate the central significance of aggression, of phantasies about the emergence of the difference between the sexes, and of (aggressive) masturbation. "Masochism" in my view is a special solution of the oedipal conflict in which the individual (man or woman) identifies with the phallus that is threatened by castration or lost. I thus assess masochism to be an independent nosological entity, one of the paths out of Oedipus to be taken nolens volens. Judging masochistic symptoms as signs of a disease or even wanting to "cure" it makes as much sense to me as wanting to "cure" homosexuality would. The only therapeutically relevant thing is to recognize and elucidate what is neurotic about masochism: secondary feelings of guilt, shame, projections, social exploitation, or implementation of the peculiar solution.

concerning (2) [a sociological theory of voluntary servitude]:

The theory of voluntary servitude relies on observations of [West Germany's] working through the Nazi era and reactions to the nuclear threat. I trace the paths the defense takes, that humans from their pulsional setup are aggressive, I look into the cui bono? The work here resembles the one in the Augean stables, since the social dominion (be it a political party, be it economic interests, sexual prerogatives of a libidinous or sadistic kind for an oligarchy) has done everything to cover the tracks of how it manipulates and channels the aggression of individuals in such a way that the aggression both remains available and yet does not turn back on the usurpers.

concerning (3) [a theory of the connection between psychology and social theory]:

This yields various approaches to thinking about the relationship between individual and society. Where do individual (unconscious) advantages and the interest of dominion coincide, where do they diverge? What then imposes itself and why and how? How can the social exert "influence" over the psychical, whose functioning, after all, is determined by the pulsional forces? (Not via the ego, not via identifications, but directly and immediately through the satisfactions taking place hallucinatorily in unconscious phantasy, by an unspoken social tendency in the service of the interests of dominion allying with the individual pulsional wish. How does the superego react to such satisfactions, which are to be condemned on the individual level but are socially effected?)—highly interesting and highly complicated questions, all of them, that cost me many a night's sleep. Since here the methodological was so difficult to handle—after all, I am myself part of this tendentious influence (which, incidentally, I finally recognize to be an "exploitation," that is to say, a further revealing and hypocritical use of language, like, for instance, employer/employee)[5]—the possible outcomes are especially enticing—and particularly speculative.

The book, as the publisher rightly noted, is a social science book; with the means of psychoanalysis, I have studied primarily the social phenomenon "masochism," have put the "voluntary servitude" on the couch, as it were. For the sake of consistency, the book would have had to be called *The Utopia of Voluntary Servitude*, a title the publisher rejected as "incomprehensible." I am still annoyed by this, because that title would have reduced what I wanted to say to the lowest denominator: if the "servitude" that today appears as a "voluntary" one were to become truly voluntary, we would have attained a utopian condition. For voluntary servitude cannot be anything other than the pleasurable satisfaction of masochistic pulsional wishes; the psychological reality, on the contrary, is that the oedipal conflict categorically demands a solution, that the masochistic outcome is as good as any other—and is equally *compelled* by the inner necessity; the social reality, meanwhile, is that the "voluntary servitude" is one imposed on the individual, not one obtained by brute force but surreptitiously, through silent subtle processes. Of course, it only appears "voluntary" to someone who wants to see the unequal alliance between interest of dominion and hallucinatory wish satisfaction as a fair deal between two equal partners. The greater share of the study is devoted exclusively to demonstrating the mechanisms between individual and society that first physically compel the servitude, then psychically establish it, and finally disguise it as "voluntary" in order to better exploit it and protect it from change.

The publisher had already typeset and announced the subtitle "Masochism *as* Morality," which I was just able to prevent *in extremis*. For that would truly have made a mockery of the content. Social masochism is as "moral" as everything that serves dominion, and while neurotic masochism is a sign of the oedipal morality, it is itself not a morality. It is completely absurd to claim, as the blurb has it, that masochism is a "protective system"—the opposite is the case: the voluntary servitude is the symptom of the oppression, where individual protection, or that of society, from power was insufficient. To speak of a "peculiar value scale" and even of an "interpretation of the world" is sheer nonsense. At least, though, the Fischer publishing house was willing to take the risk of publishing so difficult and complex a text in paperback. Another publisher (Klett!) returned the manuscript to me with the remark: the author has not understood what masochism really is ... My editor Günther Busch has contributed to the success of the project by not meddling in the content, a restraint I give him great credit for.

And you're familiar with Dr. Parin's contribution to getting the book started— ...

... schreiben Sie doch ein kleenes Büchel,'

Manuscript notes by Paul Parin: " ... why don't you write a little book?"

Notes

1 The document is preserved in the archives of the Judith Le Soldat-Stiftung, JLS-1988/89-1. The facsimile reads: "For Parin 1988/89."
2 [On these two trains of thought, what Le Soldat calls "sociogenic" and "psychogenic" masochism, see below, especially ch. II.6, "Two Paths to Masochism."]
3 [The term *Herrschaft* cuts across several distinct meanings in English: *power, rule, (pre)dominance,* to name but three. As Le Soldat uses the term and its derivates in a particular way that, more often than not, is *not* synonymous with *Macht,* "power" (see, especially, #58), the choice here has been made to keep it separate and render it as "dominion."—Trans.]
4 [This probably refers to all of part I of the book.]
5 [The German terms, *Arbeitgeber* and *Arbeitnehmer,* literally mean "work-giver" and "work-taker"—Trans.]

On the two trains of thought in the masochism book

Monika Gsell and Ralf Binswanger[1]

1 First train of thought: masochism as a psychosexual syndrome

We now take up the "first train of thought," Le Soldat's concept of masochism. We begin with an outline of the masochism concept as it emerges from the author's presentation in this volume.

1.1 Outline of Le Soldat's masochism concept

1.1.1 The starting point of the masochistic development

- The starting point of the masochistic development is a *defusion of aggressive and libidinous energies*—a traumatic event that takes place between the oral and the anal phase, at the age of about ten to eighteen months (#138). "Traumatic" is the term Le Soldat uses to designate the *internal event itself.*[2] There are no indications, in her view, that it is in every case a trauma induced from the outside, and at the very least, such an externally induced trauma is not a precondition.[3] What is decisive, rather, is a pulsional pressure lasting for a long time, which explodes the alloying of libido and aggression and leads to a sustained and irreversible *displacement of energy* from libido to aggression (#152).
- The second characteristic element of "masochistic" development is the *splitting of the genital wish* into a purely libidinous wish that is "becoming passive,"[4] and a purely aggressive-phallic wish: the libidinous share of the wish is "bound" to one's own genital, the aggressive-phallic share to the hand (#170).
- The next step in the development is the anxiety, arising as a consequence of this split, that the aggressive hand destroys the libidinously cathected genital during masturbation. The *anxiety about masturbatory self-castration* arises, which factually amounts to a masturbation taboo or a "prohibition on masturbation" (#170 and 256).

1.1.2 The turn to the mother as the first oedipal love object

- To escape the psychically unacceptable taboo, the aggressive-phallic wish is projected externally, onto the first object, the mother, and is "idealized" there (#174).[5] In the phantasy of the child, the mother is thus equipped with a phallus. The—libidinous, masturbatory—wish phantasies now revolve around the maternal phallus and the satisfactions it grants (#213). The aggressive shares are directed against the father (#181).
- Le Soldat now supposes that in the special case of the "masochistic" development, the difference between the sexes is perceived earlier as in the common oedipal development as a confirmation of the castration anxieties: "Girls reproach themselves with self-mutilation, boys fear that in watching an erection wearing off, they are witnessing the damage *in statu nascendi*" (#212).
- Under the pressure of the reality principle—the perception of the difference between the sexes and the phantasies associated with it—the phantasy of the phallic mother can no longer be maintained (#212f.)

1.1.3 The change of object

- What follows is a gradual *process of recathexis* in the distribution of libidinous and aggressive energies that will result in the change of object— and, at this stage, in both girls *and* boys. This is how Le Soldat imagines the process of recathexis: the aggression directed at the father is initially "given the goal of castrating the father and putting his penis at the mother's disposal" (#213). Both oedipal objects are charged aggressively: "reality testing," no longer recognizing the maternal phallus, "combined with the effect of fear of the father's revenge" for the intended robbing, "leads to a *double aggressive projection*" (#213). Both the mother and the father now appear aggressive-dangerous to the child.
- This state of affairs, too, is hard to bear: while it subjectively relieves the extreme internal tensions for a moment, it does so only at the price of increased anxiety about external objects. When this situation, too becomes unbearable, a phase of re-introjecting aggression sets in once more (#213).
- At the same time—supported by awareness of the real anatomic conditions— ever more "passive libidinous energies" are placed "in the cathexis of the father." Now it is the *father* who is "respected as bearer and possessor of the idealized member and admired for his taming his drives." Yet one may hardly call him a *love object*, since "the appreciation that really concerns his intact male member is merely transferred onto him. He is loved *because* he is in possession of the phallus." "This results in a constant inclination toward cathexis displacement and, ultimately, a surplus of the libidinous binding to the father" (#212f).

12 *Voluntary Servitude. Masochism and Morality*

- The threat of castration is now "definitively attribute[d] ... to the mother, and she becomes the oedipal rival for both sexes" (#214).
- The libidinous cathexis of the father aids in defending against retaliatory anxieties that have not been completely allayed by the now inverted conditions (aggressive cathexis of the mother, libidinous cathexis of the father).
- The change of object also comes with a passive turn of the sexual wishes: the child submits to the father (#213f.; 223f.).

1.1.4 The demise of Oedipus complex and the establishment of the superego

- The recathexis, however, "decays," "splits," or "falls apart"[6] once more under the pressure of the love disappointment, and an "unavoidable re-aggressivization" occurs in whose wake both parent objects are cathected aggressively once more (#223). The ego enters an uncomfortable situation: the (castration) anxiety becomes unbearable, a repetition of the traumatic early inundation. The ego deploys an emergency function: "Suddenly and radically, *all pulsional energies are withdrawn from the object cathexes and the projections are given up*"; the oedipal objects "are dismissed as far as the inner reality is concerned" (#223). We take this to mean that the psychical representation of the parents *as* oedipal, pulsionally cathected objects is destroyed.
- The aggressions previously projected onto mother and father are released in the ego and unite in the establishment of the superego.
- Since the incestuous wish was taken away from the ego already in the first thrust of repression (or of "emotional isolation"), the superego is directed not against the incestuous wish but against its substitute, masturbation. This is the first characteristic of the masochistic superego: "The establishment of the superego... reestablishes ... the preoedipal condition. *Sadism-turned-morality ruins masturbation*" (#225).
- The second characteristic of the masochistic superego is that while it is extremely cruel, it is for that very reason also *weak and deficient* (#225): precisely because it is made up of purely aggressive energies and lacks any libidinous cathexis, it "finds itself incapable of obtaining the ego's admiration and voluntary conformity. ... *The hostility of the ego is directed against the superego's missing ideal-function.* ... I go a step further and assert that the intention of the ego, and the aim of the aggression drive after the oedipal internalization, consists in eliminating the superego structure from the psychical apparatus once more" (#232).

1.1.5 The regressive resolution of the masochistic Oedipus complex

After the demise of the Oedipus complex, both girls and boys in a regressive move return to the phallic mother *but now under the new conditions* that come with the change of object: both maintain their *manifest male* choice of object but this manifest male object becomes the representative of the phallic mother; and both maintain the sexual wishes—which thanks to the change of object have been given a "passive turn"—and now imagine being "phallically" satisfied by the object. In "masochistic" women, "genital passivity and penis wish unite in the phantasy of being satisfied by the 'phallic' mother" (#223). "Masochistic" men wish "to obtain a pleasurable satisfaction in a homosexual practice from the mother who is also equipped with a phallus" (#224).

1.1.6 The "real" problem of masochism (in adult life)

In summary, we can say: the central problem of the masochistic development is masturbation. The child struggles first against the masturbation taboo, then against the diminishing of pleasure.[7] The three analysands Le Soldat introduces develop different solutions to counter this problem (#256f.). These solutions share the use of physical pain as an "aid to pleasure" (#258).

According to Le Soldat, however, the *real* problem—the masochistic neurosis—arises only secondarily, namely, when the superego interprets this pain as punishment for the castration (which internally is actively executed). Then the painful "ritual is cathected with anxiety," and the pain no longer serves "as an aid to pleasure but... to project the threat of castration. Sexual relaxation is thus no longer possible via this route. Prior to this, the lack of a connection between phantasy and physical manipulation already destroyed the psychical gain in pleasure" (#258).

This is the point, according to Le Soldat, where therapy can and must intervene: the task of therapy consists in detaching this secondary, neurotic cathexis of the ritual from the projection of the castration threat such that the masochistic form of pleasure can be preserved. It thus very explicitly does not consist in "treating away" the painful rituals—that would amount to a conversion therapy. Under the conditions of the disentanglement of the drives, the pain offers the only opportunity of maintaining access to pleasure (#258).

1.2 Nuclei of the later theory

There are many individual elements in Le Soldat's conception of the masochistic development that return in her later Oedipus theory, albeit in part on new grounds. Among the elements mentioned in our outline, this concerns for instance the concept of masturbatory self-castration; the phantasy formation of the phallic mother (as well as castrating and betraying her); the change of object, obligatory for both sexes; the castration of the father; and the collapse of the oedipal parent figures (which collapse, according to the later work, is phantasized as "murder").[8] We might say that with few exceptions (which, however, will prove to be decisive),[9] the *phantasy formations* Le Soldat will later consider characteristic of the *general* Oedipus complex—the "content

14 Voluntary Servitude. Masochism and Morality

aspect"[10] of the oedipal development—are already largely contained in her conception of the special case of masochism. What will change in the transition to the *general* Oedipus theory is, in part, the chronological sequence of phantasy formations within the oedipal narrative (for instance, she situates the castration of the father and the betrayal of the mother *before* the change of object in the special case of masochism, *after* the change of object in the general oedipal theory). More important than these chronological displacements are the theoretical assumptions that have led to them. In the next section, we take the example of the initial conflict to show that and to what extent these changed theoretical assumptions on decisive points can be called a paradigm shift that took place between the masochism book published in 1989 and the Irma book published in 1994.

1.2.1 The initial conflict: from the masturbation taboo to the problem of unfulfillable wishes, or the paradigm shift from phallic monism to constitutive bisexuality

One significant difference between the masochism concept and Le Soldat's later, general theory of the oedipal conflicts concerns the problem that stands at the beginning of the Oedipus complex and drives this complex:

- In the masochism concept, the problem of masturbation (the anxiety about masturbatory self-castration) arises from the defusion of libidinous and aggressive energies and the concomitant *splitting* of the *one* genital wish impulse into *two* genital impulses: the purely aggressively charged phallic-active wish threatens to destroy the purely libidinously charged genital. For this reason, in masochism, "castration anxiety is not one of the reasons for the solution of the conflict," as it is in the classical conception, "but the precondition" of the conflict (#213).
- The later, general Oedipus theory, by contrast, concerns two genuine, independent genital pulsional impulses: a passive-genital pulsional impulse, whose aim consists in being genitally penetrated by an object, and an active-genital pulsional impulse whose aim consists in genitally penetrating an object. The problem, too, is entirely different: neither do a libidinous and an aggressive pulsional impulse confront each other "aversively," nor do the two differing pulsional aims threaten the genital. It is much more simple and logical: for anatomical reasons, only one of the two genuine genital wishes can ever be enacted (which initially means: only one of the two genital wishes ever finds a physical correlate)—the other one remains unsuccessful all life long and thereby sustainably and irreversibly becomes a source of disruptions of the psychical balance.[11]

Thus: no "pathogenic" splitting of *one* genital drive into a libidinous and an aggressive "fission product" but *two* independent pulsional strivings, a passive one and an active one, as expressions of the entirely normal, constitutionally given bipolarity of the drive—strivings whose tragedy, if you like, is that they do not match our sexually differentiated bodies.

The perception and psychical significance of the difference between the sexes already plays an important role in the special case of masochism, just as, inversely, the anxiety about (masturbatory self-) castration will continue to play a central role in the later Oedipus theory—but the cause–effect relationships are swapped.

The decisive, *categorial* difference between the special case of masochism and the later Oedipus theory that jumps out at us, as under a magnifying glass, when we consider the different conception of the initial conflict, however, lies elsewhere: it is the *quantum leap from the phallic monism*, to which Le Soldat's thinking in the masochism book still adheres as a matter of course, to what in going back to Freud we would like to call the *paradigm of constitutive psychical bisexuality*. Le Soldat herself did not use the concept of constitutive psychical bisexuality, but in our view, it aptly captures what constitutes the starting point of Le Soldat's Oedipus theory and its radical difference from all other Oedipus theories: Le Soldat's assumption that the general bipolarity of the drive manifests on the level of genital pulsional impulses in the form of a genuinely active and a genuinely passive pulsional aim, of which, conditioned by our anatomy, only one can be satisfied in each case. In the context of Le Soldat's theoretical universe, we thus do not mean by *bisexuality* what is usually understood by it in everyday speech, namely, desiring objects of both sexes, but the *bipolarity* of the genital drive in the sense just described, of an active and a passive pulsional aim.[12]

Le Soldat does not tell us anywhere how the quantum leap from phallic monism to constitutive bisexuality came about. We suspect, however, that clearing up some terminological-conceptual inconsistencies made a non-negligible contribution. Since these inconsistencies make reading this book more difficult, sometimes quite significantly so, we would like to address them in greater detail.

1.2.2 Clarifying some terminological-conceptual inconsistencies

For those familiar with Le Soldat's later work, it is a matter of course that all pulsional wishes (not just the genital wishes, although those are at the center of Le Soldat's theory) not only have an active and a passive pulsional *aim* but each obtain their particular *quality* through their specific admixture ratio of libidinous and aggressive cathexis energies. When the libidinous cathexis qualities dominate, Le Soldat usually speaks simply of passive-genital or active-genital wishes; when large quanta of aggressive cathexis energy are involved, she especially stresses it and speaks of passive-aggressive wishes on the one hand and "active, sadistic" impulses, aims, and so on, on the other hand.[13]

This also means: the notion that both passive and active wishes are cathected with libidinous *and* aggressive energy figures among the self-evident basic assumption of Le Soldat's later theory.[14] There is no such self-evidence yet in the masochism book. On the contrary: Le Soldat practically seems to use *passive* synonymously with *libidinous*, *active* synonymously with *aggressive*, and to couple both with the *physical paths of pulsional discharge*, the *sensorial* pulsional discharge in the case of the libidinous-passive wishes on the one hand, and the *motoric* pulsional discharge in the case of the aggressive-active wishes on the other. Pulsional *qualities* (aggressive and/or libidinous), pulsional *aims* (active or passive), pulsional *sources* (the erogenous zones being cathected), and the bodily paths of pulsional *satisfaction* (sensorial or motoric discharge)—all these different aspects, which are indispensable in a differentiated description of a specific pulsional wish, seem to be interwoven so intricately in the masochism book that Le Soldat sometimes simply says *passive* or *sensorial* instead of *libidinous*, or *active* or *motoric* instead of *aggressive* (and vice versa).[15]

It is also remarkable that in the masochism book, *passive* is obviously not yet used to denote an independent pulsional aim whose discharge *can* result in a—potentially—"full-fledged" experience of satisfaction. Instead, the concept "passive" has a negative connotation almost throughout the masochism book: the "becoming passive" of sexuality comes with a loss of vitality, the satisfaction experience becomes pleasureless and bland.[16] Le Soldat, moreover, connotes "passive sexuality" with something subjectively experienced as humiliating, a dependence on and helplessness vis-à-vis the love objects to which one submits, to which one *must* submit, not because that is experienced as pleasurable but from sheer internal necessity: because one is unable to regulate the inner tensions in any other way and is threatened by the possibility of being submerged by destructive, aggressive pulsional quanta.[17]

This impression is largely confirmed by several passages in which Le Soldat spells out her understanding of these concepts: in the masochism book, she explicitly holds that libido and aggression not only prefer different paths of bodily satisfaction but, for this reason, also *cathect* different erogenous zones.[18] Thus she speaks of an "alliance" of aggression with the "motor system" to explain the girl's difficulty in *cathecting* the vagina with "aggressive" impulses (#178). And about the libido she says that it "demand[s] merely ... sensorial physical stimuli" for its satisfaction (#189). Furthermore, it appears that Le Soldat understands "passive" primarily in a descriptive sense: "We speak of active and passive pulsional wishes. *Yet no 'passive' pulsional wish exists: this expression labels an aggressively or libidinously cathected wishful phantasy whose physical satisfaction can be obtained only on the path of a sensorial excitation.*"[19]

In our view, the clarification of these categories, especially of pulsional aim (active or passive) and pulsional quality (aggressive and/or libidinous), which in the masochism book are still used undifferentiated-synonymously, likely played a decisive role in Le Soldat's "quantum leap" from the paradigm of phallic monism to the paradigm of constitutive bisexuality and paved the way toward a theoretically convincing conception of passive-genital and active-genital pulsional wishes and of the phantasies that come/or related to with them them (the phantasy of a penis of their own for girls, the phantasy of their own genital orifice for boys, and the passive-aggressive hammer blow wish for both sexes).[20] We would like to add that what against the background of Le Soldat's *later* concise terminology appears confusing in the masochism book was not simply Le Soldat's "fault": we find a similarly inconsistent confusing use of the terms *active* and *passive*, *libidinous,* and *aggressive* already in Freud, and we also find the tendency to speak of *aggressive* and *libidinous* instead of *active* and *passive* in Eissler, to whom Le Soldat refers several times.[21]

It is therefore helpful in orienting ourselves in the masochism book to think about what precisely Le Soldat means when she speaks of aggressive, libidinous, sensorial, motoric, and so on. Does she indeed mean the pulsional quality or does she thereby not designate the pulsional aim (active or passive), the pulsional source (the organ required to discharge the pulsional impulse), or the pathways of physical pulsional discharge (sensorial/motoric) instead? The use, in particular, of "aggressive" in connection with "phallic" is often to be understood in the (later) sense of "active-genital" (see, e.g., #99–100). A further, very reliable clue for "aggressive" not being used in the sense of the pulsional quality is the connection with the concept of idealization: "idealized aggressiveness" (#178) precisely has *nothing* to do with aggressiveness but, viewed in light of the later work, proves to be really a makeshift expression for the notion of the "active-genital" that was not yet available to Le Soldat (at least in the later precise sense). When we read, therefore, that the aggressive-phallic impulse is projected onto the mother and idealized there, this can be understood first of all in the narrow sense (that is to say, within the "phallocentric" logic of the masochism book) to mean: the mother becomes the bearer of one's own organ required by the child to satisfy active-genital impulses, an organ that is missed or threatened by (self-) castration. One's *own* member, imagined by girls and actually present in boys, is thus projected onto the mother to keep it safe from destruction by one's own aggressive impulse (see, e.g., #156n). The mother (as an "auxiliary ego," #149) is then to act on the active-genital pulsional impulse, substituting for the child, as it were. If we go one step further and also take Le Soldat's formula of the "becoming passive of the *libidinous* genital wishes bound to one's own body" into consideration, we can add, now founded on the later logic of the "bisexual" genital wishes: the mother does not (only) become the bearer of the child's blocked active genital wishes, but she is being phallically equipped to be able to fulfill the child's genuinely *passive* wishes.[22]

This "strategy" of discovering the meaning of difficult-to-understand passages in the masochism book by taking recourse to the differentiated vocabulary Le Soldat's *drive theory* uses later, however, does not work in all cases. It is helpful above all where nuclei of Le Soldat's later Oedipus theory are concerned, that is, pulsional conflicts and their neurotic processing in a narrower sense. Where germs of her later conception of the special, postoedipal developmental stage[23] are concerned, by contrast, the procedure for orientation just sketched would lead to misinterpretations: because different laws govern the "beyond the oedipal" (and that also means that other conflicts and strategies for working through them join the oedipal-neurotic ones), the terms *passive* and *active* have a different meaning as well. In this context, they can neither simply be understood in the sense of pulsional aims nor in the phenomenal-descriptive sense of *inactive* versus *active*. Here, however, those connotations that initially tripped us up, as it were, in the masochism book, suddenly make sense, the connotations (which are confusing in the drive-theoretical context) of *active* and *aggressive* on the one hand and of *passive* and *helpless* on the other hand. The appropriate question then becomes: am I exposed passively-*helplessly*-unable to act to a potentially traumatic event (like the inundation of the inner world with too large quanta of unbound energy)—or is there the possibility for me to protect or even to defend myself against it actively-(aggressively)-able to act? Le Soldat shows that a careful distinction between these different dimensions of the meaning of *active* and *passive* is by no means a matter of academic nitpicking but is of as it were existential significance and therefore ethically, epistemologically, and politically necessary—and in our view, a large part of Le Soldat's engagement with the relationship between individuals and social power and violence in the masochism book is due to this demonstration. This engagement concerns, simply put, the question: when is human behavior and phantasy (or imagination) primarily an expression of pulsional wishes—and when is it primarily an expression of something non-pulsional, namely, the attempt to protect or even defend oneself against helplessly being surrendered to a traumatic event or working through such an event? That this distinction is crucially linked with Le Soldat's later conception of the two worlds "this side" and "beyond" the oedipal is a point we will return to in detail in Section 1.2.4.

Next, however, we must show to what extent the nucleus of the later distinction between the two worlds "this side" and "beyond" the oedipal is already contained in the masochism book.

1.2.3 Change of object: becoming heterosexual or homosexual

The change of object lends itself to demonstrating how what Le Soldat in 1989 elaborates as the special case of masochism becomes the nucleus not only of the new, general theory of oedipal development but also the nucleus of the "border crossing" (*Grenzübertritt*) from the world of the oedipal to the beyond of the oedipal.[24]

Le Soldat's position in the masochism book on this central theorem of the Oedipus complex can be summarized as follows: unlike the conventional conception of the Oedipus complex, Le Soldat considers the turn to the mother as the first love object obligatory in all children. In the special case of masochism, however, the early love for the mother has a different function than in the "common" oedipal development: it is shaped entirely by the problem of aggression and masturbation and therefore is not really of an objectal kind (see #150 and #204).

Le Soldat considers the change of object to the father, in turn, to be in principle "optional" (#212): at least, there is *no psychical reason* for it, neither in boys nor in girls. The first love object is and remains the mother. In girls, however, the change of object is compelled by society and "coordinated with their own conflicts and aims only secondarily" (#212). As a result of the change of object, the first love object is repressed, which is why in the common oedipal development of girls, the change of object always has *neurotic character*.

In the special case of masochism, in contrast, the change of object is obligatory, and again for both sexes (#211f).[25] Yet unlike the "normal cases," it arises not from sociogenic but from psychogenic reasons (#222) and is shaped—like the oedipal love for the mother already was—by "the masochistic phantasy about masturbation" (#212).

To understand what follows, it is important not to get side-tracked by the distinction between sociogenic and psychogenic—a distinction Le Soldat was to give up later and that here merely indicates (to us) the path on which she reaches the distinctions relevant later. What is decisive here is another aspect. It concerns the question of the causal sequence. What comes first: does the early love for the mother dissolve first, and the change of object takes place subsequently? Or does the early love of the mother dissolve *as a consequence* of the change of object? The question of the sequence is decisive for Le Soldat because she associates completely different development trajectories with the different sequences and different inner vicissitudes, as it were. For the two variants in the masochism book, they look like this:

- In the *normal case* of oedipal development, the change of object does *not arise internally*. It is, rather, compelled externally and then leads to the early love for the oedipal mother being *repressed*, which is why in the normal case, the change of object has *neurotic* character. In short: first the change of object—then the repression of the first object—therefore: *neurotic* character of the change of object.
- In the *special case* of masochism, in turn, it is the other way around: the early love for the mother is given up *for internal reasons*, and this process does not take place via repression but via an isolation,[26] even before the

change of object happens. In short: *no repression*—therefore: *non-neurotic* character of the change of object.

In what follows, we would like to show the extent to which this distinction between internal and external reasons for the change of object will prove to be a significant nucleus for the later distinction between the two worlds this side and beyond the oedipal. To that end, we now bring in the question of sexual orientation or of the *choice* of object, which Le Soldat in the masochism book very directly associates with the change of object,[27] since

- girls become heterosexual as a result of the change of object;
- boys become homosexual as a result of the change of object.

This simple juxtaposition corresponds to what Le Soldat says (#211 and #214). She seems to postulate an unambiguous correlation between change of object and sexual orientation. Considered closely, however, matters are anything but simple or clear. A first complication arises from the need to differentiate the female development according to the *reasons* (social or internal) for which the change of object takes place. A further complication arises from the fact that *becoming heterosexual* and *becoming homosexual* quite obviously do not simply or do not always designate the manifest sexual orientation of the adult: sometimes they name the internal object toward which one regresses, sometimes a specific pulsional wish.[28] Connected with this is Le Soldat's peculiarly inverted use of the concept "negative" in the context of girls' change of object.[29] A further confusing aspect is that "becoming homosexual" and "becoming heterosexual" mean something entirely different depending on whether she is talking about women or men, precisely because in women, "becoming heterosexual for internal reasons" means the same as "becoming masochistic" (which is not true of heterosexual men), while in men, inversely, "becoming homosexual for internal reasons" means the same as "becoming masochistic" (which in turn is not true of homosexual women, and we should add that, as far as we can see, lesbian women cannot be assigned to any of these equations).[30]

We must add that we are familiar with these terminological difficulties from her later work, as we are with the distinctions of reasons for which one becomes homo- or heterosexual.[31] These very parallels, however, also allow for resolving the difficulties of understanding in one fell swoop and in so doing also for discovering a nucleus of the later distinction between the two worlds this side and beyond the oedipal: for what in the masochism book is designated by *becoming heterosexual* (women) or *becoming homosexual* (men) *for internal reasons* contains the nucleus of Le Soldat's later theory of the special developmental step occurring post-oedipally that leads into the *land without return* (*Land ohne Wiederkehr*) and is described by her as the "state of mind" of the "population of the beyond."[32] In short:

On the two trains of thought in the masochism book 21

the special oedipal case of masochism later becomes the special postoedipal case of the "border crossing." That is what we would like to present in more nuance.

1.2.3.1 Masochism as the nucleus of Le Soldat's theory of the "border crossing"

– What Le Soldat in the masochism book calls becoming *homosexual* for internal, namely, masochistic reasons later correspond to what she conceives of as the "gay" (*schwul*) variant of border crossing.[33] We may also assume that she considered this path of gay border crossing to be the one taken by some lesbian women as well.[34]
– What, in contrast, Le Soldat in the masochism book calls becoming *heterosexual* for internal, namely, masochistic reasons (the special case of *female masochism*) later correspond to what she names the "second variant" of border crossing.[35] Le Soldat was not able to elaborate on this "second variant" in writing, nor did it receive any "official" designation. For now, and for reasons of simplicity, we will call it the "nongay" border crossing, and we will add: in the masochism book, Le Soldat conceived of this line of development only for the masochistic development of heterosexual *women*. From the few written clues and from conversations, however, we know that she later thought that this second path is also taken by certain heterosexual men.

There is, however, one significant difference to be noted here: while in the masochism book, Le Soldat assumes that there is, for internal reasons, a causal relationship between object change and choice of object in both the masochistic-feminine and in the masochistic-masculine line of development ("becoming heterosexual" in women and "becoming homosexual" in men), in the late work, this is true only of men who become "gay": they cross the border in a way (with certain phantasy formations) that, according to Le Soldat, is necessarily—"for internal reasons"—associated with a same-sex choice of object. In the late work, this connection is as absent from the heterosexual variants of border crossing as it is from the lesbian variant. We take that to mean that the way in which the border is crossed in these cases—the phantasy formations that come with it—displays *no* connection with the choice of object manifest later.

1.2.3.2 The regular case of the female change of object as the nucleus of the new, general Oedipus theory

Le Soldat employs the metaphor of "border-crossing" to designate a developmental step that separates the inner world into "this side" of and "beyond" the oedipal development. We find a germ of this distinction in the masochism book as well: it is set up in the distinction between primarily sociogenic reasons for the feminine change of object on the one hand and primarily psychogenic, that is to say, genuinely masochistic reasons on the other. The female change of object for primarily sociogenic reasons proves to be the germ for the new, general theory of the Oedipus complex in two respects:

1 Girls' "common" change of object, which in the masochism book has a sociogenic basis, in the new theory of oedipal development is declared obligatory for all children, independent of their anatomical sex and their later sexual orientation. This generalization, though, definitively abandons the thesis of a sociogenically compelled change of object, and the "common" change of object is given a new basis in the change described earlier from the paradigm of the masturbation taboo to the paradigm of constitutive bisexuality.
2 Moreover, the common case of the feminine change of object becomes the germ of the new, general theory of the Oedipus complex insofar as the criterion of the "neurotic character" of the choice of object is generalized. While the correlation between *change of object* and choice of object is abandoned, the choice of object—now that the sociogenic factor no longer applies—has a purely psychogenic basis, like previously the masochistic choice of object: it results from the various oedipal conflict resolutions that emerge via the defense modalities of repression and regression, that therefore are of a neurotic character, and that Le Soldat calls "homo-" or "heterosexual symptom formations." As already mentioned, though, there are no criteria, in Le Soldat's view, that would allow for associating certain regressive solutions with certain choices of objects.[36] While they thus arise psychogenically, they remain random.

That is why the "gay border crossing" occupies a special place within the variants of development Le Soldat sketches: it is the only line of development she associates with "grounds for homosexuality." There will no longer be—as she still assumed for the female-masochistic variant in the masochism book—"grounds for heterosexuality."

1.2.4 Beyond the oedipal: the masochism book's contribution to a better understanding of Le Soldat's concept of the "border" between this side and beyond the oedipal

There is an abundance of clues to suggest that the masochism book is valuable not only for understanding the work Le Soldat elaborated in writing but also for that part of her work she was not able to put down on paper. We would like to take an example to show what kind of clues these are and in what direction our ideas are headed. This is also meant to invite a reading of the masochism book that is not (only) guided by its logical-contentual coherence but takes the form into account in which Le Soldat presents her thoughts. In our view, the dictum that form and content are a unity is especially true of this text. What Le Soldat thematizes on the level of content—processes of decay, processes of isolation, of reversal, simultaneity of mutually exclusive positions, and so on—presents itself in the form of the text: what belongs together thematically and systematically is torn asunder and isolated; concepts are used in contravention of their conventional meaning; apparently, contradictory positions remain juxtaposed without mediation or commentary. All this makes reading the book a sometimes painful, frustrating, highly unpleasurable process. The text's aesthetic form compels readers to go experience for themselves, as it were, what the book's content *affectively* means for those concerned. The text, however, not only *does* formally what it says contentually. In what it is *doing*, it at many points goes far beyond what Le Soldat at that point was able to *say*, that is, to capture intellectually rationally and to theorize. It thus contains a potential, and this potential is what we would now like to at least hint at with regard to Le Soldat's later concept of the border and border crossing. We do so in the format of rather free, associative theses. For reasons of space, comprehensive explanations and detailed discussions will be provided later in an independent article.

In earlier expositions of Le Soldat's theoretical work, we concentrated on those points of view that Le Soldat explicit takes herself: the pulsional-dynamic and contentual-phantasmatic aspects associated with the concept of the border (concretely: the "hammer blow zone" or the figure of "Apollo" as contentual-phantasmatic expression of the "border" of the oedipal development on the one hand; the different pulsional dynamics, conflict formations, and defense formations this side and beyond as the pulsional-dynamic aspects of the oedipal and of the special postoedipal developmental stages on the other).[37] One focus was the question whether the distinction between this side and beyond contributes to a more differentiated understanding of homo- and heterosexual conflict formations.[38]

In our view, a careful reading of the masochism book allows for studying the concept of the border in light of the structural aspect as well. That is why we begin with a thesis that might at first seem far-fetched but that will subsequently prove to be plausible: the border that separates the oedipal this side from the beyond of the oedipal is the border between ego and id, the defense structure that allows the ego to protect itself, among other things, against traumatic stimulus inundations from the inner or the outer world.[39] When we take Le Soldat's early distinction between the "common" and the "masochistic" oedipal development to be the "nucleus" of the later distinction between "this side" of and "beyond" the oedipal, we can say:

– Under the conditions of a "common" oedipal development, the border between ego and id remains intact (or: it is established as a stable border/defense structure in the course of the oedipal development in the first place) and makes neurotic forms of dealing with pulsional conflicts possible.

– In the special case of masochism (or in the hetero- and homosexual variants of the "border crossing" described later), the *construction of the defense structure has already taken place under particular conditions and displays, when compared with the "common" oedipal development, special features*.[40] The "border crossing" breaks through this particular defense structure. The breakthrough comes with the disintegration of the prior and the formation of a new defense structure, a new border.[41]

The phrase in italics, "construction of the defense structure under particular conditions …," requires explanation. Those familiar with Le Soldat's *Lectures* know that she presented matters differently there: all human beings undergo the oedipal development in more or less the *same* way and, at the end of the development, reach a border that some few cross while others do not. The lectures do not speak of "special conditions" to be considered preconditions for the border crossing or say that such preconditions are unknown.[42] In *Land of No Return*, Le Soldat speaks of possible differences in character and constitution (more impatient, more curious, and the like).[43] What thus seems to be decisive is a momentary, pulsional dynamic constellation: an "internal, pulsional dynamic overload conditioned by a chain reaction, a positive synergy of increasingly colliding aggressive and libidinous forces that do not have the usual antagonistic (mutually inhibiting) effect but … escalate equipolarly [*gleichgepolt*]."[44]

In the masochism book, by contrast, the central topic is precisely what in the books published in 2015 and 2018 is left out: the internal preconditions that in the course of the oedipal development lead to the formation of a particular defense structure. Although we cannot know whether Le Soldat would agree with our suggestion or on the contrary emphatically reject it, there is much to speak in favor, we think, of supposing that what in the masochism book she conceives of as a special case of oedipal development describes the preconditions under which, after the demise of the Oedipus complex, there is a crossing of the border from this side to beyond the oedipal—or, at least, that there can but does not have to be such a crossing. Two aspects seem important to us in this regard. First, Le Soldat saw the starting point of the masochistic development in an *early* (at ten to eighteen months of age, that is, *pre*oedipal) inundation of the child's psyche with unbound pulsional energy (#138). This is experienced as traumatic and results, among other things, in *anxiety* about the traumatic situation repeating itself being firmly anchored in the psychical system.[45] Second, we would like to recall that Le Soldat unequivocally describes the border crossing as a further—postoedipal—structure-forming step in the development.[46] In her later work, she thus thematizes a *post*oedipal process and its result, while in the masochism book, both *pre*oedipal and oedipal preconditions for this process can be found.

When we relate these two aspects to each other, we can articulate a kind of complemental series from the perspective of the defense structure:

1 common oedipal conditions: a neurotic defense structure is set up and remains intact postoedipally;
2 traumatic burdens, preoedipal or oedipal: the defense structure displays special characteristics and is primarily occupied with preventing a repetition of the traumatic incursion. All pulsional intensity is experienced as a threat and triggers anxiety about a collapse of the ego (#167–69);
3 the *post*oedipal border crossing: under certain circumstances[47] and as a kind of emergency measure, the *weakened* or in any case *changed* defense structure is first completely destroyed and then rebuilt. Le Soldat's "border crossing" can thus be understood as a progressive, structure-forming step of development that succeeds in replacing a brittle defense structure with a new one better suited to protecting against disintegration anxieties and the like.

If this hypothesis proves to make sense, we can say: Le Soldat's "beyond the oedipal" describes a special defense formation against the psychical consequence of more or less grave, internal or external, traumatic incursions that took place in the course of infantile development—preoedipally or oedipally.

To conclude our discussion of the first train of thought, let us try and account for the fact that Le Soldat describes the border-crossing *both* as a traumatic internal process *and* as a fulminant—and equally purely internal—implementation of the passive-aggressive hammer blow or Apollo wishes.[48] How are we to explain this seemingly contradictory juxtaposition of two so diverging interpretations of one and the same psychical process? We think that an explanation is possible if we bring the oedipal pulsional development back in that for Le Soldat is at the center. We can then say:

1 The character of the particular *pre*oedipal preconditions for the border-crossing, according to Le Soldat, is that of an external and/or internal trauma.
2 In the *oedipal* phase, the first development and maturation of the drives takes place, accompanied by the corresponding phantasy formations. This happens in about the same way for everybody and independently of the *pre*oedipal preconditions and the concomitant differences in the formation of the defense structure. From the *pulsional dynamic* perspective, everybody would thus reach a border at the end of the oedipal development that on the level of phantasy is represented as "Apollo"—as the sexual phantasy of an inner pulsional object. From the *structural* perspective, by contrast, the same border proves to be a defense structure.

3 This phantasy formation, in the *post*oedipal phase, allows the ego to *simultaneously* view a process, structurally, as a *renewed* traumatic invasion and trigger an emergency measure (reversal of the pulsional flow) *and* to register it as fulfilling a wish (from the point of view of phantasy), where "novelistic phantasy"[49] presents what is passively experienced and processes that unfold automatically as active action: one has confronted Apollo (has been inundated) but turned one's back at the last moment (the automatically occurring emergency measure) and has thus defeated Apollo (has evaded psychical death at the last moment, has survived the trauma).[50]—What is essential about *this* renewed traumatic process is not the destruction of structure but the formation of a new structure being established, also against the consequences of the first trauma.[51] That is why it is possible to conceive of the "border-crossing" not as a pathology but as a progressive, compensatory step.

Using different terms, we could interpret the process of border-crossing as follows: What makes the new way out of the postoedipal traumatic crisis possible is the phantasy formation produced by the drive in the oedipal development—*one risked the fight against Apollo and defeated him*. In the last moment, the *renewed*, destructive, traumatic process of the ego being inundated by great quantities of unbound energy was successfully stopped by binding these energies to a sexual phantasy. In the language of Le Soldat's masochism book, we might also say: at the last moment, one succeeded in fusing the *aggressive* (unbound) and the *libidinous* (bound) energy-quantities once more and thus to stop a psychical process that—on the structural level—would be purely destructive. That, then, would be the real triumph: "having defeated Apollo" means one succeeded in stopping a structural process of decay by binding energy to a sexual phantasy and thereby also to overcome the first, preoedipal invasion.

This concludes our reflections on the masochism book's first train of thought. We hope it has become clear that this early book is a veritable treasure trove of suggestions that allow us to see the later work—the Oedipus theory and the two special cases of postoedipal development—from new perspectives and thus not only to understand it better but to develop it further. A particularly promising avenue, in our view, is to realize the potential of Le Soldat's work as regards an integration of the psychoanalytic theory of the drives and trauma.

2 Second train of thought: "to pace out the intermediate realm that links individual and society"

In the outline for Paul Parin reproduced above, Judith Le Soldat articulates the theme of the second train of thought as follows: "'Masochism' is the symptom of a social force that acts on the individual: a socially conditioned and generated feeling and action of the individual" (above, #).

In the masochism book, she set out "to study the social conditions that can produce masochistic symptoms in the individual" (#). This would be a kind of social psychology or social psychoanalysis.

Moreover, she sought "to pace out the intermediate realm that links individual and society" (#). This evidently prompted her reference to controversies, particularly vivid in the 1970s and 1980s, about the relationship between psychoanalysis and Marxism.[52] Especially in the German-speaking countries, this discourse occupied the analysts who had emerged from the student movement in the years around 1968. They took up once more the wish "to apply psychoanalysis to society," which the Frankfurt School had explicitly abandoned in the mid-1950s.[53] Members of society were to be made to understand, "with the tools of psychoanalysis,"[54] why they so often acted against their real social interests and to be enabled to fight against the dominant capitalist conditions. The *practical* application of psychoanalysis was to be expanded in this sense. On the *theoretical* level, psychoanalysis as the "Critical Theory of the subject" was to supplement the "Critical Theory of capitalist society," that is, in this context, Marxism. The formal parallel between the two theories raised hopes about the possibility of integrating them. Helmut Dahmer interpreted psychoanalysis in general and Freud's culture-critical writings in particular as a special kind of sociology. Practicing psychoanalysts, on this view, have direct insight not into the "generally human" but—correctly—in the human "in a certain (historical-specific) expression." That could enable them to develop, as "iatrophilosophers," as healing philosophers, a "theory of the current age sufficient to orient our practice."[55]

In setting out "to pace out the intermediate realm that links individual and society," then, did Le Soldat, implicitly, assume the role of the "iatrophilosopher" Dahmer imagined? Put in these terms, she would probably have answered no. Yet she could not and certainly did not want to avoid confronting this discourse and integrating it into theory in her own special way. The theme pervades the entire book, particularly in the first part and again in the conclusion, especially in the final pages. This, in our view, makes the masochism book also a *political book*.

In this section, we trace how Le Soldat proceeds to reach the political positions that characterize her work at the time. In the first step (2.1), we define the possible directions or vectors of moving in this "intermediate realm," on the theoretical and the practical level. This yields a framework within which we present her fundamental positions in these debates. In the second step (2.2), we inquire into the way in which Le Soldat comes to assume these fundamental positions. In the third step (2.3), we follow her as she "pace[s] out the intermediate realm that links individual and society" in concrete terms. In the fourth step (2.4), we look at how her conceptions of masochism, aggression drive, and death drive can be related to those of important Marxist-oriented psychoanalysts.

2.1 How does Le Soldat position herself in the contradiction between psychoanalysis and Marxism?

The metaphor of the "intermediate realm" in which Le Soldat seeks to move is an excellent way of orienting ourselves within the contradiction between psychoanalysis and Marxism. There are two fundamental directions or *vectors* of movement to be distinguished in this intermediate realm:

1 The first vector leads from psychoanalysis to society.

   a On the *theoretical* level, one can *do social theory* and seek to enrich and change this theory by applying psychoanalytic concepts to social questions. One could, for example, trace capitalism's insatiability back to human oral greed or assign co-responsibility for its tendency toward war to ubiquitous sadism. More sophisticated than these rather trite examples are attempts to expand Marxism with something that—according to those who make these attempts—it is lacking: a theory of the "subjective factor."[56] Marxism is then understood as a "critical theory of society" and psychoanalysis as "critical theory of the subject," and one is looking for an integration of the two[57]; or psychoanalysis in general is understood to be a kind of sociology.[58]

   b On the *practical* level, the goal is to *effect change in society* by showing the exploited and oppressed the psychical mechanisms that prompt them to subject themselves and thus to act counter to their material social interests. This is to enable them to engage in a *society-changing practice*.

2 The second vector leads from society to the individual.

   a On the *theoretical* level, one can do *social criticism in theorizing psychoanalytically*. The goal is to show that how social mechanisms influence or harm the development of individuals' personalities and the way they deal with conflicts. This often happens in the oversimplification of saying that the production of surplus value and the compulsion to pursue economic growth quite generally "make us sick." More sophisticated is the formation of theoretical concepts of how the mechanisms and interests of the dominant social formation avail themselves of psychological processes of development and processing and of how, for example, they effect what Mario Erdheim calls the "social production of unconsciousness."[59]

   b On the *practical* level, the goal is to *integrate social criticism into the process of interpretation*.[60] An attitude critical of society is considered indispensable, and it is to be integrated into the process of interpretation in order to be able—as always in psychoanalysis—to discover what is unconscious.[61]

Guided by these four possibilities of moving in the intermediate realm between individual and society, let us trace what positions Le Soldat takes up.

Under heading (1a), *seeking to enrich social theory*, Le Soldat refers primarily to positions that in the search for the "subjective factor" aim to supplement or ally with social theory. Time and again, she concludes that this search cannot end in success, for two reasons. First, because "a theory capable of connecting social criticism and depth psychology is still outstanding" (#53)[62]; second, and more significantly, because such attempts at combination entail negative consequences:

> applying psychoanalysis to the social while keeping to the therapeutic position and method, however, is not only absurd, it is counterproductive. It gives rise to empty formulas such as "collectively unconscious," "social repressions," "group projections," and so on (#53).

Such empty formulas might still be harmless because they are relatively easy to recognize and criticize.[63] Things become more complex when we consider that the possibility of combining psychoanalysis and sociology in a dialectical way already exists today. Yet such a combination would not only be wrong, but it would also be detrimental in a specific way, since it

> disarms both theories in one blow—it deprives psychoanalysis of the overall conditions of its knowledge: while its theses remain correct, they are no longer relevant for the nexus of life; and social theory loses its ability to see through connections, to see that and how social and economic laws condition *psychical* misery (#65).[64]

This, in our view, applies throughout: defining Marxism as a "critical theory of society" loses sight of its aim not only theoretically to *interpret* society but to *change* it through a revolutionary process.[65] The same is true, mutatis mutandis, of psychoanalysis: it not only aims to *understand* subjects—as regards their unconscious psychical processes and conflicts—but also to provide them with the possibility to have a fundamentally new experience in an as it were revolutionary psychodynamic process.[66] Moreover, the "revolutionary" character of Le Soldat's theoretical work, too, is evident in that she does not revise Freud's central concepts but intensifies and thereby develops them.

Le Soldat thus prefers insisting on the divergence between the two branches of research which are psychoanalysis and social theory. She evidently does not consider herself an "iatrophilosopher" in Dahmer's sense, and there is no indication that like him, she conceives of psychoanalysis as a kind of sociology.

Quite logically, she rejects the aim described under (1b), to strive for *social change through psychoanalytic elucidation*:

> I recognized the thesis, in particular, that the *subjective factor*, that is, identifications and passive submission tendencies, is the motive of social processes, to be a symptom of a social amnesia. It serves to obfuscate

what is actually taking place between subject and society and effects an assignation of guilt to the individuals, whose unconscious and irrational forces are held responsible for the status quo (#261).

Yet there is a further reason why she considers an association of psychoanalysis and social theory to be counterproductive on the practical level as well: every transfer of concepts from individual psychology to society has the effect of a psychoanalytic *interpretation*.[67]

> [T]he endeavor to apply the methods of analysis to elucidate social conflicts goes beyond what is justifiable. It means wanting to proceed not only *as* an analyst, the way Freud did, but with the tools of analytic therapy, abstinent and without taking sides. That this is a mistake from the point of view of a theory of science would be harmless if it were not equally a political act, namely an unintended taking sides for the dominant ideology ostensibly to be elucidated. ... For it is a peculiarity of psychoanalysis that the very utterance of *theoretical* propositions acts on the listener *like an interpretation*. The explication of aggression theory unavoidably generates a sense of guilt because we refer what we hear to ourselves and understand it as an allusion to our own secret source of pleasure (#54–55, our emphasis).

The point could not be made more clearly.[68]

This brings us to the second vector, which goes in the opposite direction, that is, leads from society to the individual. Let's once more look at the theoretical level first, *social criticism in psychoanalytical theorizing* (2a). The aim is to get a picture of social conditions and processes generally to understand how they change individual-psychological mechanisms and avail themselves of them[69]—in a manner that individuals usually are not conscious of or that takes place "behind the back of the producers," as Marx puts it.[70]

In the following example, Le Soldat refers explicitly to Mario Erdheim and implicitly to Russell Jacoby[71]:

> A pulsional impulse whose intentions contradict the dominant ideology initially remains unsatisfied; then it is repressed; and finally, after a phase of attempts to return, it withers. It will give its energy to other pulsional aims more acceptable to power. To operate this *displacement*, cultural morality makes use of the individual conscience. The defense function is performed by the individual, but it is produced socially [explicit citation of Erdheim in a note] and supported by a collective amnesia [no explicit citation for this position advocated by Jacoby] (#19).

In talking about the contemporary social formation, Le Soldat—in the best Freudian tradition—sometimes uses the word "culture." Most often, she employs the term *Herrschaft*, "dominion,"[72] to characterize the oppression, and on occasion she also includes exploitation. Her assessment finds exemplary expression in the following passage:

> Yet as long as the *quantitative* relation of power and powerlessness is the way it is, neutrality surreptitiously turns into assent. As long as power, possessions, knowledge, and the prospect of fulfilling the pulsional demands accumulate on one side whereas on the other side, powerlessness, dependency, prohibitions on thought, and pressure to conform hold sway, ... analysts striving for neutrality and abstinence inevitably will be caught in the pleasure-promising, quantitatively greater force's pull into the sphere of influence of power. They will then diagnose frustration aggressions and an identification with the aggressor where they should perceive realistic anxiety and intentional manipulation of the pulsional vicissitudes (#29).

And thus we have reached the practical side of the second vector, *social criticism in the process of interpretation* (2b).[73] This vector brings *unconscious* mechanisms to light through which the adaptation to social forces and expectations causes psychical suffering.[74] This can be conceived of as a kind of social psychology, as a "social psychoanalysis," as it were, that is concerned not with a psychoanalytically informed sociology but with a sociologically informed psychoanalysis.

According to Le Soldat, there can be no neutrality toward power and oppression, neither within psychoanalytic treatment (vector 2b) nor outside the clinical setting, for example, when psychoanalysts make public statements: "Wrongly remaining silent, pointing, faced with the arrogance of those in power, to the pulsional wishes (masochism) and unconscious expectations of punishment, the longing for death and self-destructive rage of the victims, is not science but betrayal" (#28).

Neutrality is always a question of the social context in which we do our psychoanalytic work, and as long as this context rests on exploitation and oppression, there can be no abstinence from social *criticism*. Otherwise, psychoanalysts become accomplices of the dominant conditions instead of working in the interest of the "powerless" (see #31).

So much for some examples of the *fundamental positions* Le Soldat assumes as she "pace[s] out the intermediate realm that links individual and society." To summarize: she rejects vector 1, which seeks to understand society via the subjective-individual factor; in turn, she considers vector 2, which inversely studies how individual suffering is produced socially, to be indispensable.

2.2 What path does Le Soldat take to reach her fundamental positions?

In this section, we would like to retrace the—from the psychoanalytic perspective—most important path Le Soldat takes to reach the positions just

32   Voluntary Servitude. Masochism and Morality

presented. Central here is a matter close to her heart: to defend pleasurable aggression and the pulsionality underlying it against repression, disavowal, and taboo. She emphatically asserts that the parts of Freud's heritage that address the aggression drive, (sado-) masochism as "perversion" and as moral pressure from a "sadistic" superego, are much more subversive than the theory of the libido and the concept of infantile sexuality ever were. The zeitgeist seems to have been ready for libido theory, despite the scandalized reaction at the time. Her chief witness for this view is the revolutionary Marxist György Lukács:

> György Lukács describes the dominant interest in turn-of-the-century Europe as an interest in maintaining class societies. *This* interest promoted the development of psychoanalysis even if it turned it into a social *skandalon*. The emancipation granted the operation of the sexual drive was to attract the energies that the social conflict demanded for itself. The theater piece of sexual analysis had to be produced on the political stage since otherwise, the audience would have stormed the arena to put on its own piece (#33).

According to Lukács, the period at the beginning of the twentieth century was characterized by the imminence of the proletarian revolution, which at the end of World War I had indeed "stormed the arena" in several countries.[75] In the years after 1968, too—when Lukács's *History and Class Consciousness* from the 1920s was being rediscovered—parts of the revolutionary forces criticized the turn of large parts of the movement to psychoanalysis as counterrevolutionary. Lukács in our view names one of the more profound reasons for why that was and continues to be the case today.

In this conflict, Le Soldat first positions herself *against* "leftist psychoanalysis," namely, against the "recent psychoanalytic literature concerned with cultural criticism." She does so primarily because these approaches fail to acknowledge aggression *as* a pleasure-seeking drive: "What we look for in vain" in this literature "is the most general form of hostility, which is exclusively defined by striving for pleasure" (#26). The examples she cites include works by Otto Fenichel, Alexander Mitscherlich, and Paul Parin—authors to whom she will also, in part and under different aspects, refer positively. To illustrate the point, she anecdotally recounts the conference the Zurich Psychoanalytic Seminar organized in 1983 with the title *War and Peace from the Psychoanalytic Point of View*, whose participants "painstakingly avoid[ed] the word[s] aggression or aggression drive."[76] The views represented there shared the explicit or implicit assumption that social conditions could be explained and possibly even changed "with the tools of psychoanalysis."[77] Le Soldat has thereby reached the critique of the *first vector*: she started from the disavowal of the ubiquitous pleasurable aggression and notes now that in the leading psychoanalytic cultural critics, this disavowal prompts illusions about the compatibility of psychoanalysis and Marxism. She makes the point with reference to Fenichel—in truly dialectic fashion, given that she has just criticized him:

> Of aggression generally, we can say what Otto Fenichel says about one of its variants, the drive to enrich oneself: it is not the case that the biological drive creates the particular conditions to satisfy itself; rather, a social system makes use of the pulsional impulses and strengthens those of their derivatives that serve its special interests. Oppressing others, exploiting them and keeping them away from vital resources, forcing them into anxiety and a conflicted conscience, competition, physical and psychical violence are not genuine forms of aggressions but forms that aggression takes under very specific social conditions (#31).[78]

In this way, Le Soldat has reached the *second vector* and is able to take the positions mentioned in Section 2.1. In concrete terms, she is again and again concerned with the way in which social mechanisms and the interests of dominion avail themselves of individual *aggressive pulsionality*. When in the process, she notes that "aggressiveness in its present from must be recognized as an instrument of power and no longer as pulsional force," she will, accordingly, "tak[e] a stance against aggression" (#31).

Given how passionately she is working, we must not be surprised that—as we will see in the next section—she does not always succeed in arguing "neatly" in keeping with the positions she takes in the "intermediately realm between individual and society."

2.3 Concrete movement in the intermediate realm between individual and society

One might characterize her writing style in her own words as "bustrophedonic, aimless, all over the place."[79] "Bustrophedonic" literally means going back and forth like an ox ploughing—in our concrete case, back and forth along the two vectors. Time and again, this is confusing. In reading Le Soldat, it is thus helpful to pay attention to what side this movement *finally arrives* on: the side of society—the first vector, which she rejects in principle—or the side of the individual—the second vector, which she considers indispensable.

When in her book, the author addresses a "question that has always been waiting for answer," the question of "voluntary servitude" (#56), she is fully aware that the temptation to be drawn in by a false cultural ideology cannot really be avoided (#58). In order not to get lost, it is necessary, first, not to confuse objective power with individual dominion, and, second, to keep the pulsional cruelty of those in power and of the oppressed clearly separate, even if there are no external differences (#59)—which is of great significance in the individual process of interpretation. Both belong to the second vector.

Thus oriented, we can now turn to some examples to pursue the question whether and to what extent Le Soldat in her practical work maintains the positions she has assumed theoretically. We will see that this is usually the case and that exceptions, as the saying goes, prove the rule.

In Chapter I.7—"The ability to remain silent and the task of theory"—she points to "the different subjective positions demanded of analysts when they seek to elucidate, on the one hand, the individually unconscious and, on the other, what is generally unconscious" (#53). She thus implicitly *names* both vectors and initially *addresses* the first one in turning to a lecture that Fenichel, a Marxist-oriented psychoanalyst, gave at the Kulturverein Basel, an association that "belonged to the political left."[80] We might wonder if Fenichel was concerned with educating his listeners about the psychical mechanisms obstructing their political struggle—that is, a practical activity in the sense of vector 1b. The transcript shows him being concerned above all with a critique of psychologism—that is, with the rejection of something we designate by the first vector as well. Why, therefore, does Le Soldat cite this example? Because she wants to show that—given certain political conditions—"the very utterance of *theoretical* propositions acts on the listener like an interpretation." Had Fenichel drawn attention to what, according to Le Soldat, the lecture was about, namely, the "aggression tendency" and "pulsional pleasure" that are "in all cases associated with the idea of belligerent acts" (#54), Fenichel, "in the time of Fascism," would "have generated a paralyzing feeling of guilt in the listeners to whom [he] was speaking—as leftists, as Jews, et cetera, they had the objective social supremacy against them and not behind them" (#56). That is why Fenichel was right to avoid mentioning the fact. In other social situations, where "the priority is to communicate knowledge," such reactions, to be sure, cannot be avoided entirely, but they can be neglected (#54).

Is it necessary, though, in different political situations—in confronting the threat of nuclear war, for example—to educate members of society about psychological facts, that is, to proceed along vector 1b? In Chapter I.6, "On the necessity of lying," she overdraws the nuclear threat as the ultimate threat that makes any life in its wake impossible (#48–49).[81] In this historical situation, our task is entirely different from Fenichel's in his day. The question is, though: what is that task? At first, one is tempted to suspect that Le Soldat on this point is influenced by the No Future movement of the 1980s. At a closer look, however, the section proves to be mainly about the individual consequences of the socially produced nuclear threat and especially its consequences for conscience, which plainly corresponds to the sense of the second vector.

> Human conscience has been overrun by the historical development of the last decades; ignoring the commandments of conscience (which it

itself has posited), reality has allied with the pulsional wishes. The aggressiveness demanded by reality deprives sexuality of its force, leaves it empty, and draws all expectations of pleasure onto itself (#50).

Whether we share them or not, these reflections clearly move in the direction of the second vector. But what are we to make of her exhortation to "lie"? Is she advocating an exaggeration to counter the tendency to disavow the threat? What are we to make, moreover, of the fact that—against her position on principle—she encourages "psychoanalysis, as a partner of the *political* peace movements, [to] enter the struggle for a resilient, more intelligent conscience" (#51)?

In a different context, a remark slips in that runs counter to her fundamental rejection of the first vector: "In a system of dominion, the *individual-psychical energy joins the means of production capital, land, and labor on equal footing*" (#135). Objectively, this is not just a contribution to a *critique* of society but to a *theory* of society. As such, it misses its mark (as intuitively comprehensible as that goal might be). First, the "trinity" of the *factors*—not the *means*—of production capital, land, and labor derives from the bourgeois economics immanent to the system, and for most *bourgeois economists*, the "fourth factor of production" Le Soldat postulates, psychical energy, will remain a book with seven seals. Second, *Marxists* will insist that not *three* factors of productions but only *one*, socially organized labor, creates value and surplus value. And third, *psychoanalysts* will point out that the "individual-psychical energy" does not make individual workers ever more productive but that it can also gravely diminish their performance. The example, in our view, is evidence that the first vector is necessarily misleading—for Le Soldat herself, too.

Yet as far as we can see, this is the only occasion on which she *plainly* comes to contradict her *theoretical* position.[82] In all other cases, we consider the second vector to impose itself, as two examples, which could be replaced by many others, show.

1 In Chapter III.4, she postulates the transition from matriarchy to patriarchy as the origin of girls' change of object from the mother to the father. She thus adopts a *historical-social theory* advocated, among others, by Engels,[83] but she has no intention of enriching or changing it. Independently of whether one shares her historical derivation, she is exclusively concerned with an individual-psychological understanding of this change of object: little girls thereby react unconsciously to an "objective supremacy in the external world," similar to the reality principle (#218).
2 When she shows—as for instance in Chapter II.6—that how the individual-psychological energy of masochistically disposed people is made to serve political dominion without them knowing and wanting it, and when she characterizes this as a phenomenon to stabilize bourgeois dominion—as

36 Voluntary Servitude. Masochism and Morality

similarly is the case, formally, for racism or sexism—one might at first understand this as an attempt, along vector 1, to supplement social theory with the "subjective factor." Yet a closer look shows "Two paths to masochism" not to be about integrating psychoanalysis and social theory but about distinguishing between sociogenic and purely innerpsychical causes of psychical suffering: "the individual as well society, each prompted by different causes, with different means, and with different intentions, produce the same symptoms" (#115). The sociogenic causes clearly correspond to the second vector, the integration of social critique into psychoanalytical theorizing. The emphasis on the *divergence* between sociological and psychological research their laws is particularly clear here.

In summary, Le Soldat's statements about the intertwining of the social and the individual almost always have the character of social *critique,* not of social *theory,* and her practice remains psychoanalytic and does not enter the political stage. This corresponds to the second vector, the direction that is already plainly stated in the way she articulates the second train of thought to Paul Parin: "'Masochism' is the symptom of a social force that acts on the individual: a socially conditioned and generated feeling and action of the individual" (#).

For us, Le Soldat's radical positioning in "the intermediate realm between psychoanalysis and society" is a precondition for her proving herself a radical and innovative psychoanalytic theorist in her later writings.[84] While she does not explicitly return to this positioning, there are no indications either that she has changed anything about it or that she has given up the social-critical attitude in her practice. In our view, she in later years builds on the foundation laid here—implicitly but coherently: from here on out, the focus of her later work is resolutely on exploring psychodynamic conditions. She does not go back to the "intermediate realm"—not even where her theorizing touches on topics relevant to social criticism, such as contempt for women and discrimination of homosexuals. In the *Lectures,* Le Soldat thus postulates genuinely psychical reasons for the contempt for women and situates them equally in the psychosexual development of boys and of girls. And although she considers this psychically founded contempt for women to be universal, she does not allow herself to be tempted into deriving from that a social-theoretical explanation for the existence of structural forms of the discrimination of women.[85] She remains faithful to her rejection of what we have described as vector 1. At this point, she no longer talks about the inverse movement, the derivation of psychical conditions from social conditions (vector 2). Her focus is resolutely and exclusively on innerpsychical conflicts and defense formations; the "intermediate realm" between individual and society no longer comes up. At a different point in the *Lectures,* she addresses the "contemptible 'discrimination' of gay people."[86] She looks at this phenomenon, too, strictly from the perspective of psychodynamics, of pulsional conflicts and the defense against them, without deriving social-structural forms of discrimination of homosexual men and women. The same is true of "gay self-contempt": here, too, she resolutely focuses on innerpsychical dynamics without explaining them as the result of social conditions (as is the case, for example, of the social-psychological concept of "internalized homophobia").

2.4 How does Le Soldat's conception of the death drive link up with criticism of this concept from the left?

The political positions presented thus far align Le Soldat with a certain tradition of leftist psychoanalysts. This tradition, however, is characterized not only by leftist *political* positions. Within the framework of psychoanalytic practice and theory itself, authors of the early psychoanalytic left prefer certain concepts and reject others. In our context here, this particularly concerns conceptions of masochism, of the aggression drive, and of the death drive.[87]

Wilhelm Reich was the first prominent leftist analyst to critically engage with the death drive hypothesis. Otto Fenichel does the same in a particularly striking way.[88] We will therefore present this criticism via Fenichel's work and then show how close Le Soldat's concepts are to this view.

Fenichel begins by noting that the "task is not to prove what kinds of instincts there are, but to ask: Which classification of instincts enables us to grasp various actual psychological phenomena most easily and with least contradiction?"[89] He continues:

> The concept of an instinct, as presented in Freud's "Instincts and Their Vicissitudes" must remain our directive: instinctual need is "the demand made by the body upon the psychic apparatus." It begins in a somatic "instinctual source," which makes the psychological system excitable, and which with the aid of sensory stimuli it actually excites; the instinctual action then results in changes at this source which are equivalent to a "discharge" of the excitation—that is, to a relaxation of tension.[90]

But, Fenichel notes, a "'death instinct' does not fit in with such a definition of instinct."[91] Why not? Because in a death instinct, this process of excitation and discharge cannot unfold.

> For this reason it does not seem to me possible to set up the "death instinct" as one species of instinct over against another species. We should rather attempt to regard all the actual phenomena which are denoted by the concept "death instinct" as dependent not on a species of instinct, but on a *principle*, which originally obtained for *all* instincts,

but in the course of development has, under certain influences (in the final analysis, those of the external world), been obliged to undergo several modifications in several respects.[92]

Fenichel concludes:

the conception that in the neurotic conflict ... neuroses rest upon a conflict of two kinds of instinctual qualities, a self-destructive one, the death instinct, and an "erotic" ego which was afraid of its death instinct ... would mean a total elimination of the social factor from the etiology of neuroses, and would amount to a complete biologization of neuroses.[93]

Le Soldat nowhere explicitly refers to this criticism and yet she comes to take positions that—as we would like to show now—are essentially the same.

Freud introduced the death drive hypothesis in *Beyond the Pleasure Principle* and developed it in *The Ego and the Id*, but he always articulated it in very cautious terms and characterized it as speculative.[94] Nothing remains of such caution in "The Economic Problem of Masochism."[95] Instead, it seems that Freud has found here the field on which he could establish the death drive as a fact. Masochism appears to him as a manifestation of the death drive. Le Soldat objects to this at several points in the book. While she "consider[s] the death drive theory to be a necessary consequence of psychoanalytic reflections" (#156), she suggests "dissolv[ing] the unfruitful association of masochism and death drive again. Establishing masochistic tendencies has no need of the death drive, and the death drive can very well assert its existence without the evidence of masochism" (#109). She furthermore considers the association of aggression and death drive doubtful (#156). "At least we succeeded in liberating masochism from a heavy and foreign duty. For if aggression has nothing to contribute to the functioning of the death drive, then masochism is exonerated as its crown witness" (#164). "In the case of masochism, I see no reason to postulate a particular influence of the death drive" (#199).

In this first step, Le Soldat moves away from the association of the death drive with masochism. In the next step, she writes, "aggression is to be liberated from its being bound to the death drive, the destructive and sadistic strivings are to join the sexual libido" (#158). And finally, she denies that the death drive is a *drive*: "I think we understand Freud's death drive theory better and avoid a number of contradictions with other parts of metapsychology when we conceive of the *death drive not as a pulsional force but as a principle of psychical processes*" (#158). Not much remains of the death *drive* here: like Fenichel, Le Soldat declares the death drive to be a principle that regulates psychical processes, even if she assigns it a different content than Fenichel does. In her conception, it is an emergency mechanism of the psychical system that is activated whenever the usual ways of regulating the psychical equilibrium no longer work. Such is the case when too large quantities of unbound energy threaten to destroy the ego structures. Then an impulse in the id ensures that the usual direction of the pulsional flow is reversed, that is, that it no longer runs from the id to the ego but is pulled back from the ego into the id. The reversal of the pulsional flow relieves the ego but also entails a (temporary) collapse of the ego structures that Le Soldat describes as a "psychical death" (#158–63).

Le Soldat's conception of the death drive thus links up with the leftist criticism in that she, too, denies it the character of a drive and at the same time nonetheless holds on to it as a principle indispensable to understanding psychotraumatic processes.

Notes

1 While Monika Gsell is mainly responsible for the first part and Ralf Binswanger for the second, this introduction is the result of a close cooperation.
2 Le Soldat, in fact, writes: "I explicitly do not speak of a traumatic event because in this early phase of life, the structure of the triggering external situation seems unimportant to me, besides being impossible to ascertain sufficiently." What she is thereby rejecting—what she is not speaking of or talking about—is thus merely the conventional use of the concept of trauma in the sense of an *external* event. In the course of the book, she refers to the *internal* process described here as a trauma; see #238, 299, 304, 322, 333, 402.
3 Compare Le Soldat's conception of the "always primary pulsional anxiety" that arises "when a pulsional tension is not relaxed in time or inadequately" (#149). She understands the object-related anxieties to be "consequences and results of the defense" against the primary pulsional anxiety (#149).
4 The notion that because of the pulsional defusion the libidinous shares "become passive" plays an important role in the entire book and finds expression in different contexts in a variety of formulations; see, for example, #174: "the sexual cathexes ... become passive"; #177: "genital strivings that had become passive"; #189: "libido ... become passive"; #261: "now passive sexual libido." "Becoming passive" thus does not always seem to denote the exact same thing: at some points, "passive" refers to the sensorial pathways of bodily pulsional discharge (this presumably applies in the passage #174), at other points, it seems to refer instead to a loss of energy quanta or intensity (e.g., #189). What can safely be said, though, is that "passive" does not yet have the meaning of an autonomous, genuine pulsional wish, as it will have in Le Soldat's later work (see our more detailed terminological reflections in Section 1.2.2 of this introduction).
5 In the masochism book as in Le Soldat's later work, the expression "idealizing" usually refers to the idea of phallic intactness: objects are idealized when they are being equipped with the organ needed to fulfill one's own pulsional wishes.
6 In the masochism book Le Soldat uses the term *zerfallen*—to fall apart, to split, to decay, or to collapse—primarily in the context of the defusion of libido and aggression and to describe the consequences of this defusion: ambivalence, the "relationship of libido and aggression ... fall[s] apart" (#139; 151); the "phallic wish" is "split" into a passive and an aggressive share (#99); the object cathexes split into "good" and "bad" ones (#146); the "recathexis," the change of object, falls apart (#223); the "body-cathex[es] split into their constitutive parts" such that the sensory pulsional discharge is cathected only as "passive," the motoric pulsional discharge as "active" (#175). The concept *Zerfall* is also applied to ego structures

40   *Voluntary Servitude. Masochism and Morality*

(#157 and 163) and for "psychical structures" generally (#158). In the *Lectures*, Le Soldat uses the concept only in the first sense, by which she means that a composite entity splits into the individual components (phantasy contents, cathectic energy) from which it has been assembled. The components themselves remain intact and can make new connections (see, for instance, Le Soldat 2015, 182 and 241n7).

7 In the course of the book, several causes are being considered for the diminishing of the experience of pleasure under "masochistic" conditions, some of which are complementary; see #200 (lack of ambivalence tension); #233 (the "withered libido"); #235; 248–49; 254, and especially also note# (isolation of wish and affect); #258 ("the lack of a connection between phantasy and physical manipulation").
8 See, for example, Le Soldat 2015, 169.
9 We are thinking here in particular of the phantasy formations connected with the conception, still missing in the masochism book, of passive wishes: the colpos wish and the hammer blow wish.
10 Le Soldat views psychical phenomena and processes from essentially two perspectives, which she distinguishes as the technical and the contentual aspect of the psychical. The contentual aspect names the latent phantasy formations with whose individual derivatives we are dealing with in analysis. The technical aspect names the pulsional processes through which the phantasies are produced in the first place; see Gsell 2016, 32.
11 Vividly described in Le Soldat 2015, 128.
12 On Freud's conception of the constitutive psychical bisexuality and the significance in the formation of neuroses he attributed to it, see Gsell and Zürcher 2011.
13 See the index entries on *passive-genital*, *active-genital*, and *passive-aggressive* in Le Soldat 2015, as well as the next note.
14 See, for instance, Le Soldat 2015, 81–86.
15 One example: "The defense has compelled sensorial ('passive') wishes and aggressive impulses to be bound to separate phantasies of body areas" (#256)–*sensorial/passive* here takes the place of *libidinous*.
16 "Low in energy," she says at one point: there must be a displacement of cathexis such that "the libido appears low in energy, while the aggression in turn seems sexualized" (#188).
17 On the connection of "passive-libidinous" with submission, helplessness, and dependency, see, for instance, #43 and 260.
18 For example, #146; 147note, 150, and 210.
19 #147; Le Soldat's emphasis. Unlike elsewhere in the book, "passive" is here referred to aggressive strivings as well.
20 See Le Soldat 2015, lectures 5–7: 117–80.
21 For Freud, see Gsell and Zürcher 2011 on the concepts *active* and *passive* in relation to *masculine* and *feminine*. Our analysis of Freud's use of these concepts was already based on Le Soldat's later theory, without which it would not have been possible. For Eissler, see Eissler 1938, which Le Soldat cites as evidence for her thesis that aggression, too, cathects preferred body zones. Eissler's article is about the observation that infants immediately after birth know two different modes of oral activity: a sucking reflex and a more playful touching of the oral mucosa with the tongue. Eissler interprets this observation as evidence for Freud's pulsional dualism in the sense of "libidinous and destructive pulsional energies" (84). In fact, though, these observations would be described with more precision employing Le Soldat's later vocabulary, namely, as evidence of the pulsional dualism in the sense of *active*-oral and *passive*-oral pulsional aims.
22 The example of the following passage may serve to show just how close to this later conception Le Soldat's phrasing is already in the masochism book: "Beside

the disentanglement of sexuality and aggression, a new divergence arises between *aggressive phallic wishes* that must be projected and are *idealized* in the object, and the *passive sexual wishes* bound in one's own body" (#174). In what is called a "new divergence" here, we clearly see the later doubling of "active-genital" and "passive-genital" pulsional impulses—just with the significant difference, which we must not overlook, that in the masochism book, this doubling is not understood as primary and constitutively given but as a consequence of the defusion, and that "passive" does not designate a genuine pulsional wish but means a dependence on help from others to satisfy phallic impulses.

23 See note # above.
24 See Le Soldat 2015, lecture 9: 209–34.
25 Another difficulty in reading the book comes from the numerous passages in which Le Soldat opposes the "female change of object" with the "masochistic" = "male" = "necessary for internal reasons" change of object (that is to say, *in women, it's this way, in masochists, that way*). Time and again this prompts an uncertainty whether she does in fact refer her reflections on the masochistic change of object to corresponding female lines of development. Since, however, she presents *two* women patients as examples of the special case of masochism, we may assume that her opposition of "female" and "masochistic" change of object is a kind of shorthand—a shorthand to be read as: "common female change of object" = "not for internal reasons" vs. "masochistic, male *and* female change of object" = "for internal reasons." This reading is supported by the following passage: "Yet although I otherwise declare the change of object to be, at bottom, optional for girls as well, in *masochism*, we must postulate an *obligatory and unavoidable oedipal recathexis for both sexes*" (#212).
26 "When the most embarrassing infantile demands experience no countercathexis, they are not eliminated for consciousness but present in a particular form. They are *preconscious but emotionally isolated*. The incest phantasies do not fall prey to the usual infantile amnesia, they form a secret, pleasurable core in the ego" (#134).
27 Put in more general terms: in Le Soldat's conception, the change of object always results from the oedipal development: "The infantile conflict sets the conditions for a later choice of object and becomes the criterion for whether one will in the future acknowledge the difference between the sexes that the unconscious up to this point denies" (#127). This holds for her late work as well. There, however, it is differentiated and, as far as we can see, dissociated from the question of disavowing the difference between the sexes.
28 See, for instance, #223: "Because they regress to the binding to the mother, masochistic women appear homosexual; they seek to conquer women"—which would correspond to a manifestly homosexual choice of object—"although their *pulsional wishes*, because of the genuine orientation toward the phallus and the short phase of love for the father, rather have to count as heterosexual. Genital passivity and penis wish unite in the phantasy of being satisfied by the 'phallic' mother." In her note on this passage, she refers to one of her case studies, the acrobat, a manifestly heterosexual woman. By "heterosexual pulsional wishes," she quite evidently means that the subject assumes a passive-genital position toward the object and expect an active-genital, *phallic* "action" from the object. *Passive* is thus understood as synonymous with *feminine*, *active* as synonymous with *masculine*. In the next example, by contrast, the exact same "drive constellation" (subject: passive-genital position—internal object: phallic mother) is called a "homosexual practice": "Men, in contrast, after a period of homoerotic love for the father, return to the originary incestuous wish. We must not, however, suppose that the pulsional quality has remained unchanged. Thanks to the recathexis, the masochist,

too, now wishes *to obtain a pleasurable satisfaction in a homosexual practice from the mother who is also equipped with a phallus.* These objectal ideas are henceforth the model of all masturbation phantasies" (#223–24).

29 On #215 we read concerning the girl's change of object from the mother to the father: "This process corresponds to the *'negative' outcome of the oedipal conflict,* and I think it characterizes the *common female solution* that seems normal to us"; on #218: "the regularly 'negative' outcome of the oedipal conflict, that is to say, women's heterosexual inversion."

30 See the few passages in the masochism book where Le Soldat explicitly addresses the psychosexual development of women who later are lesbian: #211, #215note, and #221note.

31 See especially Le Soldat 2015, lectures 8–11: 181–281, as well as Le Soldat 2018, 239–40 (the distinction between "descriptively homosexual" and "dynamically homosexual") and 350.

32 Le Soldat 2018, 350 and 388.

33 On Le Soldat's use of the concept "gay," see Le Soldat 2018, 239–40.

34 See Le Soldat 2018, 218 and Le Soldat 2015, 281.

35 Le Soldat 2015, 226 and 270.

36 Thus the regressive return, for example, to early love for the mother does not automatically lead to the choice of a female object; the early-oedipal mother can also be or, rather, is preferentially projected onto a man (see Le Soldat 2015, lecture 8: 181–208).

37 See, for instance, Fäh and Gsell 2021.

38 See Fäh and Gsell 2021, as well as Binswanger 2016 and Gsell 2016.

39 This thesis accords, first, with Le Soldat's metaphorical designation, in the *Lectures,* of the boundary between the oedipal this side and the beyond as a "firewall" (Le Soldat 2015, 33–34 and 50–51). When then we also recall that the traumatic breaking through the protection against stimuli is *the* central topic of Freud's *Beyond the Pleasure Principle* (1920)—a text Le Soldat addresses in the masochism book but which later seems no longer to play a role—the scales suddenly fall from our eyes: Le Soldat's *beyond* (the oedipal) contains a tribute to Freud's *Beyond* (the pleasure principle) overlooked so far. It then is certainly no coincidence that Le Soldat's rearticulation of Freud's concept of the death drive in the masochism book quite obviously includes the "nucleus" of the later concept of border-crossing (see especially #157–59, as well as #163; the keywords here are *implosion, reversal, dissolution,* and *destruction of ego structures*).

40 These particular conditions include, for instance, an increased (when compared to the "common" oedipal development) tendency toward isolation, projection, and introjection as well as the phenomena of splitting (#205–6 and 235), the formation of the superego ("The masochistic super-ego is vicious and cruel, yet at the same time, it is *weak, deficient, and barely able to fulfill its function*" #225) and its relationship with the ego (#232).

41 Only one of these three steps of the border-crossing—breakthrough, destruction, and formation of a new border—is described in the masochism book, the aspect of the destruction of the ego's defense structure: "We must imagine the processes in the id that correspond to the collapse of the ego structures as a kind of implosion, *the pulsional forces collapse and withdraw into the id, finally withdraw from the psychical as such.* … The abatement of the pulsional energies appears to the ego as a reversal of the pulsional direction and leads to the dissolution of the structures that have become useless" (#163). "Too great an intensity annihilates the ego structures established for the defense and renders the ego helpless" (#167).—In the *Lectures*: breakthrough and destruction ("explosion") of the border (Le Soldat 2015, 218–26), formation of the new border (226–28) and of new defense formations (275).

42 See, for instance, Le Soldat 2015, 218.
43 Le Soldat 2018, 213–14.
44 Le Soldat 2018, 214.
45 What today we would designate as disintegration anxiety, Le Soldat in the masochism book calls "pulsional anxiety" (see especially #182, but also #106; #149; #234).
46 Le Soldat 2015, lectures 9–11: 209–81.
47 In *Land ohne Wiederkehr*, Le Soldat uses the English word "overload" to describe these particular conditions (Le Soldat 2018, 214 and 216).
48 For the traumatic process, see Le Soldat 2015, 263 and 277; Le Soldat 2018, y261; for the hammer blow or Apollo wish, see Le Soldat 2018, 213–14: "The drive rids itself of the contentual phantasy by fulfilling 'Apollo'—the imaginary positions of the hammer blow wish as well. Not a pulsional breakthrough, since almost nothing becomes visible in reality" (214).
49 Le Soldat 2018, 215–16. It is worthwhile, especially in this context, to cite the passage at length: "It's not my fault that all these concepts—Apollo, IRMA, robbery-murder, as well as the established superego, the id, repression—seem so novelistic. The psychical cannot help but teleologically interpret the pulsional dynamic processes, which follow their paths within like natural events, following iron laws, without sense or intention, suppose them to have feelings and motivations that they induce and generate in the first place. Inner perception cannot help it, yet reflection cannot either. As soon as it tries to capture the action of the pulsional powers in words, the forces turn into figures, acquire faces, fates. Although we always know that they are merely indifferent factors, themselves subject to laws we do not know."
50 This contentual articulation synthesizes the structural view Le Soldat describes in the masochism book in the context of her reflections on the death drive and the figure of death (#157–58) and of the description of the pulsional dynamics and the content of border-crossing in her later work (Le Soldat 2015, 215 and 219–20). In both articulations, the motif of "reversal"—an *Umkehr* as both turning around and turning away—plays a central role.
51 This suggestion accords with Le Soldat's first working title for *Land ohne Wiederkehr*, which was "The Second Time" (Le Soldat 2018, 19), and with her referring to the border-crossing, on two occasions, as a "second schism" (Le Soldat 2018, 220 and 229). The second time or the second schism would then mean: a second trauma, albeit one that overcomes or compensates for the first trauma. This compensation has the effect of a pulsional satisfaction, a point the following passage seems to make as well: "After a few weeks, it had become clear that the dream, with the help of a pleasurable phantasy, had elegantly skipped over a psychical abyss (the 'gap' in the bed). In technical terms: a traumatic memory somehow prompted by the eviction from the apartment, a memory whose content now threatened to catch fire [disintegration anxieties!]. The memory had been repressed once more, and better, underneath the dream, as it were" (Le Soldat 2018, 206–7).
52 For an overview of the history of these debates from Freud and Adler to the demise of the German Democratic Republic, see Nitzschke 1989.
53 Reiche 1995, 227 and 244 (citing Adorno [1955] 1967/1968).
54 Modena 2017.
55 Dahmer 1982, 370.
56 The term "subjective factor of history" was first used by Wilhelm Reich ([1933] 1970, 6).
57 In what follows, we use the term "subjective factor" exclusively in this theoretical context, the way Le Soldat does most of the time as well. In other contexts, we will use everyday language to describe subjective forces and mechanisms at work in the "intermediate realm" between individual and society.
58 See Dahmer 1982.

44 Voluntary Servitude. Masochism and Morality

59 Erdheim 1982.
60 Parin (1975) 1978.
61 Parin's "Is Psychoanalysis a Social Science?" too, is more specifically concerned with vector 2: "Thus, man appears as a social being shaped by a society rich in conflicts the influences of which determine his development, his social situation, as well as his mental life" (Parin 1975, 383).
62 In our view, this should read "social theory" rather than "social criticism," since Le Soldat, as we will see in a moment, considers the combination of social criticism and psychoanalysis, precisely, to be indispensable.
63 See, exemplarily, Fenichel's criticism: "If now psychoanalysts try, by falsely equating individual life with social events, to apply psychological knowledge to social events and attempt to find, say, 'an unconscious social motive force,' and in so doing overlook the material causes of social phenomena, the Marxists are right in insisting that that is nonsense" (Fenichel [1934] 1967, 301).
64 An analogous position would be advocated by Reiche (1995, 232).
65 See Marx (1845) 1970, 123.
66 See Morgenthaler 2005.
67 On this point, see Binswanger 1985.
68 The example refers to a left-leaning and in part Jewish audience threatened by Nazism, that is, potential victims whose *neurotic* feelings of guilt are easily mobilized. The psychology of perpetrators and of strata of the population that identified with Nazism and did not display *appropriate* feelings of guilt is not the topic of the masochism book. Chapter I.4, "A 'Mishap' in Germany," touches on it, but there, Le Soldat is concerned less with the psychological situation of individuals under the Nazi regime and the individual consequences of this situation than she is with analyzing a political process in postwar Germany.
69 To avoid misunderstandings: a description of mechanisms by which society avails itself of individual-psychological forces and processes can also be described as an aspect of social *theory* according to vector 1a. That, however, is not what Le Soldat is usually concerned with: instead, she is concerned with social *criticism* within the framework of psychoanalytic work. She is interested in the effects these social mechanisms have on the individual, which corresponds to our vector 2.
70 Marx (1867) 1990, 37 and 92, as well as 179 and 315.
71 See Erdheim 1982 and Jacoby 1975. By "social amnesia," Jacoby means "the application of planned obsolescence to thought itself" taking place continuously under "the pressure of society." This leads him in particular to "a critique of present practices and theories in psychology" (xviii). For him, the task is to seriously engage with subjectivity. "This seriousness entails understanding to what extent the prevailing subjectivity is wounded and maimed; such understanding means sinking into subjectivity not so as to praise its depths and profundity, but to appraise the damage; it means searching out the objective social configurations that suppress and oppress the subject" (xxii).
72 For instance on page #104: "Recall that *subjective disavowals* in particular stand in the way of elucidating the relationships between individual and society. We found these [disavowals] to be the consequence of a general prohibition on thought established by political dominion and economic profit to defend their interests." [On the translation of *Herrschaft* as "dominion," see note # above.]
73 Parin (1975) 1978.
74 These mechanisms are "unconscious" at least in a descriptive sense: a failure of reality testing, which works in a way "comparable to a defense mechanism" (Parin [1975] 1978, 40), is interpreted and thereby overcome.
75 See also #33, note #, where Le Soldat makes the reference to Lukács more concrete. Lukács did not reject psychoanalysis as such. In his review of *Group*

Psychology and Ego-Analysis, he explicitly calls Freud "a researcher of integrity" and writes in the concluding paragraph: "We did not quote this example in order to expose an otherwise meritorious researcher to deserved ridicule. We quote it as a crass example ... of how topsy-turvy the methods are with which bourgeois learning—in this case, psychology—operates" (Lukács [1922] 2016, unpaginated).

76 As I recall, the work of Melanie Klein and her school, in which aggression, aggression drive, and a conception of the death drive that diverged from Freud's (see Storck 2020, 840–43) play a central role, was practically outlawed in the circles of Parin and Morgenthaler at the time (see also Kurz 2020). That may be one of the reasons why Le Soldat never even mentions it.
77 Modena 2017.
78 The reference is to Fenichel (1934) 1953/1954.
79 Le Soldat 2018, 65.
80 #; see Fenichel's own description in the *Rundbriefe* (Fenichel 1998, 720, the letter of February 14, 1938).
81 Mao, on the contrary, holds that "[t]he atom bomb is a paper tiger ... It looks terrible, but in fact it isn't. Of course, the atom bomb is a weapon of mass slaughter, but the outcome of a war is decided by the people, not by one or two new types of weapon" ([1946] 1956, 100). In any event, the atom bomb was not used to prevent the CPC from taking power in China, nor the Communists from taking power in Cuba, even if nuclear war almost erupted there, for different reasons, in 1962.
82 Except marginally in a footnote, where she one-sidedly calls medical animal testing "a symptomatic action influenced by collectively shared individual phantasies" and does not even mention the economic reasons for which they are still being conducted (#48note).
83 See Engels (1884) 2010.
84 We're thinking here in particular of her later conception of "passive wishes" and suspect that clarifying her position toward the thesis of "voluntary servitude" was one (among several) preconditions for that later view.
85 Le Soldat 2015, 140–44 and 168.
86 Le Soldat 2015, 268.
87 Brun 1953 provides a detailed overview of the reception history of the death drive from its being postulated by Freud until the early 1950s. In a first phase, until 1931, with some delay, only thirteen original studies on the topic are published, with about half voicing approval. From 1932 to 1942, there are thirty-two, with only a third approving. In the period 1942–1952, "all ... authors uncompromisingly turned against the hypothesis of the death drive" (Brun 1953, 108)—not just the ones on the left, that is. (Brun, however, forgets about Melanie Klein and many Kleinians.) Brun himself justifies his emphatic rejection on a philosophical, physical, biological, theoretical-psychoanalytic, and clinical level, and he ultimately sees no reason either to suppose the existence of an aggression drive on the same level as the sexual drive.

This position evidently guided Paul and Goldy Parin as well as Fritz Morgenthaler, all of whom underwent their training analysis with Brun. Le Soldat's psychoanalytic roots lay in this tradition, but she later distanced herself from it in several respects.

See also the recent detailed presentation in Storck 2020, which explicitly takes up Brun's reception history of the death drive hypothesis and continues it until the present day, also with regard to the various currents within psychoanalysis.
88 See Reich (1932) 1938a and Fenichel (1935) 1953/1954.
89 Fenichel (1935) 1953/1954, 366.

90 Fenichel (1935) 1953/1954, 366.
91 Fenichel (1935) 1953/1954, 366.
92 Fenichel (1935) 1953/1954, 366, Fenichel's emphases.
93 Fenichel (1935) 1953/1954, 370–71.
94 Freud 1920 and Freud 1923b.
95 Freud 1924a, 155–70.

On the genesis of the masochism book

Le Soldat's posthumous papers contain practically no documentation on the genesis of the masochism book beside the drafts, which are archived at the Judith Le Soldat Stiftung as JLS-MASO-1 to JLS-MASO-8.[1] Le Soldat dated the earliest extant manuscript "Dec.–Jan. 85" (JLS-MASO-1). It contains the basis of the typescript JLS-MASO-2, which is also dated 1985 and contains a preface dated "Jan. 1985." This typescript or, rather, the photocopy that survives comprises the first version, about 160 pages in length, of the later book and is entitled *Zum ökonomischen Problem des moralischen Masochismus (On the Economic Problem of Moral Masochism)*. JLS-MASO-3 is essentially a copy of the text of fac*freiwilligen Knechtschaft: Eine psychoanalytische Arbeit zum Masochismus (The Utopia of Voluntary Servitude: A Psychoanalytic Study on Masochism)*. A further difference concerns an expansion of the text by about a page and a half.[2] There are several photocopies of this version; presumably, Le Soldat submitted this version to the publishing houses Fischer and Klett-Cotta in February 1985.[3] The typescript JLS-Maso-4, too, dates from 1985. It roughly corresponds to the first of the later book's three parts. The first version to contain all three parts of the later book is JLS-MASO-6. It is dated 1986 and comprises about 430 pages. Here, the three parts have not yet been separated into individual chapters. These are not added until the last version, an unbound typescript kept in two boxes marked "February 1987" (JLS-MASO-7). This is the typescript submitted to the publisher for editing (JLS-MASO-7b). It is entitled *Masochismus: Die Moral einer Perversion (Masochism: Morality of a Perversion)*. The contract with the publisher, finally, is dated January 13, 1988, and sets down the title under which the book will then appear, *Freiwillige Knechtschaft: Masochismus und Moral*.

Notes

1 Le Soldat herself did not keep the correspondence about the masochism book, and there are no relevant documents to be found in the archives of the Fischer publishing house (email message from Corinna Fiedler of the Fischer archives, March 2, 2020).

2 The expansion is an insertion that starts on page 31 of JLS-MASO-3 and ends at the bottom of page 32.
3 The papers contain a manuscript with personal notes dated October 1985 that begins with the words "I'm waiting for an answer from Busch (Fischer-Verlag)" (JLS-1985-Msc.-Prolegomena). At this point, it seems, she had already been turned down by Klett-Cotta (see above, 47).

Acknowledgments

I would like to thank the Judith Le Soldat-Stiftung and in particular the president of the foundation's board, Franz Goldschmidt, for their constructive cooperation in producing this new edition. My thanks also go to Ralf Binswanger for his specialist advice and especially for his willingness to write the introduction with me; Dagmar Herzog and Markus Zürcher for their critical reading of the introduction; Gina Domeniconi and Eva Locher for producing a Word document from the first edition; Cedric Braun for proofreading and formatting the text, for systematically revising and supplementing the references and bibliography, for verifying cross-references, and for compiling the index. I thank frommann-holzboog publishers for the smooth cooperation and expert production of the collected works of Judith Le Soldat.

Monika Gsell, Zurich, January 2021

I
Pulsional demand and wish fulfillment

1 Disentangling aggression and sexuality

If what the diagnosticians of the "triumphant calamity" of our times say is true, namely, that the intention of the Enlightenment has turned into its opposite,[1] and if we adopt the view that "the destruction of reason" shapes the destiny of our age,[2] then psychoanalysis must inquire into the contribution psychical forces make to promoting or even causing such misery. Indomitable inner powers, we are told, have taken possession of people and exploded the deceptive fetters of reason. The dichotomy between pulsional demands and culture cannot be bridged, an unstoppable regression is the price of striving for freedom and fearlessness.

While few will doubt the insight that drive and reason are irreconcilable, we will want to note that psychoanalysis knows *two* kinds of drives: sexuality and aggression. Although, like identical twins, they descend from the same psychical pulsional force, they differ in their formation, their goals, and appearance.

One reliable indication that reason and consciousness bristle at inconvenient insights has always been hypocrisy. Directed, at the beginning of our century, at sexuality, hypocrisy has recently begun to stand protectively before aggression. While sexual love has become the *enfant terrible* of modernity, the concomitant second component of pulsional energy is being ignored and passed over in silence. Hypocrisy used to want to know nothing about human beings' sexual *drive*; now it denies its constantly stimulated readiness for hostility and cruelty.

The discovery of the aggression drive does not share the comparatively harmless fate of sexuality. The reason for this, it seems, is not that a bothersome insight, insight into the pulsional constitution of human psychical life, is to be discarded once more. For in that case, it would be incomprehensible how one *share* of the drive(s) is still subject to social amnesia[3] although the other, the libido, was able to conquer a place in consciousness, [and how] the defense is now directed only against the insight's emotional consequences.

Disentangled from the psychoanalytic theory of the drives, detached from its sexual origin, the theory of sadism has become a real "non vixit."[4] Yet Freud emphasized the hostile demand of the sexual drive early on.[5] Aggression is of special significance, and perhaps even more significant than the

DOI: 10.4324/9781032666273-8

libido, because the illusion that human beings are aggressive only when they are in distress but are not originarily cruel, is much harder to dismiss than the hope that sexuality could be tamed. Freud became convinced that aggressiveness, not the general opposition of the drives, is the most "potent" obstacle to culture.[6] A dialectic that merely captures the difference between natural drives and reason will hardly be able to shed light on why culture is so selective when it finally does ascribe, albeit reluctantly at first, a right to exist to one strand of the drive but suppresses the other—and secretly exploits it.

It may still make sense to us that cruelty can be pleasurable for the individual and that it can serve the goals of political power. Nor is it difficult to understand that the success of the aggression drive means the same thing as the "law of the stronger." And since these forms of behavior do not exactly count among a culture's explicit advantages, there would be plausible reason for repressing them.

The difficulties of explaining aggression, however, are much more subtle. Freud discovered that not just physical cruelties but sadistic phantasies and dreams, too, do not stand up to self-criticism and are in any case punished by the inner censorship. Conscience is implacable and stricter than a judiciary court: it prosecutes intention and impulse as if they were deeds already done. The psychical agency of conscience is entirely ruthless in performing its function. This function is to restrict the drives, and in performing it, it itself is as distrustful, as cunning, and as cruel and uncontrollable as the drive it opposes. Yet those who think they can escape the inner reproach by means of self-control and voluntary renunciation quickly realize they are mistaken. Conscience is all the more distrustful, the more demure one is, all the more arrogant, the more one is willing to sacrifice.[7] The psychical agency—the superego—emerges in childhood because of an internalization of *pulsional demand*s. Subsequently, it can neither deny its notorious origin nor conceal that its activity still amounts to satisfying a drive. The guilty reproaches with which the superego tortures the ego share one and the same pulsional source with physical cruelty; they are nothing less than psychical sadism, turned inside.

A contradiction persists: consciousness refuses to acknowledge that there is something like a *drive* to aggression. If, then, we expect that the essence of expressions of sadism and cruelty is misconstrued, that *reason* justifies them while *conscience* will not be deceived and condemns hostility the way it condemns every other pulsional derivative, we soon find that by no means is there any inner guilty reproach. On particular conditions, conscience seems to abide aggressions of all kinds, and not only reason but conscience itself is unable to recognize the pulsional character of the impulse.

Does that mean that the theory of the drives is wrong? Or dare we surmise that there are satisfactions that conscience is unable to grasp as pulsional because they act in harmony with its own morality? Even then, the individual must turn onto itself the cruel impulses it deflects from its neighbors. The internalization of aggression is a necessary condition of human coexistence and, rather than become murderers, we suffer from the violence of our own conscience. The constant tension of the sense of guilt is the price we pay for sadism not being fulfilled. The task of the superego is to protect consciousness and the external world from the *impositions of the life of the drives*. As soon as reality demands something prohibited by the inner judgment, a subjective *conflict of conscience* arises; yet in social contexts, insofar as the interests of political, economic, or religious power are concerned, the aggressive pulsional demand of the individual no longer poses a threat to culture. When aiming for the *goals of power*, the exercise of the aggression drive is not sadism but duty and morality, its unambiguous expressions do not count as offences but as signs of courage and bravery. What we are used to seeing as a conflict between two commandments of morality, between inner voice and outer obligation, reveals itself to be a *struggle between two pulsional demands* in which conscience is not blindly hostile to the drives but indeed one-sidedly partisan. While it is correct that a social power will never seek to win the favors of the sexual drive—it would have to compete with object love and masturbation—unsatisfied sadism is its natural accomplice. Together, they form an alliance against individuals' drive *and* conscience. For, first, the interest of the social dominion is always already part of individual morality, and it takes a stringent effort to chase it out again. Conscience opposes the strivings of the drives in inner conflicts but does so always already in the service of the socially dominant morality. And second, the opposition of culture to the drives is only an apparent one, or rather, it is split. For the individual, restriction is unavoidable, and the anxiety of conscience is [culture's] instrument; yet social dominion neither can nor wants to do without the pleasurable aggressiveness of its members and subjects. Violence, coercion, and distress have long made the individual's choice in *favor* of the drive easier, justified by the social task and against one's own conscience.

Another twist seems to relieve people of the conflict, not between superego and drive but between drive and reality. While—unless one has a talent for heroism—the reaction to the embarrassing situation of being caught between inner morality and social duty consisted in the *repression of the guilt-affect* in order to act in the sense of "morality," this defense now becomes superfluous, that is, it is being replaced by another one. Where previously, the goal of all civilizing labor was to promote *internalizing morality*, now all social effort is aimed at *externalizing conscience* and ceding it to supraindividual agencies. The civilizing intention has not changed. People can be moved by the pressure of inner morality as much as by external threats of punishment. When individual conscience formation subjects itself to the interests of dominion, the super-ego works much more reliably than external coercion could ever make it. Things are different when, for some reason, the projects of individuals and the goals of dominion drift too far apart. Then conscience becomes the instrument of social resistance. Yet the origin and function of the superego cannot simply be denied, its loyalty cannot be suddenly abolished. When cultural morality incorporates pulsional satisfactions and, bypassing internal censorship, allies itself with the pulsional force, the task of conscience to keep the repressed from realization has, to be sure, become obsolete; its will to protect the subjective consciousness from the insight that what one is doing is, at bottom, something prohibited, however, has not. The defense that now appears is *introjection*.[8] The superego cannot keep fighting on two fronts, against the drive and against reality, yet it is more likely to cede to external pressure. In consciousness, the contradiction between conscience and reality disappears to the extent that the superego returns to earlier forms of external dependence. This of course does not reverse in any way the formation of conscience. Introjection, precisely, concerns only very special efforts that censorship is no longer able to recognize as pulsional. The inner judgment continues to be implacable toward sensual demands. It has, however, developed extensive "blind spots" and responds with tolerance to pulsional actions in the service of the dominant morality.[9]

An aggressive culture, however, that has come to contradict the interests of individuals cannot be content with this outcome because the two pulsional components, libido and aggression, have an irresistible inclination to fuse. Psychoanalysis knows that the two kinds of drives do not appear in the psyche each by itself but always as an alloy. It sees in this a biophysical tendency of the drives, which, to develop, depend on each other. The fusion of drives presents as an ambivalence of the effort, of the goals, and of the affects. Sexuality and aggression, the theory holds, appear as separate neither in regular cases nor in neurosis. While some exceptions are known to exist, these are characterized by seriously pathological (toxic or psychotic) conditions or are associated with the beginnings of psychical development, with infants' autoerotic, narcissistic phase. In adults, in any case, drive is ambivalent; the sexual is pleasurable through the admixture of small cruelties, and destructiveness is tempting only through the eroticism linked to it ab ovo. This fact makes it easy for inner morality to recognize an intent as pulsional by its *pleasure-quality*. Yet of course it is this very quality of the drive that balks at being oriented toward a prescribed purpose. While cruelty, hoping for satisfaction, might occasionally enter the service of an external power, libido insists on the prompt attainment of pleasure in its own body. If, however, a cultural ideology succeeded in exploding the ambivalence of the drives, committing the sadistic tendencies to itself and repressing the sexual ones, it would stand to gain a lot. Manipulating conscience or compelling the ego to adapt is not all that difficult. Changing the pulsional quality, of course, seems to me out of the question.

The radical changes of the pleasurable character, of the goals, of the modality, of the mixture ratio, in short, of the vicissitudes the drive experiences in the course of its development are largely defined by the *inner* conditions. Yet an observation sheds doubt on this thesis: our morality conceives of the two kinds of drives differently, it rebels against sexuality, in which we are unable to see anything dangerous—except its pulsional character—and secretly collaborates with aggressiveness, which arises from the same source, by denying its pulsional character. This conspicuous separation of the [two] kinds of drives presupposes a process so far unknown to us, a disentangling of the two pulsional components with apparently no consequences. Recall that conscience itself is a part of [a] drive;[10] psychoanalysis derives the emergence of the agency of conscience (superego) from an act of internalizing aggression. Under special threats, the child is to give up pleasurable sexual habits and forgo burning desires. Yet since it can neither renounce nor is able to continue being exposed to the threat, it subjects itself. The capitulation, meanwhile, does not happen without a ruse. The child makes the parental commandments its own, it introjects them, yet it by no means renounces the wish fulfillment but instead keeps it in check with the instrument of feelings of guilt. Simultaneous with internalizing a part of the aggression that now seems tied to the superego, there is a repression of the larger share of the aggression, including the disapproved sexual wishes, which can only be satisfied in the unconscious phantasies. In the future, the child turns the hostility once aimed at the opponents of the pleasure against itself. In the formation of conscience, a psychical structure has emerged from the drive. Looking at it more closely, however, we notice that a part of the aggression drive is now forced onto the detour of the superego, where it must yield its energy to the affects of unpleasure (guilt, shame, anxiety) while the larger share of sadism, tied to wishful phantasies, remains virulent in the id. From now on, conscience has a criterion whereby it can unmistakably identify pulsional satisfactions: the attainment of pleasure. The pulsional process will in every case betray itself by the pleasure that comes with it. And the efforts at denying, disguising, and justifying this pleasure just as unambiguously mark the presence of a watchful morality. When we claim that our cultural ideology has succeeded in establishing direct contact with the aggressive pulsional demands such that the *pleasurable satisfaction and conscience no longer exclude each other*, we are saying, first, that morality's "blind spots" do not suffice to explain the defense, [and,] second, that the apparently unproblematic unstitching of libido and aggression, which had to assert itself against the drives' genuine tendency to mix, may have taken place without subjective conflicts but not, in any case, without external influence. Morality and drive, meanwhile, can meet only by promoting a systematic deaggressivization of sexuality and a sexualization of aggression. A shifting of energy within the ambivalence of the drives would leave both the tendency to mix and the attainment of pleasure untouched and would help the excited cruelty triumph over conscience.

How can that happen? Although we're quick to suspect a connection between the intent to disentangle the drives and the cultural special assessment of aggression, such phenomena are hard to understand for psychoanalysis, and there is no explanation available.

Notes

1 Max Horkheimer and Theodor W. Adorno write: "Enlightenment, understood in the widest sense as the advance of thought, has always aimed at liberating human beings from fear and installing them as masters. Yet the wholly enlightened earth is radiant with triumphant calamity" ([1944] 2002, 1).

2 [Lukács (1974) 2021.]
3 "Social amnesia" is Russell Jacoby's term for the loss of a "memory driven out of mind by the social and economic dynamic of this society" (1975, 4).
4 "Non vixit" refers to a dream of Freud's he reports in the sixth chapter of *The Interpretation of Dreams*. The pedestal of a monument in the Vienna Hofburg bears the inscription "Saluti patriae (publicae) vixit, non diu sed totus," "For the well-being of his country he lived not long but wholly." Freud's dream-thought takes up this perception: "this fellow has no say in the matter—he isn't even alive" (Freud 1900, SE 5, 423 and 423n1). Telling, for our purposes here, is the explanation given for the appearance here of this *non vixit* ("was not alive") instead of the correct form *non vivit* ("did not live"): "There must have been times when he [his nephew John] treated me very badly and I must have shown courage in the face of my tyrant; for in my later years I have often been told of a short speech made by me in my own defence when my father, who was at the same time John's grandfather, had said to me accusingly: 'Why are you hitting [*schlagen*] John?' My reply—I was not yet two years old at the time—was 'I hit him 'cos he hit me.'" Freud then points to the shared meaning of *schlagen* and *wichsen*, to hit or smack, yet to the ears of the psychoanalyst, the connection is made between hitting and masturbating. [*Wichsen*, the first syllable of which is homophonous with "vix," is a colloquial term for masturbation.—Trans.]

I thus borrow from Freud the watchword *non vixit* for the disavowal that aggressiveness gives pleasure as much as masturbation does. Already the two-year-old knows that *both* are pleasurably exciting and equally prohibited; yet while there is no justification to the father for the sexual activity, there is perfect moral justification for the aggressive satisfaction: I am not to blame, he started it, I only hit back. The savings in energy expended in the service of defense that appears in the account of childish naivety and has an amusing effect is a characteristic of the "cultural" repression of a sadistic gain in pleasure.
5 Freud 1915a.
6 Freud 1930, 143.
7 Freud 1930, 125–26.
8 "Introjection" today is commonly used to mean internalization (which rather corresponds to "incorporation"). I prefer Ferenczi's original concept: "In principle, man can love only himself; if he loves an object he takes it into his ego. Just like the poor fisherman's wife in the fairy tale, onto whose nose a curse made a sausage grow and who then felt any contact with the sausage as if it were her own skin, and had to protest violently against any suggestion of cutting off the unpleasant growth: so we feel all suffering caused to our loved object as our own. I used the term introjection for all such growing on to, all such including of the loved object in, the ego. ... I conceive the mechanism of *all transference on to an object*, that is to say *all kinds of object love*, as *introjection*, as *extension of the ego*" (Ferenczi [1912] 1955, 316–17, Frenczi's emphases).

The notion of introjection as a kind of internalization is used to describe a process in the course of which the ego limits remain stable and parts of the external world intrude or are received into the ego. Ferenczi saw in this act more of an expansion of the ego, a widening of the area it claimed, to include objects outside one's own body. Freud in 1915 adopted the concept from Ferenczi, but he used it as the *opposite* of projection. In Ferenczi's originary supposition, introjection and projection were identical processes that differed only in the point of view taken by the observer. That in projection, the psychical content seems to be attached to an object of the external world changes nothing about the fact that external object *and* projected content, both as perception units (representatives), belong to the inner world. While breaking up the identity of the procedure and the result of introjection and projection does make matters easier to grasp, it does so at the expense of the insight that parts of the external world make their way into the ego with the help of *both* mechanisms.

9 In a 1965 essay, he dedicates to his students at Brandeis University, Herbert Marcuse studies the notion of tolerance in advanced industrial society. He concludes that "the realization of the objective of tolerance would call for intolerance toward prevailing policies, attitudes, opinions, and the extension of tolerance to policies, attitudes, and opinions which are outlawed or suppressed. ... Conversely, what is proclaimed and practiced as tolerance today, is in many of its most effective manifestations serving the cause of oppression" (Marcuse 1965, 81).

10 "From the point of view of instinctual control, of morality, it may be said of the id that it is totally non-moral, of the ego that it strives to be moral, and of the super-ego that it can be supermoral and then become as cruel as only the id can be" (Freud 1923b, 54; see also 48, as well as Freud 1924a, 167).

2 The identification with the aggressor is not happening

For psychoanalysis, consciousness is a sense organ that fights off unpleasant impressions.[1] Among the varied strategies, it develops to spare itself insights into contexts that, conducted by unconscious pleasure-seeking, it must avoid, *disavowal* is especially remarkable. Wholly unlike repression, whose performance requires a great expenditure of psychical energy, disavowal manages with little resources. It takes advantage of the veniality of reality-testing, separates causes from effects, and breaks up a perception's connection with its emotional meaning; it makes it possible that a fact is accepted as a fact but all the necessary conclusions from it are dismissed. Yet disavowal has also been at work when it is impossible to acknowledge a sensation of displeasure and yet its immediate source and cause is being ignored.

Those ready to share the view that cruelty is not a sexual perversion but an ordinary originary pulsional force in psychical processes will have no trouble concluding that the drive cannot simply be disavowed and avoided. Like the energy of sexuality, libido, aggression time and again finds ways and means to impose its demands. All the defense (disavowal and repression) will be left with is dealing with the embarrassing consequences of its satisfaction. It makes sense that the disavowal of the pulsional source of sadistic wish fulfillment serves the individual well; as long as it does not enter into conflict with reality, it can justify itself before the inner censorship [by claiming that] it does not pursue any intention to satisfy itself but merely reacts to external attacks. Everyday cruelties are defended before conscience as proof of courage and sincerity and are, in turn, supported by conscience in the service of "cultural" morality. The subjective illusion concerning the origin of aggression is thus the work of the pleasure principle and protects a hidden trail of pulsional satisfaction from being discovered by consciousness. On the other hand, however, it is hard to fathom why cultural morality, too, lends a hand in disavowing aggression. If psychological categories exclusively determined people's lives and their relationships with each other, the general hypocrisy would indeed be pointless. Cultural morality would have to assume the standpoint that aggression is due to the drive and stands in every case in opposition to [cultural morality's] intention to domesticate human nature. Yet what decides the fate of human beings is not the inner conditions but "socio-economic [laws] materializing over the[ir] heads."[2] Culture and society flourish according to the will of objectified forms of these laws, whose effects can also be found in the origin of the drives, in the unconscious of individuals.

The justification of the existence of the drives is of a physical nature; the body demands protection from pain and hunger as well as the relaxation of belligerence and sexual excitation. By means of the drives, the body tasks the psychical with procuring, achieving, and repeating satisfaction. The somatic pulsional source is beyond manipulation, its quality is part of the *condition humaine*; yet the development of the drives, their formation, and their vicissitudes are exposed to social influence from the beginning. A pulsional impulse whose intentions contradict the dominant ideology initially remains unsatisfied; then it is repressed; and finally, after a phase of attempts to return, it withers. It will give its energy to other pulsional aims more acceptable to power. To operate this *displacement*, cultural morality makes use of the individual conscience. The defense function is performed by the individual, but it is produced socially[3] and supported by a collective amnesia. Both profit from the new *displacement substitute*—the individual no longer has to cope with drive relinquishment as in the case of repression, while social interests of dominion have silently subjected a share in the unconscious life of the drives. Meanwhile, what the channeling of pulsional energies, the displacement of cathexis, has begun, must be finished by disavowal. The satisfaction of the pulsional demand is being supported as much as possible, yet consciousness of its existence is destroyed; through untiring *disavowals*, social amnesia generates the condition of pleasure, which now is also at the service of a special department of culture, the political and economic power currently dominating. (Only because of this groundwork does a forgetting, an "amnesia," come in later, if at all, in case the consciousness arises that while pulsional relinquishment was performed, a content-specific possibility has been lost.)

Would the hypocrisy concerning aggression thus have to be judged more sympathetically after all? Does the insight impose itself on us that we are acting against culture? Is there something like a bad conscience stirring after all? Such circumstances would save us a lot of work, and in what follows, we could limit ourselves to removing the obstacles that stand in the way of the intention to master aggressiveness and to emancipate from external seizure. That, however, is not the case. The cultural morality that produces the hypocrisy is not some kind of general or public conscience but an instrument in the hands of the dominant power; it represents the ideology of that power and, depending on current interests, is changed at short notice or, when that seems opportune, has its contents turned into their opposite. How, then, are we to explain that the individual allows itself to be saddled with further burdens in addition to its conscience dilemma? It is acting against its own interests, and although in doing so, it is determined by the drive, it destroys its prospect of future satisfactions and is not even rewarded by an increase in pleasure. What is astonishing is that [where] a culturally imposed satisfaction, otherwise the source of violent excitation and pleasure, does not give rise to burdensome feelings of guilt, the psychical fulfillment to be expected fails to come about as well. It has repeatedly been suggested to hold the defense mechanism of the "identification with the aggressor" responsible for this incomprehensible process. And it does indeed seem obvious to look for a *psychological* explanation. When people submit, without apparent need, to foreign demands, then only "irrational" forces that only psychology knows about could be at work.

In their work with children, Anna Freud and later René Spitz especially observed a psychical movement they called "identification with the aggressor."[4] They recognized it as a form of defense by means of which a child seeks to protect itself from an expected unpleasure. It feels guilty because it has transgressed a parental prohibition and in phantasy imagines how it will be punished. Yet under the pressure of anxiety, the roles are displaced. First, the little guilt-ridden one lectures himself, then he hurls abuse at his stuffed toy and beats it. If he's clever and courageous enough, he will finally assume the right of the attacker and return the threat against the opponent. The child becomes reproachful and hostile himself and thereby preempts the expected attack. That is not a bad defensive strategy. When [the child] then goes on even to adorn himself with the insignia of his "enemy," he feels their equal and acts cruelly toward them the way he feared he would be treated. This is an everyday turn of the sense of guilt that spares the individual anxiety and unpleasure.

The suggestion to use "identification with the aggressor" to shed light on those phenomena that do not occur between child and parents but in the relation of the individual to society disregards a procedural nuance. Identification is a *defense* suitable for keeping embarrassing affects away from consciousness, but without assuming a *guilt* affect, it is pointless; at a minimum, the motive of an unconscious guilt is required to get the defense mechanism going at all. The child who submits to the morality of the father and makes it his own is secretly conscious of having attacked the "aggressor" first. He even expects a punishment for his offence that seems neither to be appropriate to it nor to resemble the father's usual strictness but reproduces the extent of his own aggressiveness. One was thus compelled to postulate for the individual, too, a guilt vis-à-vis society, and there are voices enough to advocate [this view]. Individuals would thus be forced by their conscience into confessing their guilt; they would at all times be "guilty" in deeds or thoughts; they would, to exonerate themselves, project the punishing agency onto society and thus become manipulable; they would fear the social authority as they once did the father and would hold on to the projection because otherwise, they would have to endure the inner tension of a split with their superego, which seems [a] hopeless [prospect] to them.

This theory has much going for it. At a closer look, however, it is merely able to explain why it is so *easy* for the social forces to turn back the aggression against people in the form of self-punishment but not *why* it succeeds at all.

The projection of childhood circumstances and the identification of the external power with the inner punishing agency are not causes but consequences of the submission; the supposition of the psychical movement (identification and projection) describes the means, not the conditions of the defense. The motive of the defense, meanwhile, the guilt that assumes a decisive position among people, does not count in the play of forces between individual and society. When individuals feel guilty and, accordingly, become servile to authority and change as though the interest of power were their own business, then that is a *subjective* phenomenon. This is welcome and convenient for dominion; we would be all too guileless, however, if we let ourselves be persuaded that economic interests and a political power strategy could allow themselves merely to harvest the "ripe fruit" of the psychical development and did not themselves do anything to change this development to their advantage. If the subjective idea of guilt resulted "in a person limiting his aggressiveness towards those with whom he has identified himself, and in his sparing them and giving them help,"[5] that would be an astonishing coincidence, punctually arranged by the "pulsional nature" of the human for aggression to falter just at the moment that it turns against an established power. The inner censor, the superego, can be discarded as the one causing the subservience just as much as the defense processes at its disposal. There may well be a time in life when the superego is the representative of the external world, yet later, its exclusive duty is the defense of an inner reality it must protect from the violence of the drives. Although it once acted on behalf of the parental authority, it will not needlessly accept new masters. After all, it is the superego itself that produces the feeling of guilt. The subjective unpleasure of the consciousness of guilt is the weapon whereby it forces the ego into submission. Yet its own effect, the guilt, cannot at the same time be the cause of its servitude toward the external power. In short, the *objective* means, this side of physical violence and existential threat, that a social aggression makes use of to fan the subjective process of identification are not yet known. It stands to suspect that such means do their work as protected from insight as the psychical defense mechanisms do. In revealing them, we must prepare for resistance. I doubt that the source of a force that succeeds in demonstrating the subjective feelings of individuals to be the immediate and sufficient cause of social and economic events really lies in the psyche; yet that it does have psychical *consequences* is witnessed by the many kinds of *disavowals*.

The defensive mechanism of identification, which amounts to a *subjective increase in power* and *improves* the position of the attacked against their opponent *objectively* as well—the dependent do not need to relinquish their hostility and have moreover found a way to fight the fear of the other's revenge, an outcome, incidentally, usually called "courage"—thus seems hardly suited to describing a social deployment of forces that aims at and achieves the objective *strengthening* of the established power. Disavowal, this time, finds support in a psychological train of thought. Getting lost in the various dimensions and causalities in the search for the "subjective factor" at least has two advantages: the illusion of being guilty and servile but not helplessly surrendered to an agonizing manipulation, as well as the gain of pursuing, unrecognized, a violent goal.

Notes

1 Freud 1900, SE 4, 144.
2 "[T]he relationships of men today are neither determined by their will nor even by their drives but by socio-economic [laws] materializing over the heads of the individual members of society" (Adorno [1946] 2018, 638).
3 In reflecting on his work as an ethnologist and psychoanalyst, Mario Erdheim speaks of a "social production of unconsciousness": "A series of processes, to which the anthropologist is exposed both in studying the foreign cultures and in elaborating on the results in his own culture, can be described as processes of rendering unconscious [Unbewußtmachung]. Repression, disavowal, reaction-formations, isolating, and rendering undone, etc., that is to say, the familiar defense mechanisms, can be used to render the experiences had within the framework of the scientific activity unconscious. Where these defense mechanisms are supported by institutions, we may speak of a *social* production of unconsciousness [Unbewußtheit]" (Erdheim 1982, 36, Erdheim's emphasis).
4 Anna Freud (1936) 1973, 109–21, and Spitz 1957, 47.
5 Freud 1921, 110n2. *The Language of Psychoanalysis*, by contrast, describes the result of the defense as follows: "aggression at this time is still directed outwards and has not as yet been turned round against the subject in the shape of self-criticism" (Laplanche and Pontalis [1967] 1973, s.v. "Identification with the Aggressor," 208). This, indeed, fails to recognize reality, internal as well external, and turns the intention of the external world and the consequences of the defense into their opposite. Yet an unpolitical psychology—like social criticism that ignores the unconscious—cannot help reaching grotesque conclusions that incriminate the individual and justify power.

3 Remarkable alliances

> The fateful question for the human species seems to me to be whether and to what extent their cultural development will succeed in mastering the disturbance of their communal life by the human instinct of aggression and self-destruction.[1]

This *cetero censeo* concludes Freud's *Civilization and Its Discontents* of 1930. But the unambiguous warning met with broad resistance also among psychoanalysts. Freud's theory of aggressiveness became the changeling of psychoanalysis. The pulsional vicissitudes of sexuality are the subject of the "infinite" analytic discussion; aggression, destruction drive, sadism, and masochism, meanwhile, remained theoretical concepts without emotional echo. This cannot be due to a lack of experiential basis since the expressions of cruelty do not stop at analysts' doors. Were Freud's ideas on the self-destruction drive wrong, were they exaggerated, or is the rejection of the theory of aggression within psychoanalysis, too, the result of precise motives we can name?

I am quite aware of the general belief that people refused to follow Freud only once he articulated the death drive hypothesis. He himself shared that view:

> The assumption of the existence of an instinct of death or destruction has met with resistance even in analytic circles; I am aware that there is a frequent inclination rather to ascribe whatever is dangerous and hostile in love to an original bipolarity in its own nature. To begin with it was only tentatively that I put forward the views I have developed here, but in the course of time they have gained such a hold upon me that I can no longer think in any other way. To my mind, they are far more serviceable from a theoretical standpoint than any other possible ones; they provide that simplification, without either ignoring or doing violence to the facts, for which we strive in scientific work. I know that in sadism and masochism we have always seen before us manifestations of the destructive instinct (directed outwards and inwards), strongly

alloyed with erotism; but I can no longer understand how we can have overlooked the ubiquity of non-erotic aggressiveness and destructiveness and can have failed to give it its due place in our interpretation of life. (The desire for destruction when it is directed *inwards* mostly eludes our perception, of course, unless it is tinged with erotism.) I remember my own defensive attitude when the idea of an instinct of destruction first emerged in psycho-analytic literature, and how long it took before I became receptive to it. That others should have shown, and still show, the same attitude of rejection surprises me less.[2]

Not until very late, in *Beyond the Pleasure Principle* in 1920, did Freud resolve to propose an explicit theory of aggression although he had already, *avant la lettre*, interpreted hostile tendencies and cruelty as expressions of drives. When Freud later ponders why it took so long to gain insight into the *pulsional* character of the phenomena [in question], he admits to having heeded "religious presumptions and social conventions." He "hesitate[d] to make use, on behalf of [his] theory, of facts which were obvious and familiar to everyone." After all, he

> argued in favour of a special aggressive and destructive instinct in men not on account of the teachings of history or of our experience in life but on the basis of general considerations to which we were led by examining the phenomena of sadism and masochism.[3]

This reflection allows us to surmise just how great the emotional resistance against insight into pulsional aggressiveness must be, which Freud, too, initially did not escape. It is not history, not experience he allows to instruct him; only on the detour via the general *theoretical* consideration of clinical phenomena, via knowledge of sexual *perversions*, does he obtain the painful insight that humans are not only occasionally brutal, violent, and cruel but that we can no longer turn a blind eye to the ubiquity of the aggression drive. Perhaps, in the context of human aggression, we really cannot do without "auxiliar constructions."[4] Probably, however, this very detour saved Freud from hasty rationalizations.

Freud's wording suggests that aggression and destruction are identical, that in the final consequence, the destruction drive is the death drive. Would he not be pleased to see how vigorously his theses have recently been advocated?[5] While the organized psychoanalysis of the international societies almost unanimously rejects the death drive theory and won't have anything to do with sadism understood as a pulsional force, it has become fashionable in progressive circles to talk about Eros and the death drive, even to plead for rehabilitating the latter. This might at least retroactively temper Freud's ridicule: "For 'little children do not like it' when there is talk of the inborn human inclination to 'badness,' to aggressiveness and destructiveness, and so to cruelty as well."[6]

Yet I cannot get rid of the suspicion that the little children heard the message well, but all it got them was a deep bow before the *destructive* nature of the human being. Acknowledging the death drive without engaging with aggressiveness, in that case, is not only worthless but practically armors [us] against the inacceptable insight. What has been correctly recognized—the unconscious destructive force working toward our own death—is deployed to disavow something else that is just as painfully tormenting but much closer to the current emotional experience.

In recent psychoanalytic literature concerned with cultural criticism, we find much profound reflection on "blindness to the apocalypse," theses on the disavowal of the threat of nuclear war, and discussions of the human death drive.[7] What we look for in vain, though, is the most general form of hostility, which is exclusively defined by striving for pleasure. It has become common usage to reserve the term "libidinous" for the erotic pulsional forces and employ derogatory or pathologizing expressions for aggressiveness. Where denunciation does not work, the issue is played down with talk of aggressive "impulses," of frustration aggressions, and of aggressive potential. Otto Fenichel, an exceptionally committed and experienced psychoanalyst, thought that people "are not at all happy about the cruelties they are allowed to commit." Alexander Mitscherlich held that hatred does not provide satisfaction. Paul Parin calls aggressions "certain forms the ego and the superego take." Kurt R. Eissler describes aggressiveness merely as a derivative of the death drive.[8] The list of examples can be extended at will.

To illustrate this point, allow me to recount a short anecdote. In 1983, the Zurich Psychoanalytic Seminar, an association of psychoanalysts that enjoys a progressive reputation, organized a conference on "War and Peace from a Psychoanalytic Point of View." A book by the same title edited by the organizers followed.[9] While the volume's introductory essay, which summarizes and comments on the talks, does discuss pulsional wishes, the force of Eros, autodestruction, longing for death, and so on, it painstakingly avoids the words aggression or aggression drive. But that's not all, since the repressed, of course, speaks up right on cue. How? In a footnote, wrapped in a context not relevant here but telling nonetheless, and distanced as a quotation, we find in very small print the expression we are already familiar with: "little children do not like it."

But why, you will rightly ask, this demonization of aggression? What is it that makes readiness to be hostile look worse than the urge for sexual pleasure? There must be a reason that not only explains the emotional resistance, that is, the hypocrisy but also sheds light on the repression of the theory.

[Its] becoming conscious is threatened from at least three sides: first and above all from the real power and from economic dependency.[10] Second, the dominant morality must be overcome, which has settled in people's conscience. Third, the Sisyphus labor of taming the drives must be performed, because the one, the insight, cannot be had without the other, the relinquishment of the drive. If it is correct that psychoanalysis advocates attenuating the

68 Voluntary Servitude. Masochism and Morality

suppression of the sexual drive, that elucidation leads to increased tolerance of pulsionality, then what are we to make of the warning against the destructive power of aggressiveness? The path to the repressed that leads via a displacement substitute the inner censorship looks on more kindly to knowledge of hidden connections is not a bad one. What we are not allowed to know about the aggression drive, we might learn from its counterpart, masochism.

Psychoanalysis considers masochism to be the key witness for a fusion of the two kinds of drive. Introducing the new, revised theory of the drives, Freud wrote in 1933:

> It is our opinion, then, that in sadism and in masochism we have before us two excellent examples of a mixture of the two classes of instinct, of Eros and aggressiveness; and we proceed to the hypothesis that this relation is a model one-that every instinctual impulse that we can examine consists of similar fusions or alloys of the two classes of instinct. These fusions, of course, would be in the most varied ratios.[11]

This relationship of the drives one to the other is to be conceived of dynamically. Varying according to the state of conflict and the conditions of the innate constitution, sometimes sexual libido wins out in wish fulfillment, and sometimes sadism imposes itself. Undoubtedly, though, the ratio had to adapt to the inner, individual conditions. Freud does not at all envisage a socially induced disentanglement of the drives of the kind we are suspecting. When he speaks of changes in the ratio, he has pathological processes in mind:

> This hypothesis opens a prospect to us of investigations which may some day be of great importance for the understanding of pathological processes. For fusions may also come apart, and we may expect that functioning will be most gravely affected by defusions of such a kind. But these conceptions are still too new; no one has yet tried to apply them in our work.[12]

It seems we have to get used to the idea that the "grave" consequences are no longer pathological but that instead, the pathological has become our normal reality. The disentanglement in question, however, is not a mere splitting off of the sexual from the sadistic; rather, the erotic seems sluggish, dull, as if deprived of all energy, while aggressiveness seems as if, full of force and tension, it had attracted the full amount of libido.

The psychoanalytic method gains its insights through abstinence and neutrality. There is no other way than an "evenly poised attention," a "listening with the third ear," as Theo Reik called it, for psychoanalysis to come to understand unconscious connections.[13] Taking sides and making moral judgments unavoidably lead to psychological banalities. Even when we are aware of the objective supremacy of social conditions and include this knowledge in the process of interpretation on the same level as the theory of the drives, the neutrality of the analyst remains the precondition for therapeutic insight.

The rule of abstinence has also—much to the detriment of the theory, in my view—been declared to be the principle of metapsychological reflections. I think that in the analysis of unconscious psychical factors of social conflicts, the neutrality that in therapy is the *conditio sine qua non* is downright obstructive and leads to absurd results. History, not least of all the history of the Psychoanalytic Movement, has shown that abstinence in the face of social and political developments, as in the time of Fascism, is not neutrality but silent assent.[14] Wrongly remaining silent, pointing, faced with the arrogance of those in power, to the pulsional wishes (masochism) and unconscious expectations of punishment, the longing for death and self-destructive rage of the victims, is not science but betrayal.[15] With some effort, it is possible to think of a society that bridles its aggressiveness in a better or different way; it might not demand taking sides in shedding light on the oppositions of drive and dominion; the interpretation of secret machinations that evade public scrutiny might then not have to win out over the silent assent in the conscience of the analyst. Yet as long as the *quantitative* relation of power and powerlessness is the way it is, neutrality surreptitiously turns into assent. As long as power, possessions, knowledge, and the prospect of fulfilling the pulsional demands accumulate on one side whereas on the other side, powerlessness, dependency, prohibitions on thought, and pressure to conform hold sway, as long as this relation arises in the intimacy of family relationships as much as in the relationships between countries and peoples, analysts striving for neutrality and abstinence inevitably will be caught in the pleasure-promising, quantitatively greater force's pull into the sphere of influence of power. They will then diagnose frustration aggressions and an identification with the aggressor where they should perceive realistic anxiety and intentional manipulation of the pulsional vicissitudes. They will insist on the view that the ego simply isn't sovereign, that hope for the desirable satisfaction of pulsional needs is illusory. These facts, when Freud enounced them, stood in the service of insight; today, in a different age, under different social conditions, such propositions stand in the service of defense and reaction. The integrating power of a dominant ideology does not abide any benevolent neutrality beside itself. Rectitude, which is disapproved in psychoanalytic therapy because, taking sides in a moralizing way, it blocks insight into what is unconscious, now appears as a possibility of resisting and shedding light on societal blind spots. Of course, resistance cannot be the goal of scientific efforts; but it is their precondition. Human vanity has had to accept a number of affronts from science.[16] Freud introduced the illusion that psychoanalysis destroyed with the words, "Although thus humbled in his external relations, man feels himself to be supreme within his own mind." He concludes:

> But these two discoveries—that the life of our sexual instincts cannot be wholly tamed, and that mental processes are in themselves unconscious

and only reach the ego and come under its control through incomplete and untrustworthy perceptions—these two discoveries amount to a statement that the ego is not master in its own house.[17]

What hides here in a subclause—"although ... humbled in his external relations"—and supposes a polarity between the inner world and reality, namely, the conviction that the individual possesses reliable instruments for separating the misfortune brought by the environment from the misery caused by its psychical constitution, [it] arises from a historical consciousness unfamiliar with either the influencing methods of mass media or the introjection strategy of modern cultural morality. The experience that under a regime of terror, the boundaries of the ego become permeable as they otherwise do only in the most severe pathological defects teaches us not to blame all of the threat to subjective sovereignty on the life of the drives but to search for particular interests within cultural morality for whom undermining the psychical agency (of the ego) could be useful.

Russell Jacoby points to a similar reflection:

> This overpowering by a brutal reality which has left the individual numb and dumb is to be overcome, at least in thought and theory, before subjectivity can be realized: insight into the very material and social conditions that mutilate it. Before the individual can exist, before it can become an individual, it must recognize to what extent it does not yet exist. It must shed the illusion of the individual before becoming one.[18]

Against this background, the content of Paul Parin's criticism of a "social application of psychoanalysis"[19] seems to be entirely correct and, within the psychoanalytic discussion, extremely progressive; nonetheless, it seems to be too optimistic and to underestimate the real power relations:

> While the concrete powerlessness of the individual over against social forces does correspond to the situation in which the author [and] most readers... find themselves; but it does not correspond to the dialectic model of psychoanalysis. If we take this powerlessness as our starting point in a psychoanalytic investigation, we inevitably end up seeing adults as powerless children, dependent and without power, cared for or manipulated in the circles of their families, parents, and educators. Analysts, however, must think differently.... In analogy with [the notion] that every human being is not only the object of history but also a subject, that they make their history without knowing it, the "forces of the mind" (Freud) do not act in one direction alone. Only when we cleared the conflict, action, reaction, and their result that goes on to affect new conflicts, can we do psychoanalysis.[20]

It seems to be the case instead that the "dialectic model of psychoanalysis" will have to be oriented by the concrete powerlessness of subjects [and that] powerlessness is not to be left out of consideration for causing theoretical difficulties. Of course, the alternative is not relinquishing the insight into the unconscious conflicts of the powerless. Psychoanalysis, the memento of overpowering powerlessness before its eyes, must endure the contradiction between, on the one hand, knowing of the indomitability of the pulsional demands and, on the other hand, heeding the insight into the laws of reality. Humans' hostility to culture derives from the life of the drives. Yet compared to the hostility to culture on the part of a culture that has allied with aggressiveness, that free remainder of pulsionality that opposes culture serves to maintain culture. The intellect must come to terms with another contradiction, namely that the drive can be hostile to culture and at the same time opportunistically become a bearer of culture; its function, however, is not decided by the individual conscience but by the interests and current inclinations of the social power. I cannot subscribe to the moral verdict on a power-hungry, aggressive culture because the moral judgment *in globo* prohibits the psychoanalytic approach. Consciously and explicitly taking sides for the socially powerless—and not the powerless subjects—by contrast designates the "social place"[21] where psychoanalytic thinking can unfold.

Aggressiveness is a biological drive; the orientation of the drive, however, the goals it seeks out, the forms and kinds of its satisfaction, are specific phenomena shaped by a particular social form. Of aggression generally, we can say what Otto Fenichel says about one of its variants, the drive to enrich oneself: it is not the case that the biological drive creates the particular conditions to satisfy itself; rather, a social system makes use of the pulsional impulses and strengthens those of their derivatives that serve its special interests. Oppressing others, exploiting them and keeping them away from vital resources, forcing them into anxiety and a conflicted conscience, competition, [and] physical and psychical violence are not genuine forms of aggressions but forms that aggression takes under very specific social conditions. Other kinds of aggressive satisfactions are very much conceivable; other times, other cultures have actualized them.[22]

When I plead in favor of taking a stance *against* aggression, I do not thereby leave psychoanalytic terrain but draw the consequence from the insight that the complicity of power and aggression forces analytic knowledge onto a "long march." First of all, aggressiveness in its present from must be recognized as an instrument of power and no longer as a pulsional force. This ought to heighten our awareness of how much manufactured aggression has aroused and at the same time destroyed the drive. Finally, reinstated in its originary rights, aggression ought to be perceived as part of human nature and steered into new channels. This is a pious agenda that will meet with resistance the moment it is articulated. Has it not always been the case that power and aggression form an inseparable pair? Is not power in all its forms a manifestation of humans' pulsional aggressiveness? And are we justified to divide people into two categories, those in power and the powerless?

Allow me to answer with a comparison: when a truck runs over my brother, it is clear who is the victim of this maneuver and who survives unscathed. If, now, my grandmother who was driving the truck gets down from the cab, the accident may have harmed her psyche, but my brother is dead. When my grandmother gets back into the truck, again runs over somebody, gets out, laments, and cries, and gets back in again and again, we might consider her irresponsible, crazy, sclerotic; we might send her to a hospital or even to prison. If, however, my grandmother in her actions knows herself to be in full agreement with the ruling gerontocracy, if "one" thinks and acts the way she does, then *for me* she has forfeited any claim to be excused as a grandmother. I will henceforth regard her as a truck. Psychoanalytically, I will probably be able to interpret the distress, the compulsions she is subject to, internally and externally; in even the most scrupulous investigation, I won't be able to find any differences in principle between her, my, or my brother's unconscious conflicts. And yet ignoring knowledge of the "social site" of her distress, knowledge of the armoring and institutionalization of the possibility of satisfying them, would mean the loss of the truth of my knowledge.[23] They would be true in a psychological sense and wrong in every other respect, the human, the economic, and the political.

Freud is right to say that "the truth cannot be tolerant"[24]; the truth does not possess morality. The scientist searching for it, however, is conscientious; his conscience is moral. The truth thus becomes meek as a lamb or cunning, merciless or flattering, depending on who is speaking it, when it is speaking, and to whom. If it turns out that the aggression drive is innate and cannot be changed, then that is a fact we must not remain silent about. There is also no doubt about the fact that all human beings are given the same pulsional constitution.[25] Talk about what is shared, however, puts itself at the service of a perverted tolerance,[26] and degenerates into an apology of power, if it does not at the same time indicate the different forms of social intercourse and satisfaction the pulsional demand must expect [to meet with] in the external world.

There is no way around the lengthy labor: *before* it can study the unconscious conflicts, psychoanalysis must ensure that the real oppositions of interests, the material differences, are given their due in consciousness. It must also realize, however, *to what extent* distinctions must be made and how they are systematically erased from consciousness before it can set about a correct assessment of the effect of this process in the unconscious, in the conflict between drive, conscience, and reality. It does not suffice to recognize the motives and mechanisms of the inner, unconscious conflicts. Nor does it suffice to know the dialectic between pulsional forces and societal structures. If no effort is made to reach a *quantitative*[27] assessment of the effective forces as well and time and again to define this relation anew, one will end up claiming that a feather and bomb fall to the ground at the same speed, as the laws of gravity suggest.

I said that in a society nothing happens that does not ultimately serve those who have dominion. The historical development of psychoanalysis cannot be excepted from this principle. Freud's interpretation of dreams and [his] theory of neuroses initially shared a goal. The existence of sexual drives was to be made evident, the conflicts their suppression caused were to be elucidated. There must thus have been an interest of dominant morality to have facts that apparently irritate it to become conscious. Freud, after all, was able to publicly pronounce his discoveries and publish his writings with a publishing house that was by no means part of the opposition.[28]

György Lukács describes the dominant interest in turn-of-the-century Europe as an interest in maintaining class societies.[29] *This* interest promoted the development of psychoanalysis even if it turned it into a social *skandalon*. The emancipation granted the operation of the sexual drive was to attract the energies that the social conflict demanded for itself. The theater piece of sexual analysis had to be produced on the political stage since otherwise, the audience would have stormed the arena to put on its own piece.

By no means do I want to lessen Freud's merits or downplay the *inner* resistances he had to overcome? Nor do I want to play off class consciousness against psychoanalytic insights. But I do want to point out that for the collective morality of the time, the discovery of neurotic mechanisms, the elucidation of human sexual drives secretly meant a relief. Freud became a source of danger only once he started talking about the socially effective aggressions, about the conditions of culture in the unavoidable repression of pulsional forces (at a time when the incitement of people to the new National Socialist "awakening" was just beginning). Actually, though, this development of his thinking had been predictable since 1908 at the latest,[30] when he wrote in *"Civilized" Sexual Morality and Modern Nervous Illness*:

> Generally speaking, our civilization is built up on the suppression of instincts. Each individual has surrendered some part of his possessions-some part of the sense of omnipotence or of the aggressive or vindictive inclinations in his personality. From these contributions has grown civilization's common possession of material and ideal property. Besides the exigencies of life, no doubt it has been family feelings, derived from erotism, that have induced the separate individuals to make this renunciation. The renunciation has been a progressive one in the course of the evolution of civilization. The single steps in it were sanctioned by religion; the piece of instinctual satisfaction which each person had renounced was offered to the Deity as a sacrifice, and the communal property thus acquired was declared "sacred." The man who, in consequence of his unyielding constitution, cannot fall in with this suppression of instinct, becomes a "criminal," an "outlaw," in the face of society-unless his social position or his exceptional capacities enable him to impose himself upon it as a great man, a "hero."[31]

74 Voluntary Servitude. Masochism and Morality

He continued this approach of directly and openly attacking societal conditions in *Thoughts for the Times on War and Death* (1915),[32] *Group Psychology and the Analysis of the Ego* (1921), *Civilization and Its Discontents* (1930), and *Why War?* (1933). While he did not see any chance for the Communist movement to succeed, he did so not based on economic or political reflections. For him, there was no better form of aggressiveness conceivable,[33] and he considered both the given and the utopian [form of aggression] to be destructive:

> I cannot enquire into whether the abolition of private property is expedient or advantageous. But I am able to recognize that the psychological premises on which the system is based are an untenable illusion. In abolishing private property we deprive the human love of aggression of one of its instruments, certainly a strong one, though certainly not the strongest; but we have in no way altered the differences in power and influence which are misused by aggressiveness, nor have we altered anything in its nature. Aggressiveness was not created by property. It reigned almost without limit in primitive times, when property aw still very scanty, and it already shows itself in the nursery almost before property has given up its primal, anal form; it forms the basis of every relation of affection and love among people (with the single exception, perhaps, of the mother's relation to her male child). If we do away with personal rights over material wealth, there still remains prerogative in the field of sexual relationships, which is bound to become the source of the strongest dislike and the most violent hostility among men who in other respects are on equal footing. If were to remove this factor, too, by allowing complete freedom of sexual life and thus abolishing the family, the germ-cell of civilization, we cannot, it is true, easily foresee what new paths the development of civilization could take; but one thing we can expect, and that is that this indestructible feature of human nature will follow it there.[34]

In a 1932 letter to Albert Einstein—intended for a wide readership—however, he notes unequivocally:

> But may I replace the word "might" by the balder and harsher word "violence"?... conflicts of interest between men are settled by the use of violence.[35]
>
> In actuality the position is complicated by the fact that from its very beginning the community comprises elements of unequal strength-men and women, parents and children-and soon, as a result of war and conquest, it also comes to include victors and vanquished, who turn into masters and slaves. *The justice of the community then becomes an expression of the unequal degrees of power obtaining within it;* the laws are made by and for the ruling members and find little room for the rights

of those in subjection. From that time forward there are two factors at work in the community which are sources of unrest over matters of law but tend at the same time to a further growth of law. First, *attempts are made by certain of the rulers to set themselves above the prohibitions which apply to everyone*—they seek, that is, to go back from a dominion of law to a dominion of violence. Secondly, the oppressed members of the group make constant efforts to obtain more power and to have any changes that are brought about in that direction recognized in the laws-they press forward, that is, from unequal justice to equal justice for all. This second tendency becomes especially important if a real shift of power occurs within a community, as may happen as a result of a number of historical factors. In that case right may gradually adapt itself to the new distribution of power; or, as is more frequent, *the ruling class is unwilling to recognize the change.*[36]

One of his last notes, from July 20, 1938, is still concerned with the struggle—in his view, now a lost struggle—of the individual against the environment: "The individual perishes from his internal conflicts, *the species perishes in its struggle with the external world to which it is no longer adapted.*—This deserves to be included in *Moses.*"[37]

The individual's knowledge of its aggressiveness, on which those who have dominion depend, is no less dangerous than knowledge of the *real* relationships between labor power and capital. If people were to become aware of the consequences, the revolutionary potential concealed in Freud's culture-critical theories, and in his theses on the aggression drive in particular, seems explosive. Ultimately, though, what threatens collective denial is not scientific insight. The memory of the events of the two World Wars, the easily observed increase in pleasurable interest taken in brutalities, and be it just in depictions, films, or journalistic reporting, raise the suspicion even in unbiased laypeople that sadism and violence are intimately connected with human nature and [are] not simply excesses or perversions.

The defense must seek shelter in new mechanisms. It has developed something I have described as a double division of individuals' inner pulsional forces. First, the possibilities for satisfying sexuality and aggression are separated such that the two pulsional components cannot simultaneously have their say. The preferential treatment of aggression not only facilitates an increased wish fulfillment, it also promotes an energetic gradient. Usually distributed evenly, libido now preferentially flows to sadism. The erotic now seems all the less tense the more of an increase in pleasure the other side yields.

Second, for various reasons, conscience is unable to realize the pulsional character of these processes.[38] It remains silent, it neither reacts with defense nor calls on its usual aides, anxiety, and guilt affect, for help. The "liberated" aggression, however, acts like an army of mercenaries that obeys whoever is promising more pay.

76 Voluntary Servitude. Masochism and Morality

Notes

1 [Freud 1930, 145.]
2 Freud 1930, 119–20.
3 Freud 1933, 103–4.
4 [Freud 1930, 75.]
5 See, for example, Lohmann 1983.
6 The passage reads in full: "For 'little children do not like it' when there is talk of the inborn human inclination to 'badness', to aggressiveness and destructiveness, and so to cruelty as well. God has made them in the image of His own perfection; nobody wants to be reminded how hard it is to reconcile the undeniable existence of evil—despite the protestations of Christian Science—with His all-powerfulness or His all-goodness. The Devil would be the best way out as an excuse for God; in that way he would be playing the same part as an agent of economic discharge as the Jew does in the world of the Aryan ideal. But even so, one can hold God responsible for the existence of the Devil just as well as for the existence of the wickedness which the Devil embodies. In view of these difficulties, each of us will be well advised, on some suitable occasion, to make a low bow to the deeply moral nature of mankind; it will help us to be generally popular and much will be forgiven us for it" (Freud 1930, 120).
7 See Nedelmann 1982 [which features the term *Apokalypseblindheit*]; Richter 1983; and Parin 1983.
8 See, respectively, Fenichel (1938) 1981, 1061; Mitscherlich (1968) 1969; Parin (1973) 1978; and Eissler 1971.
   Something that must not go unmentioned is that Eissler is one of the few psychoanalysts who tried to maintain awareness of human aggressiveness. See, for instance, the essay "The Fall of Man" (Eissler 1975). The consequences he draws from his insights are, if I understand him right, apolitical and resigned. He reports, for example, that "Benjamin Pasamanick, the New York Health Commissioner, terms the condition in which a wealthy society such as ours does not stave off the hunger of its own members 'murderous' (Psychiatric News, April 7, 1971)." This prompts Eissler's remark, [in the German version of the essay,] that "this might be a profound psychological [!] truth ... Pasamanick's formulation almost [!] sounds like a confirmation of Freud's statement 'that we spring from an endless series of generations of murderers, who had the lust for killing in their blood, as, perhaps, we ourselves have to-day'" (Eissler [1975] 1976, 53–54 [the exclamation points are Le Soldat's addition; the reference is to Freud 1915b, 296]). See also Eissler 1971.
9 Passett and Modena 1983.
10 "Confronted with the current powerlessness of the individual—of all individuals—society and the sciences concerned with it, sociology and economy, takes precedence in explaining social processes and trends" (Adorno [1966] 1970, 55). In *Social Amnesia*, Russell Jacoby proffers the same view: "To be sure, psychologism remains false in all its forms, while sociologism at least pays respect to society as the determining structure" (Jacoby 1975, 78).
11 Freud 1933, 104–5.
12 Freud 1933, 105.
13 On the concept of evenly poised or suspended attention, see Freud 1912b and Sandler, Dare, and Holder (1973) 2018.
14 On this topic, note the embarrassing controversy about the co-editor of the journal *Psyche*, Helmut Dahmer, who aimed to strengthen the memory of the fascism-tinted past of the psychoanalytic movement within the movement itself and encountered fierce resistance from the members of the German Psychoanalytic Association. See Lohmann and Rosenkötter 1982 and Brainin and Kaminer 1982.

15 In the already mentioned conference proceedings, *War and Peace from the Psychoanalytic Point of View* (Passett and Modena 1983), the editor, Peter Passett, writes: "What is most important about this book is not the contradictions but the shared approach of the different contributions: treating the topic war and peace from the psychoanalytic point of view means looking at it from the point of view of the subject concerned. Psychoanalysis conceives of people as subjects of their history even where they act irrationally and against their interests, where they appear as manipulated, seduced, and dominated. It insists that even such action, at first sight incomprehensible, is to be explained not *only* by outside influence, overarching systems, and anonymous forces, but that it always *also* corresponds to interests of the acting persons, albeit interests that they are not conscious of and that for that very reason can be guided toward goals that contradict their real interests" (18, Passett's emphases).

These reflections, correct as they are when taken by themselves, are confused, not only in practice but already here, in their being articulated, about pulsional interests and real, material interests. The unconscious, manipulable interests can only be pulsional wishes and their derivates, while the "real" interests, which contradict the manipulated satisfactions, are material ones the subject is cheated out of. If both are equated, however, the psychoanalytic view loses its most profound insight, the insight into the contradiction between the pleasure and reality principles.

16 Freud famously speaks of three great blows scientific research has dealt humanity's self-love: the cosmological blow dealt by Aristarchus and Copernicus, the biological one by Darwin's theory, and the psychological one by the exploration of the unconscious (Freud 1916–1917, SE 16, 284–85; Freud 1917).

17 Freud 1917, 141 and 143.

18 Jacoby 1975, 81.

19 Parin 1977, S. 583 [quoting] Richter 1976.

20 Parin 1977, 585–86.

21 I adopt the term from Siegfried Bernfeld. [See Bernfeld (1929) 1996.]

22 See the posthumous collection of Borkenau's essays, *End and Beginning: On the Generations of Cultures and the Origins of the West* (Borkenau 1981), especially "Primal Crime and 'Social Paranoia' in the Dark Ages" (381–91) and "Postscriptum: The *Chanson de Roland*" (417–33).

23 I am quite aware that this concept [the concept of truth] has been relativized and discredited, not least of all by the insights of psychoanalysis. I think, however, that the risk of positivist exaggeration is worth taking if it means escaping an apologetic relativism. The latter always leads to a flattening of ideas. This in turn would be harmless if it did not foster the general dumbing down and inhibition of thinking in the service of power. To be sure, it is not prudent to let one's position be prescribed by the opponent. Even in taking the way out (which I am aiming for) that consists in enduring the contradiction between the truth that is claimed and the realization that this truth is conditioned, I get into a dilemma. This hesitation is what others, unfamiliar with such scruples, exploit. Psychoanalysis—I mean the sciences generally—however, can no longer afford being more stupid than the contemporary Machiavellians. If the social situation demands it, it must be ready to relinquish certain insights, to keep them under wraps but in the back of the mind.

24 Freud 1933, 160.

25 The pulsional constitution, of course, like all other bio-physical phenomena, is subject to certain quantitative fluctuations. We will address the consequences of the deviations below. It is not possible, however, to claim that some are constituted to be more sadistic, that others have been endowed with less aggressiveness. The individual deviations are, first, much less pronounced than one would like

78 Voluntary Servitude. Masochism and Morality

      to suppose, and second, the magnitude of the aggressiveness that develops by no means parallels the congenital equipment but results from a complex assemblage of energy distribution, defense expenditure, the effective possibilities of sublimation, and so on.

26 "The conditions under which tolerance can again become a liberating and humanizing force have still to be created. When tolerance mainly serves the protection and preservation of a repressive society, when it serves to neutralize opposition and to render men immune against other and better forms of life, then tolerance has been perverted" (Marcuse 1965, 111).

27 Freud time and again advocated quantitative perspectives (see, for instance, Freud 1909, 91–92; 1920, 62; 1923b, 27; 1926a, 153–54; 1930, 68–69; 1927b, 165; 1937, 227–28, 230, 234, and 239; 1938b, 183–84). This approach has become disreputable because those who claimed to "further develop" psychoanalysis or to refute it have appropriated it. It would not have been so easily dismissed by the psychoanalytic community, however, if economic and quantitative reflections, precisely, did not harbor a concrete explosive potential that works against the general indeterminacy (even if it draws attention to the repression).

28 The first editions of the *Studies on Hysteria* (Breuer and Freud 1895) and *The Interpretation of Dreams* (Freud 1900) were published by Franz Deuticke Verlag, Leipzig and Vienna, those of "A Reply to Criticisms of My Paper on Anxiety Neurosis" (Freud 1895) and *Sexuality in the Aetiology of the Neuroses* (Freud 1898) in the official *Wiener Klinische Rundschau*.

29 "The theory of historical materialism therefore presupposes the universal actuality of the proletarian revolution. In this sense, as both the objective basis of the whole epoch and the key to an understanding of it, the proletarian revolution constitutes the living core of Marxism" (Lukács [1924] 2009, 11–12). And: "A period's revolutionary essence is expressed most clearly when class and inter-party struggles no longer take place within the existing state order but begin to explode its barriers and point beyond them. On the one hand they appear as struggles *for* state power; on the other, the state itself is simultaneously forced *to participate* openly in them. There is not only a struggle *against* the state; the state itself is exposed as a *weapon of class struggle*, as one of the most important instruments for the maintenance of class rule" (58, Lukács's emphases). "This organization of a whole class has to take up the struggle against the bourgeois state apparatus—whether it wants to or not. There is no choice: either the proletarian Soviets disorganize the bourgeois state apparatus, or the latter succeeds in corrupting the Soviets into a pseudo-existence and in thus destroying them" (61).

30 See Freud 1954, letter 65 of June 12, 1897, 210–11, as well as the reference, in Breuer and Freud 1895, 305, to the "common unhappiness" that is "connected with my circumstances and the events of my life" which we may be "armed against."

31 Freud 1908a, 186–87.

32 "It is undeniable that our contemporary civilization favours the production of this form of hypocrisy to an extraordinary extent. One might venture to say that it is built up on such hypocrisy, and that it would *have to submit to far-reaching modifications* if people were to undertake to live in accordance with psychological truth" (Freud 1915b, 284, Le Soldat's emphasis).

33 Contrast this with Paul Parin: "Suppression and internalization have been described as the typical pulsional vicissitude of aggression. I believe to have demonstrated, on the contrary, that the suppression does not have to take place when the anal phase of ego formation unfolds under different conditions or without cleanliness compulsions. Dogon society should be considered a good example of the possibility for human coexistence to organize without internalizing aggression" (Parin [1973] 1978, 192–93).

34 Freud 1930, 113–14.
35 Freud 1932b, 203–4.
36 Freud 1933, 206, Le Soldat's emphasis.
37 Freud 1938c, 299, Le Soldat's emphasis.
38 We will learn in a later section that this inability of conscience has more than just contentual reasons. The external world is not only capable of anchoring moral principles in the internal world, it has discovered ways and means to change the quality of the *pulsional energies*, that is to say, that characteristic by which censorship can most reliably recognize pulsional derivatives.

4 A "mishap" in Germany

Some remarks on the general pulsional vicissitude of aggression in post-war Germany may serve to illustrate my theses.

The reference to psychoanalytic categories makes historical reflections that speak of a "repression of guilt" and of "disavowal of injustices committed" seem progressive. It is easily forgotten that the psychological concept of repression presupposes a pulsional wish. A *pleasurable* phantasy aims at a satisfaction recognized to be prohibited. The prohibiting agency, conscience, then introduces a counterforce, the unpleasure of the guilt affect. Mobilizing heavy psychical labor, the defense, denies the embarrassing phantasies access to consciousness. The impulses that cannot be calmed have their path to the external world cut off. When pulsional shares cannot be bridled, offenses against the law and morality are generated; when the drive is bridled too much, it returns in the neurotic conflict. The discourse of the repression of guilt thus implies a weakness of conscience, which allowed a drive to break through, but it also implies the existence of a reawakened, stricter censorship that posthumously condemns the misdeeds. Forgetting would be the visible sign of the defense function, equivalent to a neurotic symptom. Repression and forgetting would not be characteristics to be judged negatively but proof of a new, stricter morality. That, however, does not correspond to the historical facts.

If we accept a nation's jurisprudence as an organ of its cultural morality, then the postwar period, far into the 1960s, presents a peculiar picture. Citing hundreds of instances, Jörg Friedrich shows in a study that in [West] Germany's postwar history, no *forgetting* needed to be overcome; rather, the ideology of the Third Reich was seamlessly integrated into the jurisprudence of the Federal Republic.[1] He proves that injustice was prosecuted (preferably when it was "bloody" injustice) but only a vanishingly small percentage of those who were publicly and without being contradicted designated as "perpetrators" were sentenced. With justified irony, Friedrich considers this "cold amnesty" to be an *unintentional side effect* of a decision of the Bundestag, the West German parliament, which one need not be a psychoanalyst to interpret as a return of the repressed, an action guided by the unconscious:

When in October 1968, the Bundestag voted the revision of section 50.2 (today's section 28), it thereby simultaneously decided that, retrospectively, the statute of limitations had expired since 1960 for all Nazi deeds committed without base motive [*niedriges Bewusstsein*]. It decided without wanting to, entirely unconsciously.[2]

The state-imposed exculpation of everyone below Hitler and above the bestiary of the camps, however, by no means indicates something forgotten and repressed. The unconscious intervening here is not a repressed historical guilt. The parapraxis is not the success of a late-awoken public morality embarrassed about injustice committed. The motive of the parapraxis, rather, is a current intention that, at the moment of institutionalization, evades control by means of a conscious censorship. It is an unconscious, [though] of course clear, expression of the will to let aggressiveness and cruelty continue to count as *legal*. This once again seals the hitherto existing alliance between cultural morality and drive. What might seem to critics to be the repression of an embarrassing memory, for the analyst of course counts as an unmistakable sign not of the defense against a past guilt but of the *success* of an embarrassing, extremely *acute impulse*. The "mishap" is the symptom of lawmakers' unwillingness to condemn expressions of violence that accord with the dominant state ideology. The amnesty of the old perpetrators is an incidental and perhaps even unintended side effect of the legalization of their own sadistic phantasies pushing itself to the front. This "repression," rather than acknowledging injustice while rejecting guilt, performs no appreciable defense function. The offenses at issue are repeated in phantasy. In this situation, the individual conscience would have to rise up simultaneously against the inner impulse and against the injustice committed by someone else. Usually, it discharges this task with the aid of projection mechanisms and by erecting psychical barriers against the disapproved phantasy. Both measures, however, come with a considerable expenditure of energy, whose effort one gladly did without. The compromise of legalizing, in a collective consensus, brutalities without bloodshed offers momentary relief. What the individual conscience procures thereby is less freedom from a burdensome memory than an authorization, now declared to be the law in force, to [pursue] violent phantasies. If it is possible at all to speak of repression in this context, then exclusively as regards the pleasure affect that accompanies the idea of aggressive satisfaction.[3] Recall that censorship identifies the pulsional process by means of the pleasure generated. The individual motive of the "mishap" is thus to be sought in a *current relief of the defense*. The dominant interest that makes this possible in turn lies in *thwarting a censoring of censorship*; the conscience of the subjects must not appoint itself to adjudicate the usefulness of employing individual aggression for the purposes of the state. The recourse to categories of individual psychology ("repression of guilt") practically disguises the process of disavowing a current intention. Moreover, it imputes to the social a moral factor, [namely], guilt, that cannot but be the function of a collective conscience. *This* conscience does not exist.

This "getting over" Nazi crimes also affirms that those who have dominion abide only "pleasureless" aggressions. Desk murderers who live undoubtedly unconscious aggressive phantasies, military officers who functionalize their cruelty, and high finance, which profits economically from the cruelty, that is, all those who succeeded in isolating their affects, go unpunished.

Does this mean that under the form of aggressiveness rampant today, there is no guilt, no repression of misdeeds, no amnesia of the past? It would be foolish to make that claim.

Social amnesia, the process of forgetting the social past, is not a "moral" process that, tormented by awareness of its guilt, seeks to get rid of a shameful past.[4] The illusion created by those who have dominion that the current state of affairs and relationships among people is the "natural" state only stands up to individual[s'] reality testing if the bridges behind the present are systematically burned.[5] In this situation, the individual conscience is doubly obsolete. First psychologically,[6] because it can no longer fulfill its function of providing the ego, in the mediation between drive and reality, with ideals; it has become a mere duplication of reality in the internal [world]. Second socially, because the role of individuals' conscience to criticize and *renew* the social has become obsolete. Cultural morality has long dismissed the opportunistic superego and the unsuspecting ego and sought out more reliable allies.

I think this characterizes a new form of the dialectic between individual and society, new, in any case, where the relationships between reality and drive and between conscience and reality are concerned. The ego, in any case—I mean the agency "I," site and subject of the conflicts between drive, reality, and superego—is unequal to the task of emancipation and reorientation. New, in any case, are the forms of the alliance between common morality and aggressiveness. In 1961 (on the occasion of the Eichmann trial in Jerusalem), Karl Jaspers remarks that the particularity of the Nazi crimes is that they do not appear in any penal code: "These crimes are determined by a state's 'political' will. ... The *particularity of this principle, which has come into the world for the first time*, must become clear."[7] Hannah Arendt, too, distinguishes between *Verbrechen gegen die Menschheit* and *Verbrechen gegen die Menschlichkeit*.[8] That the decision of the German Bundestag to keep crimes against humanity "without bloodshed" legal was not a "mishap"[9] but the symptom of a new kind of development is, for the moment, a supposition. But it deserves looking into. What is to be tested is whether the new principle (crime without guilt) is a particular form of reifying aggression. In that case, it would have to find expression in new kinds of strategies for exploiting and defending against the drive. And it would have to be possible to discover the traces of the principle in the pulsional vicissitudes and pulsional structures of individuals.

Notes

1 See Friedrich (1984) 1994.
2 Friedrich (1984) 1994, 437. [The reference is to the *Strafgesetzbuch*, the German penal code.—Trans.]
3 The relationship between drive and repression is not as simple as it might seem. Repression can neither turn against the drive itself nor directly act on the affects. Each for different reasons, both are unable to *become* unconscious. What is repressed is only the ideational content of a wishful phantasy; affects are disavowed or shifted onto other contents.
4 The application of psychological categories to social processes generates—as does what follows—the illusion that the current state of society is the "natural" one, the soothing fallacy that the same effort by which we are used to resolving conflicts of conscience will prove viable in dealing with social factors as well.
5 Jacoby remarks that to explain the mode of production of social amnesia, it is necessary to draw on Marx's concept of reification: "Reification in Marxism refers to an illusion that is objectively manufactured by society. This social illusion works to preserve the status quo by presenting the human and social relationships of society as natural—and unchangeable—relations between things" (1975, 4).
6 The psychological concept of outdated conscience refers to parents applying standards in raising their children that correspond to the precepts of their own conscience. The superego of the child is thus constructed not on the model of the parents but on the model of the parental superego. See Freud 1933, 67.
7 See Jaspers 1966, 58–59, Le Soldat's emphasis. [The English edition, Jaspers [1966] 1967, translates only the book's third part.—Trans.]
8 Jaspers 1966, 59. Jaspers quotes Hannah Arendt's remarks in the context just mentioned. [Both *Menschheit* and *Menschlichkeit* correspond to *humanity*, the former as *humankind*, the latter as *human(e)ness*. Jaspers cites a conversation with Arendt; the formula "crimes against humanity" can be found in Arendt and Jaspers (1985) 1992, 419 (Arendt to Jaspers, December 23, 1960); see also Hans Mommsen's remark in his introduction to *Eichmann in Jerusalem* (Mommsen 2006, 24)].
9 Friedrich's book concludes with the words, "There are coincidences that everyone sees as signs. The government said flatly, 'a mishap'" (Friedrich [1984] 1994, 438).

5 Three lessons from an objective triumph

The following pages lead us into reflections that seem foreign to our topic. The detour, however, is meant to open up for us a clearer view of a peculiar symptom of masochism. When investigating the causes of a physical disease that occurs in large numbers at a certain point in time, we think of the possibility of an epidemic. It has been proven that psychical ailments, too, sprout up as if they were contagious. The *fin de siècle* was rich in hysterias, the post-war years were conducive to obsessional neuroses and depressions, and in the past decades, practicing psychoanalysts think they have seen an increase in masochistic symptoms. For the moment, there is not much we can do with that observation. And yet the affinity of an age toward neurosis must have deeper motivations than fashions or psychical reactions to historical events.

My claim is that in the neurotic diseases of individuals, a will of those in power becomes effective, indeed, that they even require the *acquiescence* of those who dominate an age. The justification of this thesis links up with the reflection that every neurosis has a particular leitmotif, an unconscious tendency, that is palpable in all its manifestations. Masochism, for example, fights against sadism, cruelty, the tendency to torment, and the prospect of suffering. The leitmotif of our age is to confront the nuclear threat. Nothing occupies people's senses more than the fear of not surviving the next general war. Such doubts of course do not leave those who have dominion untouched either, those who are responsible for the increasing number of weapons and for their development. We may suppose that their fear of the possible consequences of their own efforts has increased as well. The strategy people occasionally apply in such a dilemma is not without logic: not to give up on what has been begun (which, after all, is not being undertaken for no reason) but at the same time to prepare paths of escape.

On the one hand, then, the true fatality of the threat must be downplayed and the pleasurable pulsionality of the efforts disavowed; this notwithstanding [,on the other hand,] possible defenses and conflicts are to be given a chance. In a delicate and at the same time harmless link of the chain of collective defense, in the neuroses, the prohibition to perceive the aggression drive is eased; conflicts of conscience that arise from the pleasure taken in brutalities are made possible and immediately rejected as crazy and pathological. The observation of how individuals engage with their pulsional demands, however, provides general morality with clues about what the drive will put up with, how it can be satisfied at a profit without reflecting back on its beneficiaries. The neurotic functions as a social laboratory, elected to explore, on the small scale, the effects of a global development that has become uncanny. When individuals, driven by their striving for pleasure, seek out sadism, then there must be ways and means to transfer this tendency to others besides only the masochists. And since masochists pleasurably endure the consequences of brutalities, it ought to be possible to give one's own aggressiveness free reign without wasting any thought on destruction and death. This is seen as a way to silence the "soft voice of the intellect."[1] But in the repressed phantasies, the disavowal of the danger develops hatred and hostility all the more, because every representation of the next war can only issue in images of destruction and unavoidable suffering.[2]

Here, then, something unexpected is happening psychically. The more a phantasy induces anxiety, the more pulsional energies flow toward it. Unsatisfied unconscious tendencies detach from a different context and gather around the focus of the excitement. They come flowing in hopes of imposing their demands, too, with the greater pulsional force, underneath the general unrest. Conscience at first reacts with increased strictness but soon must capitulate. Why? Because the force of morality, too, draws its energies from the reservoir of aggression. I mentioned above that conscience arises as an internalization of sadistic wishes—hostility turning back onto the self. Yet when a tumult in the life of the drives becomes all too exciting, when the prospect of breaking through to satisfaction no longer seems absurd, then the pulsional forces prefer sticking together to leasing themselves out to morality. While conscience can hope for support from a small band of reliable faithful followers (the guilt *affect* usually remains cathected), the larger share of the internally available aggression shakes off the forced orientation against its own origin.

The result of this chain reaction is evident—the conditions of the external world block the breakthrough of the drive and the psychical forces have no other way out than the turn to passivity. People become helpless; what used to be sadistic excitement becomes longing. They can no longer imagine taking care of themselves but hope for rescue, help, and instruction. Everything they previously would have liked to do themselves they now expect [to come] from outside. Of course, under the pressure of anxiety, the brutal phantasies have not transformed into wishes to be treated cruelly oneself but into confidence in someone who in one stroke brings rescue from this distress.[3] The craving for such a dependence has the same characteristics as the aggression it replaces: pleasure[4] and pulsionality; it will also be transformed back quickly and easily. Then trust in authority and craving for passivity reconvert into hatred.

Processes of this kind cannot but be welcome to those in power in a society. Passivity is convenient, and the reverse relationship of rescue phantasies and cruelty suits their interests. But what about the individuals? Individuals should harbor a "natural" hostility against all kinds of dominion, given that at one point, in early childhood, they had to submit to their arch enemies (the oedipal rivals). All their lives, they bear the mark of this defeat: the "agency" [*Agentur*] of their conqueror, the agency [*Instanz*] "superego."[5] Freud's talk about hostility to culture would have to be supplemented with the postscript that this hostility grows to the extent that societal structures take on authoritarian traits. The projection of children's hostility toward the father onto social dependencies, where they find themselves confronting new adversaries, should generate intense wishes for revenge. The dependent, no longer helplessly dependent as when they were children, would have to do their utmost to make up for the former defeat. Aggressiveness would itself have to become the source of social liberation.

Historical experience proves the opposite. We have a number of explanations available for this contradiction: the infantile submission does not take place without pleasure, the relationship with the rival is in fact rather ambivalent; the compulsion to repeat does not permit revenge, only new subordination; the identification with the aggressor and the internalization of the aggressor's prohibition creates that inner obstacle at which oppositional impulses dissolve before they can even become conscious; finally, wishes for revenge are dashed by the real power relations, and should a revolt succeed at some point, the new lords would once more require only dependents, as long as the question of aggressiveness does not find a better solution. We now have a further conclusion to add to these arguments. As a consequence of the inner dilemma, modern humanity's hostility to culture has not increased but decreased: revenge has not become impossible, it has become unnecessary, because a *synthesis of drive and society* has formed. This, however, is not the utopia of Eros and culture Herbert Marcuse had in mind but the *suspension of the contradiction between aggression and culture*.[6]

The bombing of Hiroshima on August 6, 1945, was the first, conspicuous symptom of this development.[7] When the Nazi crimes could still be interpreted as offences by individuals against law and humanity, when under fascism, the larger share of a people could become guilty, then one cultural morality (the Fascist) entered into opposition to another (the anti-Fascist). The deployment of the first atomic bomb, however, demonstrated the victory of *one* cultural morality over all others, since this now harbored the possibility to destroy itself in the moment of imposing itself and destroy all others in the course of its triumph. The release of "Little Boy" was by no means compelled by rational considerations, since Russia, as the Americans knew, planned to enter the war against Japan at their side. Detonating the bomb in the middle of a bustling city without prior warning sprang from the not even repressed but only badly negated wish to be satisfied of cruel, exhibitionist-aggressive pulsional impulses. While on August 6, these still linked up with power-political rationalizations, that is, they at this point in time still served the alliance between drive and power interest, the release of "Fat Man"[8] over Nagasaki three days later (a day *after* the Red Army's invasion of Manchuria and Korea) shows the breakthrough of *pure* cruelty, no longer correlated with economic or political interests. It's not that the drive has escaped the spirits that called it forth; its full power and aim have now become visible for everyone. At the same time, a qualitative leap has taken place in the power versus drive dialectic. The potency of the bomb no longer corresponded to the multiplied pulsional wish of the individuals working in the development and production of the bomb. It embodied an autonomized, reified aggressive potency of its own magnitude. Reification here in a double sense. From the objectively generated illusion that the pulsional aggressiveness of individuals could be *materially* satisfied by the bomb arose (in the qualitative leap from the weapon against human beings to the weapon against humanity) a product that is no longer a means of aggressive relationships between people, a means of aggressive satisfaction, but one that objectively dominates the aggression.

After this turn, counterforces—though of course at this point in time we cannot say where these would get their energies—can prompt the drive to once again link up *more* [intensely] with the economic and political interests against the objectified form of itself. Over against the total triumph of the drive, the synthesis of culture and aggression still seems to be the lesser evil.

This designates conditions we must take into consideration when we look at special pulsional vicissitudes. The three lessons we will draw from our reflections are as follows: first, we see that in disentangling sexuality and aggression, it is ultimately sexualized aggressions that prevail over an erotism that seeks to engage in sadism. Second, we understand that in the alliance between a dominant power and the aggressive drive, it is not the power that will triumph over the drive, but the *objectivized* drive will triumph over the dominant power. And third, we are led to the insight that the goal of human aggression is always destruction; sadism, violence, oppression, [or] exploitation are already cultivated sublimation phenomena. In these forms, sexual libido recovers some of its importance.

Notes

1 One of the few passages in Freud's writings that tend toward optimism can be found in the merciless critique of religion in *The Future of an Illusion*: "The voice of the intellect is a soft one, but it does not rest till it has gained a hearing" (Freud 1927a, 53).
2 Parin 1983, 22.
3 Idealizing an authority, however, is nothing but reversing hostile impulses. When the appreciation decays, the originary aggression appears.
4 This "pleasure" does not contradict the thesis asserted earlier that aggression is socially tolerated only if it is without pleasure. Recall the discussion of hypocrisy. The pleasure affect is the most mobile part of a pulsional satisfaction and can be defended against without much effort. Pleasurelessness can just as well result from the general striving for pleasure and is not synonymous with unpleasure. The opposition arising here between pleasure and anxiety, on the contrary, is fundamental. Simplifying somewhat, we can say that psychically, anxiety operates

like an emergency break (anxiety as signal); it interrupts dangerous pulsional developments (see Freud 1926a). Yet once again, we find ourselves on social terrain. Anxiety as signal is an *ego* function. But if the ego is heteronomous, it signals the danger no longer for its own protection but in the interest of something foreign. Socially, this has long been immanent: the manipulation of anxiety joins the formation of the pulsional structures. Education *through* anxiety is well known. Less obvious but all the more effective is the *elimination of anxiety*. Obfuscation tactics and prohibitions on perception make it such that the justified anxiety as signal is at first disavowed, shifted onto replacement objects, and later, when the internal structure has changed sufficiently, is no longer recognized at all. This holds for pulsional anxiety as much as it does for realistic anxiety.

5   I am using the expression *Agentur* here instead of the correct psychoanalytic term *Instanz* to emphasize that in this regard, the superego is indeed the agent, the representative of reality. *Instanz* stresses its character as an internal structure, its function as an ideal; *Agentur* rather points to its [function of] representing *interests*. We must not pass over in silence the fact that the energies of the superego, that is, its strictness and the vehemence of the feelings of guilt, can in no way be derived from the external pressure but are fed by *its own* pulsional sources. (The literature in English, incidentally, is unfamiliar with the term *Instanz*; it has always used *agency*.)

6   See Marcuse (1955) 1956. It almost seems like a foreboding anticipation of my thesis that Marcuse changed the title of this work three times: *Eros and Civilization* (1955) became *Eros und Kultur* (*Eros and Culture*, 1957), and "Eros" finally disappeared completely, the title turning into *Triebstruktur und Gesellschaft* (Pulsional Structure and Society, 1967). Marcuse, however, takes an opposing view. Convinced that ultimately, when the tension of life diminishes, eros and destruction drive can be unified in *one* drive, he writes: "The death instinct operates under the Nirvana principle: it tends toward that state of 'constant gratification' where no tension is felt—a state without want. This trend of the instinct implies that its *destructive* manifestations would be minimized as it approached such a state. If the instinct's basic objective is not the termination of life but of pain—the absence of tension—then paradoxically, in terms of the instinct, the conflict between life and death is the more reduced, the closer life approximates the state of gratification. Pleasure principle and Nirvana principle then converge. At the same time, Eros, freed from surplus repression, would be strengthened, and the strengthened Eros would, as it were, absorb the objective of the death instinct. The instinctual value of death would have changed: if the instincts pursued and attained their fulfillment in a non-repressive order, the regressive compulsion would lose much of its biological rationale. As suffering and want recede, the Nirvana principle may become reconciled with the reality principle" (Marcuse [1955] 1956, 234–35, Marcuse's emphasis).

At first, the confusion concerning destruction drives and the principle of the death drive, initiated by Freud himself, seems to be a question of theoretical method. The inability or unwillingness to separate the two, however, turns out to be a social phenomenon. Marcuse—quite rightly—makes the Oedipus complex "the prototype of the instinctual conflicts between the individual and his society," but only insofar as "the 'sexual craving' for the mother-woman ... *threatens the psychical basis of civilization*; it is the 'sexual craving' that makes the Oedipus conflict" (270, Le Soldat's emphasis). The much more blatant threat to culture *and* sexuality posed by the former rivals, aggression and reality principle, eludes Marcuse. His opposition was to psychoanalytic revisionism, and he criticized exploitation in the form of sexual repression, the reality principle of the dominant system in "father ... domination, sublimation, resignation"; his goal, if I understand him correctly, was to change "the objective social dynamic of the period" in order to salvage individual freedom and happiness, since "in a repressive society, individual happiness and productive development are in contradiction to society; if they are defined as values to be realized within this society, they become themselves repressive" (270 and 245).

In the becoming outdated of even the most progressive opinions we can see the creeping changing of our reality. What Marcuse demands seems questionable to us because the *aggressive* happiness of the individual, insofar as it does not become critique, no longer encounters any repression. Reality principle and death drive are "reconciled."

7 *Directly* involved in the production of the atomic bomb at the time were more than 150,000 scientists and engineers, as the *dtv-Atlas zur Weltgeschichte,* vol. 2, 15th ed., p. 272, from 1966 notes [Kinder (1966) 1980]. Twenty years later, the renowned Swiss *NZZ* [*Neue Zürcher Zeitung,* a major newspaper] "forgets" 147,000 "perpetrators" and smugly writes: "The original estimate was that some thirty scientists would suffice to develop the bomb." Yet as far as personnel was concerned, one had "miscalculated by a factor of one hundred: in 1945, nearly 3000 people [!] worked and lived in Los Alamos" (*Neue Zürcher Zeitung,* 16 July 1985, 5 [Le Soldat's interpolation]). I cite these dates to show that the tacit legalization of crimes against humanity is not a monopoly of the "guilty" but a dominant trait of the current integration of what is, though without bloodshed, "without pleasure," no longer a silently passive toleration but a quite active cruelty.

8 The nomenclature shows just how much at that time, aggressiveness was freed from all constraints and even got rid of the partner it shared interests with. The production crew—with the joke's force in revealing the unconscious—called the first bomb "Thin Man," for President Roosevelt, and the second "Fat Man," for the British Premier Churchill.

6 On the necessity of lying

Reality testing is a psychical sense organ that operates on the boundary between external reality and internal world; in the service of consciousness, its task is to sort the quality of the psychical contents according to their origins. The information, for instance, whether an anxiety it feels is a reaction to an external threat or whether internal impulses have triggered the anxiety signal, is essential. It is also advantageous to be able to distinguish between psychical contents of different kinds; dream contents, phantasies, and memory shares do not betray themselves but must be distinguished by an agency. An assessment of reality, too, would of course be desirable: is an event the consequence of a law of nature or of coincidence? Who is the author of an event, whom does it benefit and whom does it harm? Reality checking usually performs its task quite well. The subject is sufficiently oriented as to the difference between phantasies, memories, and perceptions of reality.

Now, this assessment function begins to operate roughly at the same time in childhood development as the superego. Conscience arises thanks to the necessity to save indispensable infantile wishes from the paternal supremacy.[1]

For a while, the internalization of prohibitions entails confusion. The child no longer knows whether it has merely wished for the prohibited and imagined its fulfillment in phantasy or whether it has indeed given in to its impulses—in both cases, conscience rages against it equally. Nor is the child yet in a position to assess whether the sensations of guilt it feels follow from the paternal prohibitions or whether they already indicate the internal conscience. In this embarrassment, reality testing arises and creates order and security. The criterion of this order, however, is dubious. In submitting to the more powerful, the child has preliminarily lost interest in the external world; it retracts its psychical cathexes from reality. If it must relinquish fulfillment of the most ardent wishes, it wants to achieve at least an advantageous distribution of the psychical energies in its inner world for a later, new attempt at wish fulfillment. Psychoanalysis speaks of a *latency period* after the oedipal conflict has subsided. During this period, the external world is largely left to the former rival. The early reality testing produces an identity between paternal reality and reality; in later life, this equation is never fully given up.

DOI: 10.4324/9781032666273-13

The defense measures against unwelcome pulsional impulses, repression, and disavowal, take shape as if the real conditions had not changed[2]; conscience punishes the adult's wishes in the same way in which it once opposed the child's rebellious demands.[3] To be sure, the moral agency develops[4]; in the course of adolescence, it absorbs new ideals and is no longer oriented by prohibitions alone. Ultimately, though, morality understands itself as representative of the external world after all, and in this regard, it is supported by reality testing. Reality testing will of course be able to note differences in the content of the morality of the external world and that of conscience; yet it will not be able to judge the fact that the assessment of the morality of the external world is based on a projection. The illusion that this morality is identical with the morality of the father experienced in childhood imposes itself against all rational information. For the unconscious, for emotional life, which after all controls thinking and acting against conscious intention, the reality of the external world remains the one it has experienced during the profound crisis of childhood, the oedipal crisis, at the age of barely five years.[5]

Any attempt at elucidating the relationship of society and individual, every intention of changing the conditions of this relationship, must engage with the infantility of reality testing. Neurotics suffer from the insufficiency of their reality testing and at the same time use it for their purposes. If an inner conflict makes it impossible for them to relinquish a drive as demanded of them, it is quite opportune for them to be able to cede the demands of their conscience to the external world without entering into contradiction with their usual assessment of reality. This illusionary assessment of reality, however, is also welcomed by any societal power. Individuals themselves thus renounce an instrument of critique. Not only neurotics but everyone is subject to this necessity of misjudging reality. As long as *one* cultural achievement, the internalization of conscience, is not supplemented by a *second*, a revision of reality testing, there can be no change in the supremacy of a man-made reality over the wishes of individuals.

In the last section, I claimed that a society's dominant power promotes particular neurotic diseases in order to test, in their natural history, possible solutions for detrimental social developments. Now, we may suspect that this fate is met with not only by neuroses but instead is a general characteristic of societies structured by hierarchies of power. The interest of those who have dominion determines the external and internal conditions of people's lives; it influences individuals, threatening economic and social disadvantages [and] using violence; it skillfully uses the insufficiency of psychical function[s] to eliminate criticism and participates in the defense strategies thus formed.[6] The institutions of power do not abide criticism, deviant behavior, and perversions out of tolerance; opposition, rather, holds the possibility of incorporating resistance. Individuals' secret knowledge of the literal "commiseration" [*Mitleiden*] of power and the secondary gain from illness[7] it derives from the opposition to power, however, are poor substitutes for an adequate assessment of reality.

A serious activist documentary filmmaker who has made great contributions to the memory of details of a destroyed past recently showed his film recordings from today's Hiroshima.[8] In all conscience, this man has made a film concerned with the fate of the survivors, with the outsiders discriminated against today in a new society. He does not pass over the accusations, over the warnings, in silence, he does not spare viewers the sight of bodies incomprehensibly destroyed and people psychically tormented. And nonetheless, his film is scandalous. Scandalous not only in *what* it shows but because it uncovers the counterproductiveness of the truth. In truthfully presenting the objective reality, namely, that Hiroshima today prospers and thrives, that young people go jogging around the Atomic Bomb Dome and enjoy soft serve, in also showing the handful of survivors, in emphatically sharing in their fate, the filmmaker is lying. He is not being hypocritical, his empathy is beyond doubt, and yet he obviously claims that *individual survival* with and after the explosion of *reified aggression*—and not only after this concrete bomb!—is possible. That is the objective reality. That is a magnificent illusion. The filmmaker would have had to lie to tell the truth. He would have had to unmask the given reality—given by the concrete lives of the inhabitants of Hiroshima, [given] also by the personal suffering of the survivors—as an illusion to bear witness to the true reality. I do not mean by this any kind of aesthetic, artistic freedom. Nor do I mean the trivial principle that statements about reality not only can and may depict reality but always already interpret and transcend this reality. What I mean, rather, is the demand that results from reversing Leo Lowenthal's observation that in the face of terror, it would be stupid not to be stupid[9]; for activism, for the work that is to serve to abolish individual suffering, we must be *limited* in order to be smarter than reality.

The reality shows couples and playing children in Hiroshima. Not only does the individual reality of these people build on an illusion that has acquired a symptom in the disavowal and discrimination against the survivors; the *objective* reality of today's Hiroshima must be recognized as an illusion.[10] This insight must impose itself against the perception of the senses. Not only have material phenomena had to put up, since Newton and Einstein, with being corrected by theory, not only have necessarily subjective phenomena, such as feelings had to be observed critically, since Freud, and have proven to be deceptive; life itself can emerge as an illusion from the possibility of deliberately obliterating all of animate nature.

Freud's dictum still holds that "[w]e welcome illusions because they spare us unpleasurable feelings, and enable us to enjoy satisfactions instead." We notice how much the reality of our time has changed, however, when we continue reading: "We must not complain, then, if now and again they come into collision with some portion of reality, and are shattered against it."[11] Freud here is talking about the bourgeois and patriotic illusions destroyed in the war. They do not deserve mourning. For us, however, the double meaning of illusion must unfold. The disavowal of the *objective* illusion of current life in Hiroshima does not spare us, as one might think, the unpleasure of anxiety about our own possible annihilation. Rather, we enjoy the satisfaction of *illusionarily* and deeply unconsciously sharing in power at the side of the perpetrators. The one is the reversal of the other, you might say; the distancing from the victims, the downplaying of what has happened *is* the disavowal of the anxiety, is the identification with the aggressor.

That, I think, would overlook an essential, new dimension. Since the terror has become the one described everywhere in the world, since the state systems themselves have come to be threatened by the general atomic terror, processes of becoming conscious can take place individually only on the *condition* of gaining insight into how much every word and every action is *objectively* part of *this* terror. This requires, at any moment, a conscious double-entry accounting in the inner [life]. The objective illusion of reality, the illusion of possible survival after the nuclear bomb, must be made to pass for a *subjective* illusion of those who have dominion. That is objectively wrong. But if we do not do what is wrong, if we do not present the illusion as truth, we further the lie that life after the atom bomb is indeed possible. This absurd situation arises when there is no other reality beside the reality of the aggressor, when the reality of the aggressor is identical with *objective* reality. The other reality, the one that I mean, in which the reality of the aggressor would be a subjective reality, must first make space for itself in the reality objective today. It not only appears as an illusion, today it *is* an illusion.

Human conscience has been overrun by the historical development of the last decades; ignoring the commandments of conscience (which it itself has posited), reality has allied with the pulsional wishes. The aggressiveness demanded by reality deprives sexuality of its force, leaves it empty, and draws all expectations of pleasure onto itself. Reality testing neither is able to distinguish between inner and outer reality nor is it capable—not psychically and not objectively—of recognizing the illusion generated by those in power for what it is. The innerpsychical coalitions that the system of no longer repressive but integrating dominion forces onto individuals are no longer the ones that arise in childhood. Reality testing and its emotional signals (anxiety, feelings of guilt, pleasure) that people develop in the course of childhood and adolescence are not the ones that can guarantee their physical survival.

Anna Freud reports: "I am reminded of something my father said ... when he spoke of how we bring up our children. He said we supply them with a map of the Italian lakes and send them to the North Pole."[12] I do not presume to judge how much Freud knew about in whose service and to what ends this kind of education is conducted; certainly not in the interest of parents, or of the oedipal rival.

We do not talk about drives and defenses. We do not talk about the unconscious, about emotional movement and becoming conscious. Worse than that, we militate for furthering morality, for strengthening conscience—a faux pas that not even enduring engagement with the causes and consequences of the aggression drive can make up for. Not to mention [the circumstance] that we seriously encourage lying, demand an absurd assessment of reality

94 Voluntary Servitude. Masochism and Morality

that everyone could easily recognize as psychotic. I even think that this is the point where psychoanalysis, as a partner of the *political* peace movements, must enter the struggle for a resilient, more intelligent conscience.[13] What I have said so far was meant to define my standpoint, my platform,[14] and to present my intention.[15] The work of psychoanalysis can begin only there, not somewhere and everywhere.

Notes

1. Even in the "society without the father" (as Alexander Mitscherlich calls it in his eponymous book, [1963] 1969) and the change Horkheimer observed of the function of the family in the process of socialization, a change in which the father objectively loses power and his power increasingly becomes illusory and irrational, psychologically, the morality of the oedipal rival—however deficient it might seem to us—counts as *the* given form of power. That this is the one of the *father* also applies, in my view, based on psychological, not on social-critical considerations, to the little girl as well.
2. For a more precise account of the difference between repression and disavowal, see Freud 1915c and Freud 1938b, 203–4. Grossly simplifying, we may say that in a repression of what is embarrassing and unacceptable, no memory remains in consciousness, whereas in disavowal, the memory and the perception are untouched while the emotional content—anxiety, pleasure, joy, wrath, terror, etc.—is missing. Repression, on the individual level, abolishes history, social repressions annihilate it. Individual disavowal makes emotionally adequate action—escape, curiosity, combat, etc.—impossible; socially incisive disavowals effect adequate—adequate *in their sense*—attitudes in the first place.
3. On this point, see Parin (1969) 1978. Parin explicitly talks about how interest in political events takes place "via sublimated libido and numerous autonomous functions of the ego." The fact that these autonomous functions of the ego repeat essential earlier conflicts, resuscitate oedipal phantasies, mobilize tested defense formations—that they are, precisely not "independent" from the infantile experiences—renders the "best possible handling of new burdens 'in an emergency'" possible in the first place (28 and 31).
4. Harold Lincke thinks that the superego is "essentially a symptom- or compromise-formation" and "itself unassailable," [such that] the defense can be directed "only against its consequences" (Lincke 1970, 381–82).
5. Part III below further discusses this problem.
6. I think that civilized human beings conduct absolutely unproductive, in no way justifiable "medical" tests on animals in thousands of "laboratories" not *only* to satisfy sadistic cravings. I see in this institutionalized animal cruelty a symptomatic action influenced by collectively shared individual phantasies. Through the identification with the aggressor, what is psychically done to one in order to keep *power* healthy is physically repeated on the animals. Power, in this case the chemical industry, does not profit from these experiments economically, on the contrary; why it keeps them alive is most likely explained by the fact that—without reflection—it knows about their *symptom* character. When a symptom is prohibited, the aggression bound up in it is freed and turns against the one who prohibits it. Examples like this one can be found everywhere.
7. On this point, see Freud 1905b, 43–44 and 43n1; Freud 1916–1917, SE 16, 381–84; Freud 1926a, 98–99.
8. The filmmaker is Erwin Leiser, the documentary is his film *Erinnern und Verdrängen* [*Remembering and Repressing*—the actual title, though, is *Hiroshima—Erinnern*

oder Vergessen, Remembering or Forgetting]. There, he used selections from another film he made in Hiroshima, *You Must Choose Life* (1963).
9 Lowenthal (1945) 1990, 2: "Thinking becomes a stupid crime; it endangers [the individual's] life. The inevitable consequence is that stupidity spreads as a contagious disease among the terrorized population. Human beings live in a state of stupor—in a moral coma."
10 The point is not to designate the life of the people existing there today as an "illusion." Neurotic anxiety that arises from the reversal of mourning, too, is anxiety actually experienced. With these formulations, I am pointing to a new category of thought: the power [*Potenz*] to extinguish life *as such* compels the idea that concrete life, life suffered could be an illusion. This *life* appears in toto as a defense against an objective reality (the possibility of annihilating all life).
11 Freud 1915b, 280.
12 [This is the epigraph in Sandler 1983, 35.]
13 The already mentioned conference, *War and Peace from the Psychoanalytic Point of View*, took an opposite stance. The preface to the proceedings concludes by noting: "The psychoanalytic approach to the topic is of course not the only legitimate one and it is certainly one-sided: but it is central and, in its one-sidedness, indispensable. It is the only one *able to see the human being as the subject of its history without restrictions* because it does not reduce the motives of [human beings] to their conscious shares and is therefore *not compelled to take recourse to foreign influences where this action makes no more discernable sense* (Passett and Modena, 1983, 20, Le Soldat's emphasis).
14 "Our platform" is the term Otto Fenichel used to designate the general point of view of his circle of Marxist psychoanalysts. See Dahmer 1982, 239–365.
15 Freud referred to psychoanalysis as the *Sache*, the cause; see the twenty-fourth of the *New Introductory Lectures* in Freud 1933 (GW 15, 163). [The phrase is rendered as "my ideas" in SE 22: 152.—Trans.]

7 The ability to remain silent and the task of theory

In a lecture he gave in Basel in 1938, Fenichel named two reasons in response to the question why people let themselves be incorporated into a war machine. Every person who resists the public power is threatened. Prison, criminalization, punishment, and social and physical death await them. They perform the function the system assigned them even if it obviously goes against their interests because they are afraid; their anxiety is real and rationally founded. The second reason is psychological:

> the factor that cruelly destructive drives that at other times had to be repressed may now express themselves may certainly play a role. (I don't believe this role is very great; for most combatants are not at all happy about the cruelties they are allowed to commit).[1]

Coming from an experienced psychanalyst like Fenichel, this is a rather remarkable statement.[2] He seems to postulate what is psychoanalytically untenable, [namely], that pulsional actions are a matter of the will, that being "happy" is a criterion of pulsional satisfaction. In the context of the sexual drives, Fenichel would never have let such formulations slip in. They stand in stark contrast to Freud's views, which Fenichel knew and shared; they also run counter to all clinical and practical experience. Following the elucidation by Freud's discussion in *Civilization and its Discontents*, no psychoanalyst could have doubts about the quality of aggression. We wonder, therefore, whether Fenichel, and Reich along with him,[3] *had to* turn against the thesis of a general pulsional aggressiveness of the human being in a personal defense or out of political considerations.

The argument that they did not want to provide Fascism with a psychological alibi is certainly not sound. *Every* scientific and philosophical insight can be used or abused to justify a social system that functions with or without it. Even if it had been unwise at the time publicly to advocate the aggression theory, there would have been no need for Fenichel to restrain himself before the Basel Association, which belonged to the political left. I much more suspect that he had other reasons to do without Freud's theses. Although he does not elaborate on it in this context, I think that he was preoccupied with a fundamental difference between psychoanalytic method and psychoanalytic theory. I mean the different subjective positions demanded of analysts when they seek to elucidate, [on the one hand,] the individually unconscious [and, on the other,] what is generally unconscious, for example, disavowed social conflicts, negated social functions, repressed history, and the like. The psychoanalytic method cannot simply be applied to the social. Analysts lack all the necessary instruments for it: the setting, the "evenly suspended" attention, and the emotional transference relationship. This of course leaves analysts, who are used to working with people's unconscious and with their own, free to make use of *this* experience to think about the social. Freud seized that opportunity from the beginning. It is absurd for psychoanalysis to abstain from social criticism. Applying psychoanalysis to the social while keeping to the therapeutic position and method, however, is not only absurd, it is counterproductive. It gives rise to empty formulas such as "collectively unconscious," "social repressions," "group projections," and so on. A theory capable of connecting social criticism and depth psychology is still outstanding. Just this much for now: since it would not otherwise be able to establish a transference relationship and gain insight into the unconscious, the method must start from the individual as the subject of its history. Every psychoanalytic interpretation conveys some insight into how and why people defend against the knowledge that *they* steer their own fate. The central conflict, the Oedipus complex, shows, in the account of the genesis of conscience in particular, that what determines the severity of conscience is *not* the introjected prohibitions, *not* the real strictness of the feared rival, the father, but exclusively the power of *one's own* aggressions.[4]

The attempt to interpret the pulsional vicissitudes in the psychoanalytic cure [by starting] from heteronomous influences merely leads to conscious psychological banality. Psychical changes can be achieved only to the extent that people understand *how much* they are the subjects of their history. I say "how much" on purpose, not "that." Even if an individual is a victim of contemporary history, a victim of power, of violence, and oppression, psychoanalysis will insist on rendering those *subjective* motivations that caused one's own fate to take this course and no other.

It is, however, momentous to confuse a methodological instrument (the therapeutic positions) and the essence of a theory, *criticism*. Insofar as it is the case that in psychoanalysis, the theory is part of the method, the attempt to redeploy the method as part of the theory amounts to a defense against its theses.[5] And the endeavor to apply the methods of analysis to elucidate social conflicts goes beyond what is justifiable. It means wanting to proceed not only *as* an analyst, the way Freud did, but with the tools of analytic therapy, abstinent and without taking sides. That this is a mistake from the point of view of a theory of science would be harmless if it were not equally a political act, namely, unintended taking sides for the dominant ideology ostensibly to be elucidated. The correctness of this claim is easily illustrated by Fenichel's strategy during his lecture tour through Europe, at the time assailed by Fascism. Had he acted correctly according to the theory of technique and not left the methodological standpoint, he would have pointed to the unconscious wishes of the people going to war. In that case, he could not have remained silent about the aggression tendency and he would also have drawn his listeners' attention to the pulsional pleasure that—albeit repressed, and overgrown by anxiety about suffering from violence oneself—is in all cases associated with the idea of belligerent acts. That way, Fenichel would have told the truth scientifically and psychoanalytically but would have had a paralyzing and dejecting effect on his audience. Applying the psychoanalytic method in theoretical reflections in the face of real danger would have meant nothing else than taking a stance *against* those endangered. Of course, an interpretation or exposure of the unconscious was not even needed. For it is a peculiarity of psychoanalysis that the very utterance of *theoretical* propositions acts on the listener like an interpretation. The explication of aggression theory unavoidably generates a sense of guilt because we refer what we hear to ourselves and understand it as an allusion to our own secret source of pleasure.[6] This reaction cannot be avoided, and it can usually be neglected when the priority is to communicate knowledge; to risk it among people already in danger anyway and, in the dominant opinion, "guilty," however, would have been a sadistic, political act.

Precisely because he had correctly grasped the objective situation, Fenichel had to relinquish an essential part of the theory and *in this moment* pass over the subjective unconscious motivations in silence. He concluded that what "can explain wars for us" is "not the psychological study of the combatants" but that we must explain, "inversely, the psychical situation of the combatants from the real societal function of wars, which acts on combatants in manifold ways, and namely, in a way that covers up the true state of affairs."[7]

Why did Fenichel not point at least to a dialectic between individual pulsional wishes and societal functions? Is it justified to leave a central thesis of the theory (the pulsional aggression) and an essential principle of the method (the interpretation of subjective motivations) aside to promote a process of becoming conscious of societal processes?

Interpreting the objective situation and *simultaneously* naming the subjective motivations does indeed mean depicting a correct dialectic between individual and society; yet neither the correctness of the theoretical insights nor the method correctly applied but only the *quantitative* relationships of this dialectic define the meaning, the effect, and the social consequences of what is being said.

I set great stores by the *quantitative assessment of forces prior to any analysis of content*. In our case, it will always lead to simply noting the supremacy of the social. This may seem trivial. Yet what is *physically* a matter of course for us in the *social* [domain] must first be learned. The supremacy of the social that in psychoanalytic reflections we assign little methodological value compels us to cede theoretical ground as soon as we seek to *communicate* our insights at a specific time, under particular political conditions; what ground we cede is decided not by us but by the current interest of power. There is only one way to make up for the loss, namely, *consciously* to give up *even more* parts of the theory in order to clear a platform for insight into the real conditions. This thesis is based on the fact that psychoanalysis must recognize when and where and through what changes it can hold on to its substance. When the dominant ideology of the thirties forces the elimination of aggression theory, psychoanalysis remains behind as a comparatively harmless psychology of sexuality; when, however, [psychoanalysis] intentionally gives up its claim to propagate the dialectic between individual and society and insists on *neglecting* (and precisely not emphasizing!) the subjective factor, it gets another chance to continue having an effect as a method for studying the unconscious and not as an apologetic psychology.

It should now no longer come as a surprise that an exclusively libidinous theory of sexuality or the theoretical emphasis on the subjective leads to innocuousness. It is just as important, though, to understand that holding on to aggression theory and the dialectic would, in the time of Fascism, have generated a paralyzing feeling of guilt in the listeners to whom Fenichel was speaking—as leftists, as Jews, et cetera, they had the objective social supremacy against them and not behind them.

Today, we cannot hope to once again successfully use the strategy with which Fenichel defended against the Fascist threat. What was right in facing the Fascist danger, today, fifty years later, in facing the nuclear threat, seems practically to deflect from the true state of affairs.

Fascism at that time was a deadly danger for certain countries and certain people. Fenichel's very own fate, indeed, shows that it was possible to escape the danger. In early 1938, he was traveling across Europe (with the exception of Germany) to give a series of psychoanalytic lectures, and some months later, he was forced, like Freud himself, to save his life from the Fascists and flee. He was, however, able to continue working, having emigrated to the United States.

If in 1938, there was good reason to analyze the danger the better to *fight against* it (this is also the thrust of the efforts of the exiled Frankfurt School),[8] our task today is entirely different.

People are being forced into wars that neither promote their interests nor procure them any kind of advantage. Clear and simple though it may be, people do not acknowledge this fact. The denials of the profiteers are understandable. On the one hand, they can have no interest in the truth being discovered. On the other hand, they can claim no more weight than the assurance of a notorious thief that the thousand-dollar bills just flew into his pockets by themselves. The question that has always been waiting for answer, an answer that has much more than just psychological significance, is the question of "voluntary servitude."[9] How do those in power manage to have so many collaborate in their plans? What external and what internal conditions, what drives, what fears force people to let themselves be subjugated in blind docility? Do people not know enough to be able to judge their situation in accordance with reality? Are they being systematically disoriented? Can they do nothing because distress and violence force them? Or can they not get rid of power, no matter how much they want to, because unconscious assimilations, internalizations, keep them captive? Are not all people, powerful or dependent, equally aggressive, is the pulsional constitution not the same in all human beings, such that everyone enjoys aggressiveness as soon as there is a chance? Does it not render our criticism of objective power invalid when *everyone* strives for power and violence? Self-destruction drive, masochism, are they not forces inaccessible to reason whose results must ultimately appear equally irrational and absurd? Given how serious the situation is, should we not rather turn to the causes of the *defense*, the "disavowal of danger," as Paul Parin says?[10]

In psychoanalysis, we know that interpreting and working through the resistance, the forces, that is, which oppose the becoming-conscious, is the precondition of change. Without lengthy work on and with the *emotional* resistances, there is no consciousness; without consciousness, no real change. Psychoanalysis also knows, however, that working through the defense remains without effect when the *theory* that orients the interpretation is incomplete or wrong. The history of psychoanalysis itself, which developed via the mistakes of its theories, is its own witness here. That is why I postulate to revise the psychoanalytic theory of aggression and, where necessary, to renew and supplement it. We saw above that great internal resistances act against the direct observation of the aggression drive. That is why in these pages, preference is given to the study of masochism, a form of defense against aggression.

One of the basic ideas of psychoanalysis is that what is pathological is not really distinct from what is healthy,[11] that what is neurotic affords us an insight into the way the psychical works, an insight that the all too smooth functioning of the normal prevents. Masochism, according to Freud's thesis, is a particular pulsional vicissitude of aggression. That is my starting point in considering the possibilities of defending against aggressive pulsional impulses via the example of masochism. I begin with an observation and a reflection.

The reflection is simple. If the assessment of popular wisdom is correct that masochists are people who voluntarily accept suffering, then investigating the conditions of this suffering must provide us with a number of clues as to how, in what way, and why pain and suffering are seemingly voluntarily endured and sought out. We must not hope to obtain conclusions about the conditions of abiding societal suffering, but we expect information about the forces with which an external power that brings suffering can ally. Perhaps we reach the conclusion that what we already know is all there is, namely, that power links up with anxiety, feelings of guilt, and the pulsional pleasure of aggressiveness. That external power makes use of internal allies (parts of the superego, functions in the ego, or direct pulsional forces) is not unknown. Freud says that masochism is destruction turned inward.[12] What could be more evident than basing "voluntary servitude" on a double internal mechanism? Individuals would participate in the aggressions of those in power and thus satisfy their own destructiveness; simultaneously those in power would use the internalization of the aggressor for their own purposes and, in one blow, turn subjects' unused aggression back onto them to oppress them.

That's how it could be. But I want to quickly note an observation. Psychoanalysis, which since its inception has devoted itself in detail to almost all psychological topics with theoretical reconsiderations and rearticulations, has trouble with the question of masochism. It is no exaggeration to say that in the years since Freud's 1924 essay, that is, more than sixty years ago, there is, in the spate of work on neurosis theory, hardly a monograph on masochism that gives a new account of the *theoretical* problems. The exceptions are quickly listed: these are, above all, Theo Reik's *Masochism in Modern Man* (*Aus Leiden Freuden*, 1940) and Wilhelm Reich's *The Masochistic Character* (1932).[13] Since research interest is not something that turns to this or that topic on a whim but is very much part of the general ideology, I must suppose that it cannot be in the interest of the morality now common to elucidate the mechanisms of masochism. I will hardly [be able to] avoid the temptation to be drawn in by a cultural ideology. I will be content, however, should I succeed, as I look at the phenomena more closely and in a more differentiated manner, as I seek out nuances that would correct or better justify our view of the whole, in not falling prey to *two dangers*. (1) Objective power, which I have been talking about so far, must not be confused with individual dominion. Objective power is a social and historical entity. While it feeds on the aggressiveness of subjects, it is not identical to it. Objective power *acts* through the aggressiveness of those in power *and* of the oppressed but is of course not exhausted by it. It takes complex transformations, which are subject not just to psychical conditions, for either power or dominion on the one hand, or, on the other hand, powerlessness, voluntary servitude, or masochism to arise from pulsional aggression efforts. They are the result of processes in the tricky and enigmatic transitory zone between what is individual and what is social. After all, we must postulate the same pulsional constitution for all human beings. What is decisive, however, is the pulsional vicissitude imposed by socialization—and the present or absent (as the case may be) degrees of liberty of this vicissitude. (2) The fact that while it is possible to distinguish objective power from dominion (the power exerted *among* people), it is not possible to separate out the pulsional cruelty of those in power and of the oppressed, must not deceive us. The slap in the face that Beate Klarsfeld gave Dr. Filbinger is not identical with the slap in the face Erich Mühsam had to abide from someone in power in his day.[14] Both nonetheless are expressions of the same pulsional impulse.

Notes

1 Fenichel (1938) 1981, 1060–61. Fenichel gave the lecture at the Kulturverein Basel on January 17, 1938. We owe the publication in 1981 of the manuscript to Russell Jacoby and Randi Markowitz.
2 Fenichel is the author of what remains the best, most vivid textbook (Fenichel [1945] 1996).

102 Voluntary Servitude. Masochism and Morality

3 See Reich (1932) 1938a; Bernfeld's reply, (1932) 1938; and Reich's counter-critique (1932) 1938b.
4 See Freud 1923b, 53–55.
5 To view, as has become popular again in recent years, the emotional experience as *the* analytical agent [*Agens*] is to turn necessary conditions into sufficient ones.
6 Freud by contrast says: "In point of fact psycho-analysis is a method of research, an impartial instrument, like the infinitesimal calculus, as it were" (Freud 1927a, 36). Let me also point out here that Freud was right to employ the procedure he did *in statu nascendi* of psychoanalysis, namely, to deploy the therapeutic method as a research method to develop the theory. The strategy necessary to develop the theory, however, turns into its opposite when it is made the principle of *communicating* the theory. Unless one heeds the special rules of its communication, the emancipatory research tool becomes an involuntary means of oppression.
7 Fenichel (1938) 1981, 1062.
8 See Jay (1976) 1996, ch. IV, "The Institut's First Studies of Authority," 113–42.
9 The concept goes back to Étienne de La Boétie [see La Boétie (1574) 2012].
10 "*Activism on our part against the disavowal* of a reality full of dangers, however, takes courage" (Parin 1983, 34; Le Soldat's emphasis).
11 Freud 1938b, 283.
12 Freud 1924a, 165.
13 I am explicitly not referring to the therapy-oriented clinical studies by Wilhelm Stekel, Karen Horney, Edoardo Weiss, Sacha Nacht, Bernhard Berliner, Ludwig Eidelberg, Anna Freud, Franz Alexander, René de Monchy, Marie Bonaparte, Wolf-Dietrich Grodzicki, and others. It also seems to me that the clinical work is limited to the years from 1925 to about 1945. In more recent literature, masochism features merely as pointing to the source of a resistance, the so-called negative therapeutic reaction, as "feminine" [masochism] (for instance in Janine Chasseguet-Smirgel), or as sexual perversion (in Fritz Morgenthaler or M. Masud R. Khan).
14 [This seems to be a confusion of names: In 1968, Klarsfeld slapped the then-chancellor Kurt-Georg Kiesinger to show "that a part of the German people—its youth in particular—revolts against a Nazi heading the federal government" (quoted in Frohn 2008).

Hans Filbinger, a former Nazi navy judge, succeeded Kiesinger as Minister President in the state of Baden-Württemberg (an office that corresponds to that of a governor in the United States) when the latter became chancellor in 1966. Public debate about Filbinger's Nazi past did not occur until 1978, following statements by author and playwright Rolf Hochhuth against which Filbinger sought an injunction. It seems likely that news reports about this affair also evoked Kiesinger and the slap he received from Klarsfeld, which might have led to Le Soldat's confusion. There is, to our knowledge, no public criticism of Filbinger on Klarsfeld's part until after his death in 2007 (see Oswald 2010).

Erich Mühsam (1878–1934) was an anarchist writer and activist arrested by the Nazis in February 1933 and murdered in Oranienburg concentration camp.]

8 A disarming contradiction

Affect inversion and affect suppression are convenient means to bar unpleasant psychical contents from access to consciousness. In sleep, too, during dreaming, feelings can disguise themselves and transform into their opposite; the motor of the events is the intention to regard disturbing conflicts as resolved, unfulfillable wishes as satisfied, to be able to go on sleeping unworried.

The Hungarian psychoanalyst [Sándor] Ferenczi reports an impressive example of affect inversion in dreams:

> An elderly gentleman was wakened at night by his wife, who was alarmed because he laughed so loudly and unrestrainedly in his sleep. He explained later that he had had the following dream: "I was lying in my bed; an acquaintance came in; I wanted to turn up the light, but could not do it. I tried again and again—in vain. Thereupon my wife got out of bed to help me, but she could not manage it either; but because she was embarrassed before the gentleman at being in her *négligé* she finally gave it up and went back to bed again; all this was so comical that I had to laugh exceedingly at it. My wife said, 'Why do you laugh, why do you laugh?' but I only went on laughing,—till I wakened." The following day he was very depressed and had a headache—"from laughing so much that I was exhausted," he thought.
>
> Considered analytically the dream seems less cheerful. The "acquaintance" who entered is, in the latent dream thoughts, the figure of death evoked on the previous day as the "great unknown." The old gentleman, who suffers from arterio-sclerosis, had on the previous day had occasion to think of dying. The unrestrained laughter takes the place of weeping and sobbing at the idea that he must die. It is the light of life that he can no longer turn up. This sad thought may have become associated with recently intended but unsuccessful attempts at cohabitation, in which not even the help of his wife in her *négligé* was of any avail; he was aware that he was already on the downward path. The dream work was able to transform the sad idea of impotence and death into a comic scene, and the sobbing into laughter.[1]

This inversion of affect is only too understandable. Especially at an advanced age, individual death is a law of nature. Humans are usually not in a position freely to decide their death and the moment of their death. We do not regard the illusionary transformation of compulsion and necessity into joy and freedom, and doing so in a life-situation in which there is nothing left but acknowledging nature, as crazy but as the sign of a stoic, serene attitude.[2] Clinicians would prefer seeing insight and mourning rather than dejection and headache, but they will never suspect this defense against affects to be a pathological process.

Affect suppressions that concern the collective death of many, at a moment that a few decide, should not be able to count on similar forbearance from psychoanalysis. Collective, weapon-made death isn't a natural law. But why do people act toward the possibility of their mass death like the old man in the dream—they don't want to know?

We have already expressed some conjectures. We pointed to the possibility that the *psychical* defenses worked so well and smoothly, the adaptation to the dominant morality had advanced so far, that people no longer perceive the danger or, when they do thematize it, as in the world-wide peace movements, the *objective* conditions now appear qualitatively unchangeable.[3] We have also, however, considered the possibility that a genuine pulsional force of the human could be at work that collaborates with the preparations of the human's own demise, the aggression that destructively falls back on the human. We may safely declare the first two conjectures to be certainties. Robert Oppenheimer was not wrong when on July 11, 1945, as the third movement, *Élégie*, from Tchaikovsky's *Serenade for Strings* was playing on the local radio station, he remembered the line from the Hindu holy text, the *Bhagavad Gita*: "Now I am become Death, the destroyer of worlds." Since that hour, history has become less makeable. Geographic escape, collecting the forces of resistance, and fighting the enemy, as could still be practiced in facing the Fascist danger, is and will be no longer possible. It is also correct that the disavowal of the danger must function all the more seamlessly the greater the trauma to be expected is. We cannot indulge in representations of the destruction of life on Earth the way we might play with prohibited sexual representations in phantasy. Pulsional impulses usually are repressed; the representation of the apocalypse, however, releases triumphal aggressions: *I, I alone will survive, even if millions die!*[4] The representations are isolated from the affects: deprived of their context, they can be treated like indifferent rational reflections.

What, then, about the third reflection? I think we have a right to demand of psychoanalysis that it answer the question whether humans do indeed go about their own destruction based on an unchangeable, "natural" pulsional constitution. We must ask whether the theses about the destruction and death drive belong to the uncomfortable truths humanity has to accept from psychoanalysis. It would then be up to us to work for *this* truth becoming conscious and to promote strategies for sublimating and taming the drive. The opposite, however, has also been claimed, namely, that the theses concerning the human death drive are part of a power-political campaign of obfuscation and intimidation. The discussion of these fundamental positions is not new.[5] The lack of novelty, of course, should not prevent us from turning to the problem once more. At every age, every social critique must examine the givens anew, reconsider its theories, and take a stand once more. One thing, however, should give us pause: polar oppositions, dichotomies (death drive yes/death drive no) are figures of thought to which knowledge flees when prohibitions block its dialectical path.

I said earlier that both the insistence on the death drive and the rejection of drive theory can be signs of a defense.[6] I interpreted both positions as consequences of a disavowal or of a displacement to an acceptable substitute. To escape the insight into the tempting force of pleasurable cruelties, we make up the illusion of peaceableness or rush ahead to the abstraction of the death drive. Am I thus going to postulate a dialectic between psychoanalysis and social theory?

The conflict of the opposing efforts of the human drives and the, in turn, differing interests of humans as social individuals recommend that theory adopt a dialectic method. The alluring prospect, however, of conveniently linking what is contradictory by pointing to its irreconcilability, mistakes the path for the goal.[7] While we avoid the danger of one-sidedly ignoring the "subjective factor" in sociology or social critique in drive theory, observing the contradiction is a way of evading the task of investigating the *causes* and *conditions* of the opposing interests.

Before this labor can begin, we must clear up the relationship between psychoanalysis and social critique. Neither the statement that they are irreconcilable nor the suggestion that each looks at "different aspects" of human life is satisfactory.

Psychoanalysis has developed a method that allows for obtaining insight into *unconscious* states of affairs. It makes use of "freely suspended attention"[8] to follow the flow of associations undisturbed. In so doing, it is interested less in the development of thought contents than in the emotional movement; this movement repeats repressed experiences that had traumatic effects and gets wishes going that unavoidably lead to conflicts. The therapeutic goal is to interpret the consequences of these conflicts for the personal vicissitude as the result of unconscious pulsional wishes. Yet the unconscious can never be grasped *directly*, by whatever method. Writing "that everyone possesses in his own unconscious an instrument with which he can interpret the utterances of the unconscious in other people,"[9] Freud names a necessary but not sufficient condition of psychoanalytic understanding. Only *theory* teaches conceiving of otherwise disconnected phenomena as manifestations of something else that itself cannot be experienced. The effects of the unconscious remain unrecognized if they do not receive, from theory, connection, and definition.

Psychoanalytic theory limits itself to looking at individuals. Freud's writings in cultural critique assume a contradiction between individual pulsional demands and social necessity. Even where psychoanalysis is socially engaged, it seeks to bring about a change, through limiting [itself] to what is individual, that will mediately have effects in the society as well. Critical theory shares this intention. Adorno says: "Subject itself must be brought to its objectivity, its stirrings must not be banished from cognition."[10] The chances, it seems, are not bad for a psychoanalytic [and] social-critical exploration of the individual.

The treatment of the death drive thesis in the history of the two theories, though, suggests that a shared enterprise is out of the question; the divergences in outlook, method, and goal are too great. The principle of the death drive is where the good intentions of changing situations of suffering for the individual separate.

The thinking that is necessary for knowing objective oppositions turns out to be of no use in observing unconscious processes. Simultaneously, the neutrality and abstinence, which prompt the unconscious to open up in the first place, are a deceptive expedient in exploring social mechanisms. Where, then, is the site, which is the instrument, where a dialectic of the two methods can develop for both theories to be able to work together? [To quote Adorno once more:]

> Without psychology, in which the objective constraints are continually internalized anew, it would be impossible to understand how people passively accept a state of unchanging destructive irrationality and, moreover, how they integrate themselves into movements that stand in rather obvious contradiction to their own interests.[11]

Psychoanalysts who have not yet become wary of the thesis of identification with the aggressor in the context of history, who moreover view the death drive theory as dubious, will welcome such concessions. I, however, prefer insisting on the divergence of the two kinds of research. The relationship that exists between individual and society today requires a thinking in antinomies and polarities. A world where oppositions are not being mediated but where an objective supremacy of a few over many exists, a social power that satisfies its demands through strategies of integration, can only be captured by a thinking that clearly brings out the obfuscated oppositions. The *consequences* that these processes leave behind in the individual and that are rendered unconscious can be elucidated only by the "freely suspended attention" that tracks the emotional movement in detail. Measuring the expansion of the sphere of influence of social dominion to people's unconscious with psychological yardsticks would mean nothing but concealing it with such anthropomorphous categories of thought.[12]

Nor can I see any advantage in trying to connect the two methods dialectically. I rather consider the cooperation of psychoanalysis and social theory to be something obvious. As far as the relationship of the two theories with each other is concerned, I think that *social-critical insight is in every case the condition of psychological thinking*. The method of psychoanalysis can unfold only when it has become conscious of its own conditionality through the contentual elucidation of social oppositions. Social analysis, the thinking in dichotomies, must precede psychological analysis, the thinking in conflicts. An—albeit desirable—dialectic of the two principles of thought is excluded as long as the current objective supremacy of the social endures. This is true equally of therapeutic efforts and of the intentions of theory. As far as Adorno's demand is concerned to conceive of the "psychological factor" by way of the psychology of individuals, we will have to learn later that this idea itself stands in need of critical analysis.

The dialectic that confronts us develops the contradiction between death principle and pleasure principle *within* individuals and [the contradiction of] power/dependency *between* individuals. Postulating a transverse contradiction, namely, between death drive thesis and social critique (such as the discussion cited has undertaken) means nothing but negating that this is not an antinomy between two theses but the discrepancy between knowledge and the condition of this knowledge.

Let me say it again: social critique is the condition of psychoanalytic insights, not their antithesis; at the same time, it is the goal of psychoanalytic work. While the reflection that there already is a dialectic between drive theory and sociology today does not let itself be deceived by hope for a reconciliation of the different approaches, it does assume that the two contradictory theories could supplement each other. It thereby disarms both theories in one blow—it deprives psychoanalysis of the overall conditions of its knowledge: while its theses remain correct, they are no longer relevant for the nexus of life; and social theory loses its ability to see through connections, to see that and how social and economic laws condition *psychical* misery.

Notes

1 Ferenczi (1916) 1950/1952, 345, quoted by Freud in chapter six of the *Interpretation of Dreams* (Freud 1900, SE 5, 472–73).
2 Specht analyzes a dream reported by Plato's Socrates in the *Crito* (44a–b) [and, earlier, by] Homer in the *Iliad* (9.363) as a similar consoling phantasy: three days before his execution, a beautiful woman in white robes comes to him and says, "Socrates, may you arrive at fertile Phthia on the third day" (Specht 1972, 656).
3 Günther Anders has called our age "The Last Age": "However long this age may last, even if it should last forever, ... there is no possibility that ... the possibility of our self-extinction can ever end—but by the end itself" (Anders [1959] 1962, 493).
4 Compare, by contrast, Parin 1983.
5 See Sandkühler, ed., 1970, which includes the studies by Bernfeld, Reich, Jurinetz, Sapir, and Stoljarov that are otherwise difficult to find.
6 Compare, for instance, the diverging positions of Wilhelm Reich [(1932) 1938a] and Ashley Montagu [1968], who ultimately reach the same conclusion, namely, to discard the aggression *drive*.
7 "The path is the goal" is a formula popular among analysts. See Blarer and Brogle 1983: "*everything* can better structure or disturb the concrete psychoanalytical field; this is because by its very nature, it is defined by the all-encompassing process of endless socialization as well as by the two personalities that are the

analysand and the analyst. Seen this way, for analyst and analysand, *the path remains the goal*" (83, Blarer and Brogle's emphasis).
8 Freud 1912b, 111–12 [Le Soldat writes *freischwebend*, "freely suspended," whereas Freud, as cited earlier (#), has *gleichschwebend*, "evenly suspended"]. See also Reik (1948) 1949.
9 Freud 1913a, 320.
10 Adorno (1969) 2005a, 251.
11 Adorno (1969) 2005b, 271.
12 Jacoby, too, rightly criticizes this tendency (1975, 46–72).

9 From sadism to the death drive

In the seventh chapter of *The Interpretation of Dreams*, Freud calls wishing the "primary activity of the unconscious."[1] Years before he will recognize in the pulsional forces the motivation of wishes, he sketches a "schematic picture of the psychical apparatus"

> There can be no doubt that that apparatus has only reached its present perfection after a long period of development. Let us attempt to carry it back to an earlier stage of its functioning capacity. Hypotheses, whose justification must be looked for in other directions, tell us that at first the apparatus's efforts were directed towards keeping itself so far as possible free from stimuli; consequently its first structure followed the plan of a reflex apparatus, so that any sensory excitation impinging on it could be promptly discharged along a motor path. But the exigencies of life interfere with this simple function, and it is to them, too, that the apparatus owes the impetus to further development. The exigencies of life confront it first in the form of the major somatic needs. The excitations produced by internal needs seek discharge in movement, which may be described as an "internal change" or an "expression of emotion." A hungry baby screams or kicks helplessly. But the situation remains un altered, for the excitation arising from an internal need is not due to a force producing a momentary impact but to one which is in continuous operation. A change can only come about if in some way or other (in the case of the baby, through outside help) an "experience of satisfaction" can be achieved which puts an end to the internal stimulus. An essential component of this experience of satisfaction is a particular perception (that of nourishment, in our example) the mnemic image of which remains associated thenceforward with the memory trace of the excitation produced by the need. As a result of the link that has thus been established, next time this need arises a psychical impulse will at once emerge which will seek to re-cathect the mnemic image of the perception and to re-evoke the perception itself, that is to say, to re-establish the situation of the original satisfaction. An impulse of this

kind is what we call a wish; the reappearance of the perception is the fulfilment of the wish; and the shortest path to the fulfilment of the wish is a path leading direct from the excitation produced by the need to a complete cathexis of the perception.[2]

The entire *Interpretation of Dreams*, we might say, stands for demonstrating the thesis that every dream is a wish fulfillment. Freud discusses, and substantiates with his own dreams and those of others, his assumption that what can regularly be discovered in the *latent* dream content is the *pleasurable* fulfillment of an unconscious, repressed wish. This of course makes those dreams look all the more exciting that seem to contradict the wish fulfillment hypothesis: anxious dreams, dreams of punishment, and dreams with embarrassing and unpleasant contents. Some are easily interpreted as distorted wishful dreams. Inversions of affect and other defense measures make the dream appear as uncomfortable while thorough analysis proves its latent, unconscious intent to be a wish fulfillment after all. Freud admits only two kinds of dreams as counter-wish dreams in a narrower sense. One kind is subtended by an obviously aggressive moment; their pulsional force, he says, is undoubtedly

> the wish that I may be wrong. These dreams appear regularly in the course of my treatments when a patient is in a state of resistance to me; and I can count almost certainly on provoking one of them after I have explained to a patient for the first time my theory that dreams are fulfilments of wishes.[3]

Rather than recognize in these dreams of his intractable patients the fulfillment of an unconscious *aggressive* transference wish, he sets them aside without discussion. By contrast, he highlights *another* kind of counter-wish dream. The *other* motive of those unpleasurable dreams

> is so obvious that it is easy to overlook it, as I did myself for some considerable time. There is a *masochistic* component in the sexual constitution of many people, which arises from the reversal of an aggressive, sadistic component into its opposite... . It will at once be seen that people of this kind can have counter-wish dreams and unpleasurable dreams, which are none the less wish fulfilments since they satisfy their *masochistic* inclinations.[4]

This introduction of masochism is doubly telling. We see how difficult it is to recognize evident manifestations of aggressions as such when these disguise themselves with rational arguments. It seems more "obvious" to unmask a masochistic *defense* against the aggression than [to unmask the aggression] itself. In the smallest of spaces we find, at the very first mention of "masochistic inclinations," the entire conflict that was to characterize Freud's efforts on this topic later.

The "masochistic component" arose as a defense against aggression and sadism—arose in an indeed equivocal sense: genetically in the psychical development [and] in terms of the history of ideas through the defense against insight into the ubiquity of sadism. At the time of *The Interpretation of Dreams*, Freud may not yet have attributed any profound significance to the pleasure taken in cruelty, but there can be no doubt that he observed it. The patient's pleasure in proving the professor wrong, Freud's own pleasure in teasing his analysands, to be sure, are harmless derivatives of aggression; yet defiance and mockery unmistakably are pulsional derivates that indeed, under different conditions, have the potential psychically to destroy someone. Freud plays down his suspicion with a humorous turn of phrase and thereby turns to the *masochistic* phenomena with all the more focus.

[The fact] that Freud took little interest in masochistic sexuality as well, that the topic instead remained for him a problem of theory, once again strengthens the assumption that the early concept of masochism is a displacement substitute for knowledge of sadistic drives. Aggression theory would be articulated *expressis verbis* only twenty years later. Another four years later, in 1924, Freud developed theses that treated masochism and sadism on the same level; yet despite insight into the sovereignty of the aggression drive, he could never resolve to leave *genuinely masochistic strivings* out of consideration.

As the first example of masochism, we encounter the dream of "a young man who in his earlier years had greatly tormented his elder brother, to whom he had a homosexual attachment." After the psychoanalytic cure has prompted "a fundamental change" in his character, he dreams "the following dream, which was in three pieces: I. His elder brother was chaffing [*"sekkiert"*] him. II. Two grown men were caressing each other with a homosexual purpose. III. His brother had sold the business of which he himself had looked forward to becoming the director." Freud reports that the young man "awoke ... with the most distressing feelings," yet "nevertheless it was a masochistic wishful dream, and might be translated thus: 'It would serve me right if my brother were to confront me with this sale as a punishment for all the torments he had to put up with from me.'"[5] The example illustrates Freud's early conception of a masochistic sexual *component* that would result from the defense against the aggressive one. The expectation of punishment is seen as the driving force and the motivation of the reversal into the opposite. Masochistic inclinations would thus arise secondarily, based on originary sadistic wishes.

Now, how are we to understand this "reversal into its opposite"? Does it concern the pulsional object or the pulsional aim? Are aggressive pulsional aims being replaced by masochistic ones or does the very quality of the drive change? As we can see, after the "fundamental change" in character, neither the forbidden love object, the brother, nor the forbidden sexual aim of sadistically "chaffing" him are given up but rather are held on to unchanged in the dream-thought. The only turn we can discover is the one from activity to passivity. That, however, does not contain the sexual component but the *kind of satisfaction* being phantasized. Feelings of guilt cause the new wish fulfillment to be passed for a punishment ("it would serve me right …").

We would hardly know anything about this dream if the precision of the dream labor had worked. The "most distressing feelings," however, betray the not entirely successful defense against a *current* wish impulse. The distress must refer to the originary phantasy that between him and his brother there is a business in which they both caress *and* chafe each other. *Now*, however, the "brother" undoubtedly is Freud, the "business" is the analysis. In the old wish as in the new, the libidinous pulsional aim remains untouched. We cannot state exactly what in the manifest dream gives the impression of masochism. I think it is the turn to passivity in holding on to the aggressive pulsional aims—and the "most distressing feelings" that can hardly disavow their erotic source.

Based on these first elaborations, masochism is to be conceived as a reversal into the opposite that *changes the pulsional aim* in a particular way.

In the sixth chapter of *The Interpretation of Dreams*, Freud brings up "masochistic impulses in the mind":

> As a young doctor I worked for a long time at the Chemical Institute without ever becoming proficient in the skills which that science demands; and for that reason in my waking life I have never liked thinking of this barren and indeed humiliating episode in my apprenticeship. On the other hand I have a regularly recurring dream of working in the laboratory, of carrying out analyses and of having various experiences there. These dreams are disagreeable in the same way as examination dreams and they are never very distinct. While I was interpreting one of them, my attention was eventually attracted by the word *"analysis,"* which gave me a key to their understanding. Since those days I have become an "analyst," and I now carry out analyses which are very highly spoken of, though it is true that they are *"psycho*-analyses." It was now clear to me: if I have grown proud of carrying out analyses of that kind in my day time life and feel inclined to boast to myself of how successful I have become, my dreams remind me during the night of those other, unsuccessful analyses of which I have no reason to feel proud. They are the punishment dreams of a *parvenu*, like the dreams of the journeyman tailor who had grown into a famous author. But how does it become possible for a dream, in the conflict between a *parvenu*'s pride and his self-criticism, to side with the latter, and choose as its content a sensible warning instead of an unlawful wish fulfilment? As I have already said, the answer to this question raises difficulties. We may conclude that the foundation of the dream was formed in the first instance by an exaggeratedly ambitious phantasy, but that humiliating thoughts that poured cold water on the phantasy found their way into the dream instead. It may be remembered that there are masochistic impulses in the mind,

which may be responsible for a reversal such as this. I should have no objection to this class of dreams being distinguished from "wish fulfilment dreams" under the name of "punishment dreams." I should not regard this as implying any qualification of the theory of dreams which I have hitherto put forward; it would be no more than a linguistic expedient for meeting the difficulties of those who find it strange that opposites should converge.[6]

We know that [Freud] later acknowledges this kind of punishment dreams (when, for example, not boisterous ambitious phantasies but shamings make it into the manifest content) to mark the success of the superego motivation. In keeping with Freud's second conception, meanwhile, masochistic tendencies replace the dream censorship or self-criticism. They would be the *motivating force of an affect-defense* and would also characterize the result of this defense. Forbidden pleasurable phantasies would be reversed *through* masochism into phantasies tormenting the self.

In *Three Essays on the Theory of Sexuality* (1905), Freud presents masochism as a *perversion*. In so doing, he advocates a conception we are already familiar with from *The Interpretation of Dreams*. Masochistic tendencies, he says, never occur genuinely, but rather "invariably arise from a transformation of sadism." What is new, however, is the qualification

> that masochism is nothing more than an extension of sadism turned round upon the subject's own self, which thus, to begin with, takes the place of the sexual object. ...
>
> The history of human civilization shows beyond any doubt that there is an intimate connection between cruelty and the sexual instinct; but nothing has been done towards explaining the connection, apart from laying emphasis on the aggressive factor in the libido... .
>
> But the most remarkable feature of this perversion is that its active and passive forms are habitually found to occur together in the same individual. A person who feels pleasure in producing pain in someone else in a sexual relationship is also capable of enjoying as pleasure any pain which he may himself derive from sexual relations. A sadist is always at the same time a masochist, although the active or the passive aspect of the perversion may be the more strongly developed in him and may represent his predominant sexual activity.[7]

While the sexual aim, which can be satisfied "in two forms,"[8] an active and a passive form, remains unchanged here, masochism is to be sought in the turn against one's own person. Masochism would once more be a *defense against the drives, but a defense that concerns not the pulsional aim but the pulsional object*. (Recall that in the first example, we saw the characteristic feature to be the turn from activity to passivity, especially when the homosexual pulsional object, the "brother," was *maintained*.)

The thesis continues to be that masochism is a derivative and defense substitute of sadism, that is, it is genetically and economically subordinate to sadism. In the years 1907 to about 1910, it undergoes a variation that Freud, however, abandons again later. In [his] interpretation of Jensen's *Gradiva*, aggressive and masochistic pulsional aims are exchangeable. Sadism can be replaced by passive, masochistic wishes. Inversely, however, sadism can appear as the counterpart of masochism that can become conscious.[9] In the fourth of the *Lectures on Psycho-Analysis*, we find a formulation that juxtaposes masochism and sadism as *equals*, as a pair of opposite pulsional components

> Alongside these and other auto-erotic activities, we find in children at a very early age manifestations of those instinctual components of sexual pleasure (or, as we like to say, of libido) which presuppose the taking of an extraneous person as an object. These instincts occur in pairs of opposites, active and passive. I may mention as the most important representatives of this group the desire to cause pain (sadism) with its passive counterpart (masochism).[10]

After all these rather incidental indications, Freud in *Drives and Their Vicissitudes* (1915) for the first time decides to undertake a "more thorough investigation" of the "pair of opposites" sadism–masochism. As earlier in *The Interpretation of Dreams*, sadism is the originary pulsional aim, masochism is derivative, secondary. Freud puts it unambiguously: "Whether there is, besides this, a more direct masochistic satisfaction is highly doubtful. A primary masochism, not derived from sadism ... seems not to be met with."[11] Masochism now appears as a *particular pulsional vicissitude of aggression*. Like any pulsional vicissitude, it is a consequence of defense, the result of a compromise between drive and reality. The transformation of sadism into masochism is said to have three stages: the originary object of sadistic wishes is given up and replaced by one's own person. With the turn against the own person, the active pulsional aim transforms into a passive one. This, however, would only turn sadism into self-torment and self-punishment. Only when a new object can be cathected as a projection substitute for the former sadistic ego has masochism emerged from sadism.

The substitute object for the sadistic ego can of course also be the former pulsional object. Such was the case in the example cited from the *Interpretation of Dreams*: "It would serve *me* right if my *brother* were to confront *me* ... as a punishment." We see, Freud's implicit thesis is one that diverges from his prior conception. Masochism is not a pulsional component but a particular *form of object relation* that is the *result of the sadistic pulsional vicissitude*. Characteristically, the object changes while the sadistic pulsional aim remains unchanged. The originary object is given up, the sadistic pulsional wish [is] projected and identificatorily satisfied. The libidinous share of the pulsional wish, we must suppose, remains unchanged and blends with the passive pulsional components. The latter assume the place of the projected pulsional wishes. In any case, we note one nuance of the defensive labor: sadistic and libidinous wishes can be subject to different vicissitudes, connect with different modalities of satisfaction, take different objects as their aim—and yet represent the same wishful phantasy.

In this work, Freud for the first time attempts a diagnostic delineation. Obsessional neurosis and masochism share a starting point, sadism against others. In obsessional neurosis, sadism is being directed against one's own person, yet without the passive wishes having to look for a new object. When a projective identification comes in to supplement the obsessional neurotic pulsional defense, masochistic symptoms arise. In 1915, Freud still has no doubt that genetically, active pulsional aims are to be situated earlier than passive ones: masochistic tendencies occur only in "someone who was originally sadistic."[12]

Freud explains the ambivalence of the drive, the side-by-side of different developmental stages of the same drive, of active and passive pulsional components, as follows

> With regard to both the instincts which we have just taken as examples, it should be remarked that their transformation by a reversal from activity to passivity and by a turning round upon the subject never in fact involves the whole quota of the instinctual impulse. The earlier active direction of the instinct persists to some degree side by side with its later passive direction, even when the process of its transformation has been very extensive.[13]

The development of the drive is to be conceived of in waves, somewhat like successive eruptions of lava

> We can then perhaps picture the first, original eruption of the instinct as proceeding in an unchanged form and undergoing no development at all. The next wave would be modified from the outset-being turned, for instance, from active to passive-and would then, with this new characteristic, be added to the earlier wave, and so on.[14]

Yet at this point, theoretical difficulties appear. What is being cited here (in the theory of drives) to support the thesis of an originary sadism comes to contradict another (genetic) concept, that of narcissism.[15]

If the originary pulsional aim is sadistic and active, then consequently the originary pulsional object in the first autoerotic phase of development must be the individual itself. At least with regard to the pulsional object, masochism would be older. The transformation of sadism into masochism would be a *return* to the narcissist object. That would mean "that the instinctual vicissitudes which consist in the instinct's being turned round upon the subject's own ego and undergoing reversal from activity to passivity are dependent on the narcissistic organization of the ego and bear the stamp of that phase."[16] Freud uses the auxiliary construction of a "preliminary narcissistic stage of sadism." [17] It remains unclear, however, what we have to imagine by this. Is this a sadism directed against the narcissist self?

Recall that in *Three Essays on the Theory of Sexuality*, masochism was described as "an extension of sadism turned round upon the subject's own self,"[18] and that [in *Drives and their Vicissitudes*, 1915] the close connection with the libido was never in doubt: "of course, it is not the pain itself which is enjoyed, but the accompanying sexual excitation."[19] At this point at the latest, it is obvious that the problem of masochism is a complex one, that its relationship with sadism is not as simple as it seemed at first.

Freud of course suspected as much ten years earlier, writing in the *Three Essays*: "Clinical analysis of extreme cases of masochistic perversion show that a great number of factors … have combined."[20] Although even in the *Lectures* (1917), he still presents masochism without further ado as the counterpart of sadism and does not enter into the topic any further,[21] we may assume that at that time, the insight imposed itself on him that the problem of masochism was not going to be solved by any theoretical concepts then available. When the topic is mentioned in Freud's writings of the following seven years until the publication of the 1924 monograph, it is always in a clinical context. It seems that Freud, without explicitly mentioning it, wanted to test various new hypotheses.

The young wolf man's "masochistic purposes"[22] express themselves in screaming fits. The father is to be seduced into assuaging the sense of guilt with a beating and satisfying the passive sexual wishes at the same time. Here a connection between masochism and homosexuality is suspected for the first time. The boy's masochism develops as a consequence of the "suppression of the beginnings of genital activity," after being rejected by the Nanya. Simultaneous with the submissiveness, violent strivings appear in him. In his sadistic phantasies, he is identified with the father while his masochistic tendencies want to make him the sexual object of the father. He is denied the advance toward the genital organization since that would mean "transform[ing] his masochism towards his father into a feminine attitude towards him—into homosexuality." This result, however, is opposed by castration anxiety. That is why his sexual excitation, aimed at the father, is split into a repressed homosexual and a dominant masochistic inclination. The two, though, are identical insofar as they derive from the same source and pursue the same goal. A masochistic attitude, we now understand, is a *substitute*, capable of becoming conscious but *regressive*, for homosexual pulsional wishes. Yet it owes its existence to castration anxiety, not to sadism. For the first time, Freud here speaks of a "masochistic ideal." In the identification with a suffering figure (Christ), "sublimation" succeeds, that is, a desexualization, compelled by the defense, of masochistic tendencies.[23]

The study "A Child is Being Beaten," published in 1919, situates masochism temporally in the psychosexual development.[24] Masochism is being located genetically at the boundary between pregenital and genital organization, in the phallic-exhibitionist phase. In the analysis of the wolf man's infantile neurosis, the connection between sadism and masochism was mentioned only in passing. Now, Freud attaches great importance to *genuine sadistic pulsional aims* that are transformed into masochistic ones exclusively with the help of the sense of guilt. Masochism can develop above all in "children in whom the sadistic component was able for constitutional reasons to develop prematurely and in isolation." That is why, when the genital organization is affected by repression, the path toward a regression to anal-sadistic modalities is made particularly easy. The idea of "being beaten is now a convergence of the sense of guilt and sexual love. It is not only the punishment for the forbidden genital relation, but also the regressive substitute for that relation."[25]

Freud attempts a comprehensive hypothesis that integrates genetic, structural, and economic reflections. Masochism is a conversion of sadism; the defense takes place coming from the superego under pressure from the sense of guilt. It occurs in children who for constitutional reasons experience a premature and isolated emphasis on the sadistic component in their sexual lives. Fully formed masochism is the regression product of genital incestuous strivings and draws its energy from precisely this libidinous source. Simultaneously, it satisfies the sense of guilt's need for punishment, which had set the regression into motion. While previously Freud spoke of masochism or masochistic strivings, now the concept of "masochistic phantasies" appears. On their basis, "an elaborate superstructure of day-dreams, which was of great significance for the life of the person concerned," develops.[26] Masochistic phantasies serve for masturbation or, on the contrary, bind the sexual excitement and make relinquishing masturbatory acts possible. The idea of masochistic phantasies already appeared in *From the History of an Infantile Neurosis*, albeit as a masochism that "found expression in phantasies."[27] The difference between the two articulations, but also the novelty of the idea of masochistic phantasies, is not fully evident at first sight, yet it is of broad significance for understanding Freud's subsequent reflections.

While earlier, masochism meant *the modality of pulsional wish, a pulsional aim changed by the repression* or by another defensive process (which of course expresses itself in phantasy activity as well), we are now being confronted with a completely different implicit idea. To the extent that they build on a repression and usually remain unconscious, phantasies that acquire significance for the lives of those concerned cannot be anything but *neurotic symptoms*. They are expressions as well as attempts at solving a hidden neurotic conflict. They bind anxiety and are accompanied by a restriction of the ego. This, finally, paves the way toward what will later be called "moral masochism."

The problem of masochism now rests for five years. Freud turns to his great works, *Beyond the Pleasure Principle* and *The Ego and the Id*. When the monograph *The Economic Problem of Masochism*—which is entirely under the sway of the new insights concerning the death drive and the theory of interstructural conflicts—comes out in 1924, the problem of masochism becomes a criterion for the theory as a whole. Masochism and the action of the pleasure principle, it seems, exclude each other. "[I]f mental processes are governed by the pleasure principle in such a way that their first aim is the avoidance of unpleasure and the obtaining of pleasure, masochism is incomprehensible." Yet "if pain and unpleasure can be not simply warnings but actually aims," then the pleasure principle seems to be abolished. [28]

At first, the contradiction cannot be resolved. The entire theoretical construct anchored in the idea of the pleasure principle threatens to be undermined by a clinical observation. One should think that Freud, confident in his theory thanks to decades of practice, would doubt the phenomena and his observation, that he would lay out the manifestations of masochism more broadly and that—in keeping with the psychoanalytic tradition—by examining the nuances, he would obtain, beyond the obvious contradiction, deeper insights into the phenomena and corrections for the theory. We can only surmise why he chose another path. A closer engagement with the topic would only have brought to the light of day once again what he had known for a long time, what for years he had also articulated theoretically in definitive terms, what nonetheless he did not want to believe in—the ubiquity of the aggression drives. It seems as if Freud here, in a niche of analytic theory, as it were, sought a way out in order not to have to recognize the full extent of human sadism. Would he have thought differently had he known Auschwitz and Hiroshima? The attempt at postulating a third, genuine pulsional force beside sadism and sexual libido, masochism, looks like an attempt at salvaging the honor of humanity, which cannot after all be exclusively destined to pursue a pulsional quest for pleasure. I see Freud's next theoretical step, the articulation of the death drive hypothesis, to be grounded in this inclination toward an implicit rehabilitation of psychical life. Since 1920, it has been beyond doubt that the death drive is an indispensable foundation of psychoanalytic reflections. For a while, however, the Nirvana principle that belonged to the death drive was "unhesitatingly" identified with the pleasure/unpleasure principle, a conception no longer tenable in 1924.

> However this may be, we must perceive that the Nirvana principle, belonging as it does to the death instinct, has undergone a modification in living organisms through which it has become the pleasure principle; and we shall henceforward avoid regarding the two principles as one.

The clarification follows:

> The *Nirvana* principle expresses the trend of the death instinct; the *pleasure* principle represents the demands of the libido; and the modification of the latter principle, the *reality* principle, represents the influence of the external world.[29]

None of the three principles can be excluded by another. In case of conflict, however, the principles can reciprocally change, diminish, or temporally postpone each other quantitatively and qualitatively. This provides the metapsychological justification for why the pleasure principle, while it can never be abolished, must, for example, put up with a temporary postponement. That would manifest in an increase in the unpleasure tension.

In *Beyond the Pleasure Principle*, the pleasure principle was still being subordinated to the Nirvana principle, sometimes also identified with it. Reflection on the problem of masochism had to make it obvious for Freud "that there are pleasurable tensions and unpleasurable relaxations of tension."[30] The affects pleasure and unpleasure cannot refer to the increase or decrease of a quantity, the tension due to stimulus, but must be characterized by a particular *quality* of the tension. If the supposition is that the Nirvana principle, in the service of the death drive, strives for diminishing and finally using up the energy quantities of the psychical system, then the pleasure principle is concerned with stating the conditions under which a stimulus tension qualitatively becomes pleasure. In other words, we must wonder in what way "the libido, … alongside of the death instinct, seize[s] upon a share in the regulation of the processes of life."[31] The solution of this task, however, presupposes the concept of a *possible conflict between the psychical regulatory principles*. Neither the clinical material, that is, neither the manifestations of masochism nor the theoretical problem of the contradiction between masochism and pleasure principle could be grasped correctly as long as the abstract principles' capacity for conflict was not presupposed. Through the mediation of the investigation of masochism, the thesis of the death drive and the idea of an innerpsychical conflict (between ego, id, and superego) have been joined by the idea of an interference of the three psychical principles.[32]

The phenomena of masochism seemed to throw one of the cornerstones of analytic theory, namely, the pleasure principle, into question. The newly gained insight that the psychical principle (and not only the forces on the level of pulsional wish versus defense) are capable of conflicting with each other has abolished the contradiction between quest for pleasure and masochism. The masochistic expressions henceforth count as evidence of the Nirvana principle and the death drive to which the striving for pleasure must at times subordinate itself. Freud's subsequent efforts aimed at supporting these theses via clinical observation. Masochism appears to observation in three different forms: "as a condition imposed on sexual excitation, as an expression of the feminine nature, and as a norm of behaviour."[33]

For Freud, "feminine masochism" is a diagnostic category to designate masochistic phantasies or perverse activities of *men*. They thereby place themselves "in a characteristically female situation; they signify, that is, being castrated, or copulated with, or giving birth to a baby."[34] The manifest content expresses, among other things, a sense of guilt related to forbidden infantile masturbation. As we will see later, Freud does not call "feminine" the syndrome that we today would more likely entitle "feminine masochism," a submissive, seemingly self-sacrificing attitude, but considers it a variety of moral masochism.

A first explanation that offers itself for erogenous masochism takes recourse to ideas from the *Three Essays on the Theory of Sexuality*, where we read:

> Indeed, as Freud points out, 'it may well be that nothing of considerable importance can occur in the organism without contributing some component to the excitation of the sexual instinct.' In accordance with this, the excitation of pain and unpleasure would be bound to have the same result, too.[35]

This would be the physiological basis on which erogenous masochism would be built as a superstructure. Freud later rejects the hypothesis as inadequate because "it throws no light on the regular and close connections of masochism with its counterpart in instinctual life, sadism."[36]

The *relationship* between sadism and masochism seemed so obvious and self-evident to Freud that it required no further discussion. It also formed the core of his earliest thesis in *The Interpretation of Dreams* that masochism is the repression product of sadism. Although now, in 1924, he comes to hold the opposite view, that masochism is more originary, not derived from sadism, he nonetheless has not abandoned the notion of "regular and close connections" between sadism and masochism.

The foundation of the ideas that follow is the death drive theory. For Freud, what is happening in masochism is incomprehensible without the influence of the death drive. The libido encounters the death drive, which dominates *ab ovo*; its task is to render [the death drive] harmless and use its energy for its own purposes. Both forces, libido and death drive, blend and strive, after the first phase of development, the autoerotic or primary-narcissistic phase, toward the pulsional objects. The idea relevant in our context is that the *libido* channels large parts of destructive energy off to the outside with the help of the muscular system. The destruction drive directed at the objects is always already infiltrated by libido. A share of the drive enters directly into the service of the sexual function—that, [for Freud,] is "sadism" properly so called. [He continues:]

> Another portion does not share in this transposition outwards; it remains inside the organism and, with the help of the accompanying sexual excitation described above, becomes libidinally bound there. It is in this portion that we have to recognize the original, erotogenic masochism.[37]

Masochism subsequently is assigned the status of a *partial drive*; it "accompanies the libido through all its developmental phases and derives from them its changing psychical coatings."[38] Masochism is thus an autonomous drive—a genetic sediment from that developmental phase in which the alloying of death drive and libido was taking place. It is an unconverted share of the death drive acting intrastructurally that, like the originary destructive pulsional forces (although [it is] caught under the dominion of the libido), knows only its own organism as its aim and object. That is the definitive articulation of 1924.

The consequences of these theses are not immediately evident. For if masochism is a part of the death drive not channeled to the outside, then we must suppose masochism to be identical with the death drive working inside the organism, the "originary sadism." On the level of the content, this interpretation is not objectionable; it does, however, endow masochism with a psychological significance Freud is unwilling to grant it. Although the theory of the death drive would have suggested at least the equivalence of sadism and masochism (in the sense, for instance, of a shared source from which the two pulsional strands would develop differently), sadism remains primary and masochism can't seem to shed its connotation as a symptom. [Masochism] remains something effected, something assembled instead of an autonomous driving force.

We may surmise with more certainty that the discrepancy between theoretical knowledge and clinical understanding on this topic is not a coincidence. The difficulties, however, cannot simply be attributed to the inadequacies of psychoanalysis; what becomes visible here, rather, is one of the synapses where the social intervenes in the scientific knowledge process. Only the ideological current then dominant can have had an interest in driving metapsychology and neurosis theory apart on the question of masochism that also intended to disavow pleasurable aggressiveness.[39] Maintaining the general illusion contributed to forming the false consciousness that ultimately declared the consequences of the aggression of the ones to be the aim of the "masochistic" submission of the others.

The final chapter of Freud's masochism book is devoted to a topic that in the years that followed was to become particularly significant for the concept of the superego and the theory of technique. In *The Ego and the Id*, he assumed a "'moral' factor, a sense of guilt, which is finding its satisfaction in the illness" to be the cause of the so-called negative therapeutic reaction.[40] [The latter] reaction is a curious process in the transference relationship. It appears as a need to hold on to suffering and willfully to evade convalescence. What up to now was visible as a *neurotic symptom* now makes its way into the current transference to the analyst and "constitutes one of the most serious *resistances* and the greatest danger to the success of our medical or educative aims" of the therapy.[41]

In *moral masochism*, the "ultramorality," a "heightened sadism of the superego," is opposed by the ego's need for punishment, which [Freud calls] "the ego's own masochism."[42] The ego tries to obtain from the superego, from the objects, or from the powers of fate a punishment that would satisfy its "masochistic trend." The ego submits to the sadistic superego like a masochistic person to their love object. Freud notes on the short-circuiting conclusion according to which moral masochism is nothing but erogenous masochism that moral masochism is usually *unconscious*. Conscience and morality arise from the desexualization of oedipal wishes: "through moral masochism morality becomes sexualized once more ... and the way is opened for a regression from morality to the Oedipus complex."[43]

It is not entirely clear whether a part of the oedipal wish that remained virulent makes use of masochistic tendencies or whether masochistic wishes follow regressive oedipal tracks. This secret connection, however, explains why the sadism of the superego is mostly loud and conscious but moral masochism remains larval. Repression would [thus] apply not so much to the masochism as rather to the forbidden *oedipal wishes* reinvigorated via this detour.

A supplementary explanation comes from an entirely different, wholly unexpected side. What is now being called secondary masochism is the turning back of sadism onto one's own person. It is not identical with genuine masochism but once more a pulsional vicissitude of aggression. It is equally a consequence of cultural pulsional suppression, which "holds back a large part of the subject's destructive instinctual components from being exercised in life." This draws our attention. Can we find something to make our problem easier here?

> We may suppose that this portion of the destructive instinct which has retreated appears in the ego as an intensification of masochism. The phenomena of conscience, however, lead us to infer that the destructiveness which returns from the external world is also taken up by the super-ego, without any such transformation, and increases its sadism against the ego. The sadism of the super-ego and the masochism of the ego supplement each other and unite to produce the same effects. It is only in this way, I think, that we can understand how the suppression of an instinct can—frequently or quite generally—result in a sense of guilt and how a person's conscience becomes more severe and more sensitive the more he refrains from aggression against others. One might expect that if a man knows that he is in the habit of avoiding the commission of acts of aggression that are undesirable from a cultural standpoint he will for that reason have a good conscience and will watch over his ego less suspiciously. The situation is usually presented as though ethical requirements were the primary thing and the renunciation of instinct followed from them. This leaves the origin of the ethical sense unexplained. Actually, it seems to be the other way about. The first instinctual renunciation is enforced by external powers, and it is only this which creates the ethical sense, which expresses itself in conscience and demands a further renunciation of instinct.
>
> Thus moral masochism becomes a classical piece of evidence for the existence of fusion of instinct. Its danger lies in the fact that it originates from the death instinct and corresponds to the part of that instinct

which has escaped being turned outwards as an instinct of destruction. But since, on the other hand, it has the significance of an erotic component, even the subject's destruction of himself cannot take place without libidinal satisfaction.[44]

These words conclude Freud's book—and leave us at a loss.[45] It is up to us to note how much Freud's *premises* and ours differ. We recognize the "cultural suppression of the drives" of sadism he is talking about first in today's education and family morality. We can no longer follow him, by contrast, when Freud says that a good conscience, a milder censoring of the ego, is the reward for "avoiding the commission of acts of aggression that are undesirable from a cultural standpoint." For us, *this* "cultural" has split into two strands, an oedipal individual [culture] and an aggressive-triumphal social culture. The sadism the former prohibits, the latter demands. A socially secured good conscience can only be had by following the particular aggressiveness command of the current ideology. Where the oedipal conscience still decides, in adolescence for instance, where it rejects common cruelties in the sexual, the profession, at work, in looking for a job, and so on, it is soon set straight by the assimilating ego (where censorship is immediately effective).

For Freud, at the end of the book, the new conception is certain. Masochism is a direct derivative of the death drive to which it also owes its virulence. It belongs to that share of the death drive that in the blending with the libido did not participate in the death drive's being turned toward the outside world. Although one might thus speak of an identity of death drive and masochism, that would not quite be correct because the intrastructurally effective part of the death drive associated with libido and masochism thus finds satisfaction in libidinous aims and together with libidinous aims. The pulsional object of masochism, of course, remains that of the death drive: the self.

Masochistic and libidinous aims interpenetrate such that it cannot be decided whether the libido makes use of masochistic pulsional energies or whether masochism uses libidinous facilitations for its own aims. Saying that masochism concentrates in the ego as a need for punishment, what is called *moral masochism*, does not at all mean what common sense might suggest, a particularly sensitive morality, but on the contrary a regressive invigoration of the Oedipus complex, a renewed *sexualization of morality*. The masochistic wishful phantasies do not demand suffering and punishment for moral reasons but because they represent prohibited, once pleasurable and now repressed pulsional wishes from the sphere of the Oedipus complex. In the course of the development of psychoanalytic theory, Freud moved from his original conception of masochism as the product of a transformation of sadism to the opposite notion [of] masochism as the genuine, first pulsional force. Identical with the death drive working inside the organism, it alloys in the psychical with the libido. What is conceived of as sadism now is that part of the destruction drive stemming from the originary that is channeled toward

124 *Voluntary Servitude. Masochism and Morality*

the outside. In one of his last writings, *Analysis Terminable and Interminable*, a reconsideration of masochism leads Freud to remark that

> we shall no longer be able to adhere to the belief that mental events are exclusively governed by the desire for pleasure. These phenomena are unmistakable indications of the present of a power in mental life which we call the instinct of aggression or of destruction according to its aims, and which we trace back to the original death instinct of living matter.[46]

This idea is the starting point of the reflections that follow. I ask whether aggression drive and destruction drive can really stand in for another without further ado, whether the thesis that the aggression drive contradicts the psychical's striving for pleasure stands up to renewed scrutiny, whether not even the power of the death drive might be nothing but the power of, precisely, a *pleasurable pulsional satisfaction*. I also take up the explanation that moral masochism "becomes a classical piece of evidence for the existence of fusion of drives."[47] After everything we have said so far, *we* can claim it only as a witness for the opposing party, for split-up pulsional strivings: sexuality here, aggression there. Masochism—this is the thesis I start from—is so scheming because its symptoms seek to bridge the constantly [yet] imperceptibly growing gap between sexual satisfaction and aggressive strivings. The "opposing party" might then turn out to be the one that, obeying a new reality, had to change its position; rather than bear witness to the fusion of drives, it is an expression of the fragmentation of drives. It would be nothing extraordinary, after all, for a neurotic symptom to remind us of what has slipped from our consciousness.

Notes

1. [The phrase is, in fact, the header on page 571 of GW II/III, and thus probably not Freud's.—Trans.]
2. Freud 1900, SE 5, 565–66.
3. Freud 1900, SSE 4, 157–58.
4. Freud 1900, SE 4, 159, Le Soldat's emphasis.
5. Freud 1900, SE 5, 159.
6. Freud 1900, SE 5, 475–76.
7. Freud 1905a, 158–59.
8. [Freud 1905a, 157.]
9. Freud 1907, 93.
10. Freud 1910a, 44.
11. Freud 1915a, 127–28.
12. [Freud 1915a, 129.]
13. Freud 1915a, 130. In a vivid image, this was later referred to as the "telescope principle." [It is not clear whom Le Soldat has in mind here. The image of the telescope is used, however, by W. H. Gillespie (1971, 159).]
14. Freud 1915a, 131.
15. The theory of narcissism, however, is an indispensable part of the theory of the drives itself.

16 Freud 1915a, 132.
17 [Freud 1915a, 132.]
18 Freud 1905a, 158.
19 Freud 1915a, 129.
20 Freud 1905a, 158.
21 "Next come the sadists, puzzling people whose tender endeavours have no other aim than to cause pain and torment to their object, ranging from humiliation to severe physical injuries; and, as though to counterbalance them, their counterparts, the masochists, whose only pleasure it is to suffer humiliations and torments of every kind from their loved object either symbolically or in reality" (Freud 1916–1917, SE 16, 306).
22 See Freud 1918, 28 [modified].
23 Freud 1918, 63–65.
24 Freud 1919a.
25 Freud 1919a, 189.
26 Freud 1919a, 190.
27 [Freud 1918, 109.]
28 Freud 1924a, 159.
29 Freud 1924a, 160, Freud's emphases.
30 Freud 1924a, 160.
31 [Freud 1924a, 160.]
32 The significance of this insight is not sufficiently appreciated in the literature, and it has gained no influence over [psychoanalytic] technique. In their work on the topic, Heinz Hartmann, David Rapaport, and Kurt R. Eissler hardly mention it. This might be due to the fact that Freud later only rarely makes the distinction between Nirwana *principle* and death *drive* and that the *reality principle* is lost in the dichotomy death drive versus Eros. It may also have played a role that Freud is reluctant to distinguish between the effects and manifestations of a principle and the principle itself. He employs the pleasure principle, for instance, clinically, in economic and structural observations, as well as in phylogenetic articulations. (This prompted Max Schur, for example in Schur 1966, to spell out two different pleasure and unpleasure principles.)
33 Freud 1924a, 161.
34 Freud 1924a, 162.
35 Freud 1924a, 163; see also Freud 1905a, 158–59 and 203–4.
36 Freud 1924a, 163.
37 Freud 1924a, 163–64.
38 Freud 1924a, 164–65.
39 Recall that in the interwar years, fascism striving for dominion sensed these connections and did not hesitate to "bundle" pulsional forces that are unconscious for the individual and employ them for its own purposes. Freud was working on the problem of masochism when Hitler's Beer Hall Putsch took place in Munich in 1923, while domestic affairs in Austria in the years 1922–1927 amounted to a latent civil war. The tendency of the times, however, is best seen in developments in Italy, where on May 30, 1924, following the Fascists' election victory, the Socialist deputy Giacomo Matteotti was murdered for his parliament speech about the dominion, the "regime of violence" (Matteotti 1924).
40 Freud 1923b, 49.
41 [Freud 1924a, 166, Le Soldat's emphasis.]
42 [Freud 1924a, 169.]
43 Freud 1924a [169; the passage reads in full: "through moral masochism morality becomes sexualized once more, the Oedipus complex is revived and the way is opened for a regression from morality to the Oedipus complex"].

44 Freud 1924a, 170.
45 Freud later never explicitly discussed masochism [in detail], although his further, partly contradictory remarks suggest that the problem was far from settled for him. When we organize his various remarks from the years after 1924, two directions his ideas are taking become clear above all. On the one hand, and primarily when he addresses clinical problems, Freud sees in masochism a *neurotic* development (in connection with regressive, passive tendencies). On the other hand, in metapsychological reflections, masochism remains a dangerous *originary pulsional force* characterized by its immediate link with the death drive.

Thus a footnote in "Inhibitions, Symptoms and Anxiety" initially bears out the second idea: pulsional anxiety arises when the ego shies back from satisfying a (masochistic) pulsional demand, the destruction drive aimed against one's own person. Yet only two lines further, we read: the "hidden feminine significance" of phobias of heights ... is closely connected with masochism" (1926a, 168n1).

In "Dostoevsky and Parricide," "masochistic" stands for "passive in a feminine way" (1928, 185). The *New Introductory Lectures* tell us what this means metapsychologically: "One might consider characterizing femininity psychologic ally as giving preference to passive aims. This is not, of course, the same thing as passivity; to achieve a passive aim may call for a large amount of activity... . But we must beware in this of underestimating the influence of social customs, which similarly force women into passive situations... . The suppression of women's aggressiveness which is prescribed for them constitutionally and imposed on them socially favours the development of powerful masochistic impulses, which succeed, as we know, in binding erotically the destructive trends which have been diverted inwards. Thus masochism, as people say, is truly feminine. But if, as happens so often, you meet with masochism in men, what is left to you but to say that these men exhibit very plain feminine traits?" (Freud 1933, 115–16).

We now finally understand the puzzling use of "feminine" in this context. In the thirty-third lecture on "Anxiety and Instinctual Life," we learn about Freud's final conception, that masochism is older and more originary than sadism: "It really seems as though it is necessary for us to destroy some other thing or person in order not to destroy ourselves, in order to guard against the impulsion to self-destruction" (Freud 1933, 105).

46 Freud 1937, 243.
47 Freud 1924a, 170.

II
The economy of excitation

1 The Drummer's dream

A patient recounts the following dream to me:

> I get to a huge cathedral. I see you enter it, clad in a black robe, holding a red tambourine in your hands. You [*Sie*] are being chased. I must distract your pursuers, and decide to seduce them [*sie*]. A man comes, I chat him up. It works. But the next one is already coming. You, however, are walking back and forth; I'm thinking, you should hurry, you're in danger, after all. The next one I must seduce is wearing a floppy hat, he's not that easy to get. He pushes me into the cathedral, and that's when I know that they already got you and you are being tortured. I'm being carried up to a gallery and tied to a chair, my eyes are being ripped open with clamps (like in the movie *Clockwork Orange*). I must watch you being tortured. I'm terribly scared, and I'm thinking: If I don't want to, I don't see anything. Then I hear your voice: Hey, you! You've got to try a little harder! Thank God, I'm thinking, you're cynical as always, they haven't broken you. But suddenly they say to me: Fine, it's your turn then! I try to throw myself into the depths, still tied to the chair. I'm thinking, if I'm dying, I want to take some of them down with me, but as I'm falling I know that was a mistake. It is by far not deep enough, I won't die. Arrived at the bottom, I see, as I'm lying on the ground, a long line of men. They rape me, one after the other. It doesn't impress me. But then it's the turn of a really big one, a prize fighter, who grins and says: I will hurt you [*Dir*]! He, too, rapes me, and it really hurts. I'm crying and he says mockingly: *I* finished you [*Sie*] off! But I pick myself up, I say: You're a monkey. Then I'm thinking the worst is over now. I look over to the others still waiting in line: you can't finish me off anyway![1]

The dreamer, I'll call her Stephanie, is a still youthful woman who has been in psychoanalytic treatment for four years. She is a teacher at the municipal *Gymnasium* and spends her free time on an unusual occupation: she wants to become an *acrobat*. The thought of wresting from her body, through exercise, feats that seem impossible has excited her whole phantasy. Every day after class, the intelligent woman with a sense of humor who, despite her conspicuously attractive appearance, lives alone, hurries to her training. There, with dogged diligence, she practices the most difficult figures. She came into analysis because the complete control over her body she had in mind did not succeed after all. Shortly after the beginning of the treatment, the young woman was caught up in a fulminant regression. She gave up all activities, stopped training, and also refused to continue teaching. She fully withdrew from her few friends and her family, locked herself in her room for weeks on end, and succumbed to drugs.[2] She began neglecting her external appearance and lost weight, to become just a bag of bones. Yet she never thought of giving up her analytic cure. On the contrary, even when she was in the most miserable condition, she showed up on time for her sessions; she demanded pity and help from me. The more I made her understand that I was neither willing nor able to "help" her, the more desperate her condition became. She seemed to be very clear about what kind of help she wanted—affection, love, support in her striving for control of her body—but I insisted on continuing to explore the unconscious phantasies. If there was something she so urgently demanded, then it could not lie within what had already been talked about but must have had to do with the hidden wish of an as yet unconscious conflict. In this situation, Stephanie made a suicide attempt that failed. With injuries that were slight but impressive by their terrible appearance she then came to the analytic work.

At first sight, the diagnostic judgment seems to pose no difficulty. The young woman is a masochist. She has assumed the same defiant position toward her analyst as she does elsewhere in her life. She demands help from the analyst with the same doggedness with which she tried to force her body to perform impossible feats. Yet the answer "masochism" sheds no light on either the aim of her longing or the inner conflicts. For it is not unimportant that during the time of years-long crisis, Stephanie could no longer pay the fee for her therapy.[3] Only a few days prior to the dream she had paid off a significant part of her debts. Since I never left any doubt that I expected payment for the sessions sooner or later, the analyst is easily recognized as the "prize fighter" in the dream. On the other hand, "the worst" now really does seem to lie behind her. She has succeeded in escaping a great danger; she did not die in her suicide attempt. One might be inclined to believe the dream to have served a reparation function of the kind that often occurs after accidents. There, the danger is conjured up again and brought to a good end. One might also consider it a reproach to the analyst: *I* would have saved you had you been in danger; you, however, are only cynical and coarse, watching me as I toil away and even asking to be paid for it! All these interpretations have something going for them. A simple psychoanalytic rule, however, says that a dream, a symptom, and every expression of the unconscious cannot be understood without further ado, that is, not without profound interpretational labor. What has been repressed from consciousness for reasons cannot, or can only under very specific conditions, as in jokes, for instance, reappear in consciousness naked, as it were, without having to put up with multiple and varied disguises and redistributions? We may not hope to be able to infer the unconscious (because embarrassing) content already from the manifest dream text, from what pulsional pressure has brought to the light of day.[4]

We have already come to know the significance of hypocritical affects in the first part.[5] We will do well here, too, to remain skeptical toward the obvious emotional movement. The acrobat wants to save me; in so doing, she gets into trouble herself and experiences anxiety, terror, pain, and powerlessness. Her report ends where defiance and contempt boil up. The dreamer awoke at that point and was full of horror and anger, she assures [me]. We know that dreams are wish fulfillment phantasies. Should we see in Stephanie's dream the realization of a genuine masochistic wish fulfillment? According to death drive theory, we would have to pay most attention to her wish to die. Failed in reality, this wish [c]ould remain virulent and would, once it blends with passive sexual impulses, provide a good reason for the dream. We could also claim that the dream celebrates an orgy of revenge and gloating. By paying the fee, she has performed a loathed duty and now, in keeping with talion law,[6] expects the reward for years of suffering. Yet as nothing changes in the attitude of the analyst, she considers herself deceived and settles the scores with her. In the manifest dream text, it is difficult to distinguish between *Sie* [(= you)] and *sie* (= the men) anyway.[7] To her, the analyst seems to be someone conniving with the men; she herself is being used and raped.

Plausible arguments can be cited for both hypotheses. We must be prepared, however, for the dreamer's associations to lead us onto wholly unexpected paths.

And indeed, the young woman's elaborations on her dream are rather astonishing. After years of silence about her sexual habits, she suddenly reveals to me that she has never experienced an orgasm with a man. She likes sleeping with men, [she says,] gets excited as well, but there is no shared climax. She is vaginally insensitive, only her clitoris is excitable, and even that only when she stimulates herself. She considers this to be infantile. But then she takes her last statement back and reveals to me, not without shame but rather reproachfully, that there is, however, another possibility to reach an orgasm. In puberty, she developed a sexual practice but later *dropped* [*fallenlassen*][8] it again. Back then, she had a little cat lick her vulva, alone in her room, later in playing with other children as well. Enouncing the next idea seems to demand even more of an effort from her to overcome shame. For a while, already in analysis, she waged a desperate struggle against masturbation. She worked night and day, did weight and strength training, tried to sleep with men as often as possible only to escape [her] phantasy. [In this phantasy,] she is tied into a masturbation machine, her hands and feet bound. The machine moves a lever stroking across her vulva. The movements of the lever are neither predictable nor controllable. She is completely helpless. The machine is giving her one orgasm after the other. She is writhing and resisting but cannot evade the slowly, then again quickly moving lever. Finally, she is very wet down there, as if she had wet her pants. That is when the machine suddenly stops. She stoops to wipe up the wetness or investigate it, but that movement sets the machine in motion again, and the whole thing starts from the beginning.

Of course, we ask: why this sudden readiness to recount something embarrassing? We are unlikely to be wrong if we see in the report the dreamer's wish to sexually excite and seduce the analyst. Everything she enumerates is to be done to her. The analyst is to replace the torturers, the rapists, the little cat, and the masturbation machine's lever and *genitally satisfy* her. She is willing to let herself be tormented and tortured if only the analyst is willing to see what "comes out" of the masturbation. So strong an inclination toward passivity, meanwhile, makes us even more skeptical.

The multiplication of the pursuers and rapists in the dream, the confession of a series of sexual practices previously shamefully passed over in silence substitute for a still hidden wish that is more obscured than revealed by the provocatively displayed passivity.

We cannot remain in doubt for long about what the patient really wants now: she wants to *rescue me*. In her phantasy, *I* am in danger. The rescue, however, does not succeed; she must watch something terrible and then becomes the victim of violence herself. We know from the analysis of male patients that rescue ideas about a woman usually have the meaning of wanting to have sexual intercourse with the woman. We recognize in this an allusion to oedipal wishes, where "rescuing a woman" had the meaning of taking the mother away from the father, saving her from his sexual advances and—exposing her to one's own [advances]. Rescue phantasies about a man, however (the idea, for instance, of rescuing a friend from danger), regularly turn out to be examples of a danger one is wishing for, reversals of hostile impulses.[9]

For the unconscious, "rescue" is synonymous with killing or with coition and sexual possession.[10] When in consciousness, *one* phantasy (the rescue) must represent two irreconcilable impulses, to love or to kill, that is to be understood as a success of the defense. To obfuscate a prohibited impulse, its aim is labeled as the opposite. With the same intention, one can disguise an egotistic sexual demand by making it pass for altruistic, for being in the interest of the "rescued." The defense is also accommodated by the pulsional energies' inclination to blend with one another; a natural ambivalence of the emotions seems to promote the exchangeability of erotic and aggressive aims. In reality, however, it is a single, namely, a *phallic impulse* that allows for reversing rescue and killing. To children, sexual acts often seem like sadistic attacks.[11] The sadistic coitus theory is a regular part of infantile sexual phantasies. Children imagine that during the parents' sexual intercourse, something terrible is happening; bits and pieces of sense perceptions and phantasies (the "primal scene") seem to confirm to them that the father beats the mother and treats her sadistically. The difference between the sexes is being explained by the child imagining that during coitus, the father castrates the mother; it also projects its own excitations when later it thinks that in bed, the mother takes revenge for the castration, that is, that a fierce struggle is taking place between the parents. Beating and abusing then stand for coition. At the age of four to five years, the demands of the oedipal conflict transform the sadistic fears into phallic impulses; these [impulses] then unite the intention to kill with particular incestuous wishes. Yet we would make it too easy for ourselves in our task of shedding light on the problem of masochism if we simply blamed the striving for suffering on the ambivalence of repressed pulsional wishes.[12] While the ease with which aggressive and erotic aims replace each other in Stephanie's dream—the drumming, the rescue, the torture, and the rape all seem to serve the same intention—cannot be overlooked, the suggestion that she wants simultaneously to rescue and to kill *me* does not clarify her burning wish.

Notes

1 I have modified, by elisions and abridgments, the biographical data and [the narrative of] the course of the analysis of the three patients discussed in what follows. Relinquishing nuances "very definitely diminishes" (Freud 1900, SE 4, xxiv) the material presented, [but] the patients' right to the analyst's discretion permits no alternative. I must confess, though, that this restriction posed no difficulty for me. Masochism aroused my curiosity not so much because of the secret sexual phantasies, which occur in other neurotic conditions as well; my scientific curiosity, rather, was awoken by the intriguing relationships between pleasure principle and death drive, by the seeming reversal of all values that usually apply to the psychical. The masochistic conflicts demand a comprehension that goes beyond restoring repressed memories.
2 These drugs were barbiturates or amphetamine-type medications; alcohol or intoxicants were out of the question for her.
3 Unlike in Germany, psychoanalyses in Switzerland are not covered by public health insurance.
4 "Two separate functions may be distinguished in mental activity during the construction of a dream: the production of the dream-thoughts, and their transformation into the [manifest] content of the dream" (Freud 1900, SE 5, 506, Le Soldat's interpolation). The *dream work* changes the latent dream thought into manifest content; in doing so, it makes use of the mechanisms of condensation, displacement, the consideration of presentability, and a secondary, rational revision. The *work of dream interpretation* must reverse this process. It does not suffice, however, to guess what has been defended against. The course of dream formation, the form and the contents of the defense are, like the conditions of a dream's being reported, essential supports of the interpretation.
5 See Chapter I.8 above [#60–61].
6 On talion law in the unconscious, see Freud 1910c, 216–17.
7 [In German, the formal second person singular pronoun and the third person plural pronoun are homonyms and take the same verb declensions. In addition, *sie* is the third person singular feminine pronoun.—Trans.]
8 The allusion to "letting herself fall" [*sich fallenlassen*] in the dream is unmistakable. In reality, she *dropped* a sexual habit; in the dream, it is her who is "dropping." Flying, falling, swimming, and so on, are common means of representing sexual pleasure. The case of rhythmic movements, like the expected abolition of gravity in flying (=orgasm), poses no difficulties of interpretation. I cannot agree with the opinion, however, that ascribes dreams of falling particularly to women and points to the pleasure expected of *afterward* being "picked up and petted"

(see Freud 1900, SE 5, 395). I see in the symbolism of falling an excellent example of the prevalence of aggressive drives in sexuality. The defense against guilt (I'm not doing it, it's being done to me) allows for complete abandonment to a linear, irreversible movement. The result of the falling, be it pain or humiliation, does not serve to justify the association (like someone who has fallen, I want to be taken care of; because I have fallen, I am to be helped) but—thanks to the reversal—once more to defend against the reproach of having been aggressive (I haven't hurt anyone, rather, I've been hurt). The indication of the rhythm of the excitation must remain unelucidated here; see, however, part III below. [The passages are listed in the index entry "rhythm."]

9   See Freud 1910b, 172–73; Abraham (1922) 2018.
10 To avoid a banality some authors adhere to when they seek to blend love and death, we had better not combine pulsional qualities, pulsional aims, and the ambivalence of the pulsional wishes in a *mixtum compositum*. The association of love and death creates a clever double illusion. If love has something to do with death, then it cannot be all that pulsional and guilt-ridden; if on the other hand death is linked with sexuality, one deprives the end of some of its terror and projects pleasure and transience where the opposite is imminent.
11 Infantile sexual theories that phantasize a sadistic coitus, Freud says, are "the expression of one of the innate components of the sexual instinct, any of which may be strongly marked to a greater or lesser degree in each particular child" (Freud 1908b, 221).
12 See, for example, Stekel (1925) 1968 and Bataille (1963) 2012.

2 A female rescue phantasy

In a short essay, Karl Abraham reports the dream of a nine-year-old girl. Waking up screaming in anguish from a dream after having observed parental sexual intercourse, the girl tells her mother: "A man wanted to murder you in your bed but I rescued you."[1]

The central thesis of psychoanalysis is the infantile Oedipus complex. In early childhood, humans must undergo an agitating inner conflict, as research has confirmed without exception.[2] The child chooses a love object that it desires sexually and that it wants to possess. At the same time, it confronts a rival whom it wishes to eliminate through murder. We usually have to assume that the libido is oriented toward the other sex, the aggressiveness toward the same sex. Men desire women as substitute of the formerly loved mother and compete with other men. The negative outcome of the oedipal conflict, that is, the inversion of the object choice, is an alternative to the more common solution. In the common solution, the identification with the rival and—in relinquishing the desired love object—an internalization of impending punishments occur that put an abrupt end to the passionate courtship. In inversion, by contrast, the rival is adopted as the love object, and the identification takes place with the former object; in this case, one wants to be loved by the same-sex partner the way the mother should have done. In every case, however, psychoanalysis presupposes an originary, a *first heterosexual love choice*. The oedipal boy desires the woman who used to feed him; the little girl, by contrast, to satisfy her genital-sexual wishes (as distinct from the "pre-genital" wishes of early childhood) seeks a male love object whose anatomical constitution promises sexual satisfaction.

What are we to make of this little girl who, long after the oedipal crisis, obviously still desires her mother? For the rescue phantasy in no way serves to defend her from hostile impulses against the father.[3] To interpret the dream, all we have to do is replace the little word "but," which does not exist in the unconscious, with "and."[4] A man wanted to do it with you in bed (or rather, has already done so, as the little girl observed), *I want to, too, I do as he does*. Are we dealing with a future lesbian? Or does the little girl turn to the mother *regressively*? There can be no doubt that the little girl desires the mother—as if to affirm the dream wish, roused from sleep she calls the *mother* from the parental

DOI: 10.4324/9781032666273-19

bed to her own. The anxiety affect, however, comes from the insight that she wants something dangerous; in the anxious visions of the following days, she punishes herself for the almost successful fulfillment of the embarrassing wish in the dream. She wanted to have sexual intercourse with the mother; now snakes that want to bite her leg appear to her and black men who wag their fingers at her.[5] The anxiety upon awaking, *after* she allowed herself the complete realization of the oedipal wishes in the dream (*I do in bed with mother what usually father does, I do it in his place and better!*), can only be interpreted as expression of the frightening knowledge of penislessness, of the castration phantasy. The subsequent "signs of illness" are signs of anxiety, sense of guilt, and shame. That is coherent because, after all, by demanding the place in bed beside the mother, she would expose herself to the revenge of the father. The tormenting ideas are symbols that are to remind her of the power of the father.

A second source of concern is also quite evident. In imagining to do it with the mother like a man, she must confront the embarrassing insight that she does not have anything and does not possess an appropriate sexual organ, with which she could satisfy the mother. She has nothing to match the father's phallus. The genital wishes that in this context are to be identified as phallic have found an object, but they have not found a physical correlate. The phantasies that follow the dream, a snake crawling into her bed, men wagging their fingers in the toilet, are to be seen as compromise formations between anxiety and wish. The penis symbols remind her of the paternal power and demand renunciation and submission from her, but at the same time, she hopes to find (in the most propitious places, in bed or on the toilet) a member she might *appropriate*.[6] We are compelled to suspect, underneath the oedipal constellation, an older but no less rich layer. In the little dreamer's masturbation phantasies, there seems to be a connection between her penislessness and her wish for coiting. "You," the mother she desires and whom she calls over for consolation, are names for her own excited vulva that can become conscious. The personification of body parts is nothing extraordinary. While the first sentence of the dream presents the sexual wish as fulfilled, the second sentence negates what has happened. The link is the sadistic coitus idea. "The father 'murders' you, and I 'murder' you better!"

Might it be possible to find a similar oedipal construction in the acrobat's dream? She wants to rescue me from the advances of the men, and she sacrifices herself in my place. Does that mean that she wants to deal with me the way the little girl does with her mother? Does the initial rescue phantasy change into a rape scene because her phallic, active wishes yield to regressive, passive strivings as soon as she gets to *see* something specific? Her incantation "If I don't want to, I don't see it" points in that direction. Like the little girl, she would be missing something to be seen on her body. The unconscious conflict could form around her penislessness and could make the current vindictive, phallic impulses—she wants to *show* me!—appear particularly painful. We must, however, test another hypothesis as well. Stephanie wants to do it with me "like a man." The "sloppy hat," however, the thought of her factual genital anatomy, forces her into scorn and mockery. She thereby tries to escape the fatal insult by her phallic "impotence." Instead of conquering me, she must submit and demand for herself what she had wanted to do to me. At this point, the question whether it is the consequences of her *penislessness* or not rather *genuine passive wishes* that transform the rescue phantasy into submission is of secondary importance beside the fact that she attributes her awkward situation *to her own fault*. The "drumming" (masturbation) was how it began, such that today she is so dependent on others for the satisfaction of her genital wishes. With cynical mockery, however, she not only disavows her own helplessness but also turns her reproaches against me. She cannot forgive me for watching her crisis, as she thinks, without doing anything, "tied to a chair," with "eyes open." She heaps insults on me, mocks me for my inaction, for my inability to "really" help her. She can see only two explanations for my behavior. Either I am a sadist, want to diligently humiliate her, force her to pay, to labor by the clock ("clockwork"), or I am just as helpless, powerless, and *castrated* as she is.

One detail, however, excites our curiosity. At the end of the dream, she says: "You're a monkey," a rather odd name for a rapist. "Monkey," she enlightens me, is the correct name for the heavy military knapsack soldiers carry on their backs. On that point, she remembers a long-forgotten scene with her first boyfriend, whom she had seduced into having anal intercourse with her. After unsuccessful attempts to reach orgasm genitally, she talked him into trying it with her "from behind." This association, too, cannot be understood otherwise than as asking me to dance. The allusion to my name (Soldat [= soldier]) is unmistakable, and during the analysis, I am sitting *behind* her.

The acrobat's dream has revealed its homosexual and vindictive components, it allows for surmising passive and anal-erotic impulses, but it does not reveal which inner movement characterizes it. The inclination toward passivity, the sexual tendency to seduce, castration anxiety, as well as scorn and mockery to defend against helplessness are traits that are too general for us to permit ourselves using them to justify her "masochism." The most obvious, the manifest content of the dream, about torture, rape, sexual pleasure, bondage, and longing for death, seems the least apt to justify the predicate. "There needs no ghost, my lord, come from the grave to tell us this," we hear in *Hamlet*.[7] We must summon our patience, therefore, and look for further authorization to call a phantasy or a behavior masochistic.

Notes

1 Abraham (1913) 1982.
2 Psychoanalysis continues to claim general validity for the Oedipus complex, maintaining that it is an *unavoidable* crisis of the psychosexual conflicts in human development among all cultures and in all ages. Evidence for this thesis is provided not just in everyday practice but by psychohistorical and ethnopsychoanalytic research as well.

3 Karl Abraham, of course, takes a different view. He cannot grant the little girl a homosexual choice of object, sees her sexual wishes to be aimed at the father, and thinks that the child's secret wish concerns an "attempt on the life of the mother" (Abraham [1913] 1982, 182).
4 There is nothing in the unconscious one might equate with a negation or an objection. See Freud 1933, 74.
5 If Abraham's thesis were correct, if the mother were the oedipal rival and not the incestuously desired love object, it would be incomprehensible why the child would associate her expectations of punishment with men, not least of all with Abraham himself, who must calm her down with "psychotherapeutic measures."
6 The paternal phallus the child hallucinates everywhere is as much the memento of her defeat, as a threatening warning of further punishments, as it is the phantom-like fulfillment of her hope to make up for the anatomical "lack" after all.
7 Freud cites the line [*Hamlet* 1.5.131–32] in his presentation of associations and allusions in *The Interpretation of Dreams* (Freud 1900, SE 4, 175).

3 The physicist's dog

An example of a dream that might at first sight appear as "sadistic" was told to me by an aging homosexual:

> I am being pursued, surrounded by three young guys. I strike down one of them, he remains lying on the ground, dead. I then abuse him, fuck him in the ass. He doesn't move, since he's already dead, done and done for. I squeeze his breasts, tear his shirt off. I want to see his ass, fuck him with my fist; he is dead, but he plays along.
>
> Suddenly, I'm in a restaurant. The waiter is cheeky, spills champagne. I get mad at him, too, I hit him, scream: You fucking dog!

The dreamer is being driven to desperation by his lover. The lover lives off him, torments and humiliates him cruelly. My patient, a physicist by profession, a quiet, occasionally curt person, and broad-shouldered and tall, has in fact recently fallen in love with a young waiter to get away from his tormentor, albeit without success. His phantasies return again and again to the heartless boyfriend. For nights on end, he waits in the cold in front of [the lover's] door, smashes windows out of jealousy, and risks his professional career just to be close to the beloved. The thesis that masochism is a defense product of an originary sadism seems to find confirmation here. In dreams, the hostile impulses that are fended off less than in waking life garner strength. Those who in everyday life are masochists allow themselves angry and coarse satisfaction during sleep, when their inner censorship is attenuated. It is peculiar, though, that the lover does not appear in the dream. The attacks are directed not at him, the constantly present tormentor, but at three young guys that surround [the dreamer], and finally, the waiter who is spilling champagne.

The physicist reports this dream with pride and satisfaction. He thinks he has finally let his justified aggressions toward his boyfriend run freely; for him, it is settled that the abuse of the three guys in the dream is really aimed at his boyfriend. I, by contrast, think that his satisfaction derives from his succeeding, in the dream, in hallucinatorily coping with an *acute anxiety*. The three guys who assail him are none other than his genitals.[1] The breasts he is tugging at, too, stand as a symbol for his male member.[2] My patient feels

DOI: 10.4324/9781032666273-20

entirely exposed to the violence of his sexual desires. His penis, which in reality is everything but dead, sovereignly rules him and forces him into the role of an attendant, a waiter. He is the servant of his member whom he must serve whether he wants to or not. The "spilled champagne" recalls (through the allusion to ejaculation) the seminal fluid that is produced in his obsessive nightly masturbation. In the dream, however, he is not powerless and his member—like his young boyfriend—is beautiful and desirable, [the member] is in his power and he can do with it as he pleases. The dream pleasurably inverses the servitude experienced every day vis-à-vis the alliance his sexual excitement has entered into with his nasty lover, the subordination to his two masters.

Yet here, too, a detail draws our attention. The "restaurant" he "suddenly" finds himself in and where the words "fucking dog" are said, these details, like the acrobat's "monkey," do not seem to fit in with the rest of the dram. The incongruence, though, is quickly cleared up. On the ground floor of the house in which I have my office, there is a bar, a sort of eatery that serves fish.[3] Knowing also that my patient has a habit of regularly bringing his dog to the analytical sessions, an interpretation imposes itself. The glaring sexual content is meant to obscure the fact that he has come to be acutely dependent on me. The physicist fears to find in me an agency as strict and condemning as the one he carries within him in the form of his conscience. Yet it is the relationship with his superego, it's *devastating judgment* on his servitude, that forces on my patient a "masochistic" maneuvering among two, three, including me now four masters. Unlike the bedraggled impression left by the physicist's lax working and sexual habits, his inner morality is implacable. We might even say that the inner agency's unusually strict judgment of his wishes for sexual satisfaction produces the struggle with masturbation and the ambivalence toward his boyfriend in the first place that make him seem so shabby. He desperately defends himself in order for the conflict in which he is crushed between sexual wish, superego, and his lover not to be transferred onto the analyst as well. In the dream, he identified with me. He wants me to feel the same kind of angry excitation to which he is incessantly exposed.

When we compare both dreams, some shared features stand out. The acrobat and the physicist both participate in a sadistic sexual phantasy they want to satisfy voyeuristically, and both *shy away from the sight of the difference of sex*. Stephanie, imploringly: If I don't want to, I don't see it; the physicist stresses hypocritically boldly: I want to see!

We may suppose that when "pursuers" appear in their dreams, both feel *assailed by their own aggressive, genital-phallic impulses*. Stephanie directs her wishes at the analyst and is horrified by the insight into her penislessness. The physicist attempts to satisfy his sexual excitation masturbatorily; what the "analyst" is in Stephanie's dream, for him is the killed "guy," his member. In his phantasy, he abuses him the way Stephanie is abused by her tormentors. For both, the sexual excitation seems to be a process driven by aggressive energies. What stands out is not so much the phantasies' sadistic content but this *quality of wish cathexis*. The phallic excitation is not, as it usually is, narcissistic-exhibitionist but angry (she is "drumming," he is "hitting").

Both also share a similar defense process. The castration anxiety splits the phallic wish. The wish breaks into two parts, a passive, powerless share that remains attached to the phallus, and an aggressive share that is initially ascribed to the ego, then projected. Split and projection can choke anxiety. When in his everyday life, the physicist worships his young boyfriend as the incarnation of an unscathed member, he doubly insures himself against its loss. The physicist's phallic sexual wish does not seem to know of any other object than his own body. But a peculiar recathexis has taken place in him—not his genital organ is excited but he himself is charged with anger and abuses the young "guy." The aggressiveness displayed provocatively and loudly, meanwhile, covers over the helplessness and powerlessness of the ego, which finds itself locked in between aggressive sexual wish and anxiety. It would be misguided, however, to suspect the upheaval of the ego to be an identification with the condemning agency, the superego. The economy of the internal forces demands that the sexual excitation be treated *before* the feelings of guilt are engaged with; *quantitatively*, the aggressive-phallic energies in the case of the physicist are to be estimated to be greater than the aggressions the superego has at its disposal. The former thus have priority in the defense; they are shifted to the ego, and the ego functions are being sexualized. Censorship is thus no longer directed against the original cathexis of the genital (or only in dreams). The ego and the object relations have attracted the full quantity of the excitation. The alleged love object is, at bottom, no longer a person but a displacement substitute for the genital. It must fulfill this function taking turns with the ego; the undiminished sexual *quality of the cathexis* betrays the origin of the projection. The ego is as sadistic and dangerous toward the genital, the object as sadistic and dangerous toward the ego as the aggressive phallic sexual excitation used to be. Neither the physicist nor the acrobat fears a punishment (castration) for nonpermitted sexual cravings, yet both suspect that through their genital wishes, they mutilate themselves or have already injured themselves.

The defense is thus aimed neither at the embarrassing wish of object (homosexuality) nor at the content of the wishes (the incestuous phantasies during masturbation) but, in this first phase, at the *aggressive component of the strongest, phallic impulse*. This [impulse] is associated with the *idea of autocastration*. Only in the second phase of the defense does mechanism of compensation and disavowal set in that become responsible for the impression of masochism.

Both dreamers must constantly protest their innocence: I haven't destroyed "him," I wanted to save him, I worshipped him, and so on. In the dream, Stephanie gets back what she is painfully missing "by the dozen." What for her is the "monkey," for the physicist is his "fucking dog"—from the analyst he hopes for and in the dream receives the "fucking dog" back, although of course not the invective but a cheeky and lively member that belongs to him and is subject to him as uncontestably as his faithful four-legged companion.

Notes

1 "In any case the number three has been confirmed from many sides as a symbol of the male genitals" (Freud 1900, SE 5, 358).
2 It seems less intuitive that breasts, too, an undisputedly "feminine" trait, are marshaled to represent the penis. Psychoanalytic experience, however, leaves no doubt. The association breast–penis is established via a series of intermediate links, for instance via cows' udders, which perform the function of the breast but look like the male member, or fellatio, where the member is sucked like the mother's breast, as it were.
3 The "physicist" later reported a dream in which he sees the analysis as a "fish farm" and a "wastewater treatment plant." See below, II.13, #.

4 Somebody's late

As my third example, I would like to recount the dream of an analysand, a successful, enterprising, and funny businesswoman who spends every spare minute taking care of her kitchen and her home. She cooks and she cleans, she bakes, and comes up with new recipes, so I'll refer to her as the kitchen fairy. On a day on which, as always, she shows up on time for the session, she reveals she dreamt in the night that she came too late for the session, that I was "pissed off" [*stocksauer*] at her, but that I looked very unusual, much younger than in reality, like a fat girl, and was wearing a white night gown.

This dream, too, is incomprehensible if we do not know the circumstances that led to it. My patient, a beautiful, sociable, and candid woman, well over thirty, who has for years been living in the same household with her boyfriend, a vivacious craftsman, is *virgo intacta*. She recounts the dream early in her analysis.[1] It does not seem difficult to interpret it. My patient hopes that it is not too late for the analysis and that she can still have a wedding (long white gown) and have a child (become fat).

Why, though, does this all too understandable wish, which she could have communicated to me in other ways, become the trigger of a dream? Why does she not present her fear directly? And what could her longing for a husband and a child have to do with the question of being late? Incomprehensible, too, for the moment, is the choice of the expression "pissed off."

When we learn that in the course of her analysis, the patient develops symptoms that can only be called masochistic, we are being exhorted to look for a *particular conflictual structure* in this dream as well. She, who is unchallenged at work, popular among her friends, constantly feels disadvantaged. She unconditionally submits to her boyfriend, whom she loves and worships. She atones for even the smallest inconvenience she must cause him with feelings of guilt and new miracles in the home and in the kitchen. I could discover no signs of excessive ambivalence in her feelings for him. She really wanted to appeal to him; yet as soon as the smallest erotic tension appeared between them, the "kitchen fairy" entered a subdued, spiteful irritation.[2] We do not overlook that, rather than communicating a fear to me or complaining, she constructs a situation in the dream in which she herself is the guilty one. This process corresponds to her habits in the waking state. When she

DOI: 10.4324/9781032666273-21

felt unloved and rejected, she neither tried to change her boyfriend's mind nor complained. She did not plead and made no reproaches. She took all responsibility upon herself, blamed herself for her appearance, her fat legs, and suspected herself of impertinence or more likely too much reserve. The way she is, she cannot appeal to anyone, [she says]; it is only right that her boyfriend wants nothing to do with her.

Psychoanalysis recognizes this emotional movement to be a defense process. Reproaches against others are transformed into self-accusations. This is a particular form of identification.[3] Yet this process, too, cannot be claimed for masochism either. It applies too generally. We might perhaps explore the self-accusations to understand what is being fended off, the origin of her complaints, and fears that it might be too late for her happiness. Yet the triumphalist and satisfied tone in which she presented her modesty blocked this path for the associations. I was compelled to conceive of the fact that no man desired her as an unconscious triumph, as a privilege successfully fought for.

In her lonely nights, she masturbated regularly and pleasurably by imagining cruel scenes of torture. In these, she was being tortured herself or had to watch someone else being tormented. She reached orgasm whenever a long longed-for relief for the tortured precisely did *not* arrive but the tormentors instead escalated their treatment in a particularly brutal way.

Sometimes also an unexpected turn of events that led to a more painful ending caused excitation. I succeeded in finding genetic explanations for the content of her phantasies but I could not at this point discover the reason why she took as the source of her pleasure the divergence and not the congruence of wish and satisfaction. That she was suffering from the effect of unconscious feelings of guilt seemed evident. There were connections to be found in her biography that made it far less painful for her to presume the fault for her unhappiness to lie with her than [to accept] being defeated by unchangeable conditions. In what follows, however, I omit the larger share of the analysis. My intention here is not to present a detailed case history. As long as there is still confusion as to whether masochistic strivings are to be conceived as genuine pulsional demands or rather as results of pulsional defense, we cannot turn our attention exclusively to phantasies; we would not be in a position to contribute anything worth mentioning to their elucidation. What obstructs insight, however, is not conceptual ambiguity. [Insight] is also hindered by the fact that in masochism, more unanimously than is usually the case in the psychical, inner impulses and social influence appear to combine to produce the same effect. *Curiosity* is inhibited and appears as a dangerous impulse. It is turned away psychically because it is directed at sexual contents that thanks to their connection with sadism lead to an unacceptable result (anal or genital rape, castration). In the social context, their excitation is prevented because *emotional* curiosity especially could contribute to elucidating the violent reality. Under such conditions, we will have to take recourse to collecting individual observations. By claiming a causal connection between "dark" symptoms on the one hand and a for the moment unknown pulsional dynamic on the other, to which social intensions are attached—we do not know yet how and what for—I will try to bring the observations into a definitive relation with each other.

Notes

1 The first communications and dreams in an analysis are particularly significant. Like good books, people tend to characterize themselves already in the first sentence, in the very first remarks. They silence conflicts whose real depth and foundation can become conscious only much later. In addition, in the initial communications, it is wishes that tend to take the spotlight. The defense asserts itself in the development of the transference when the wishes are rejected as too embarrassing and the conflicts return to their usual place in the psychical assemblage.
2 I do not know for what reasons her boyfriend lived in physical proximity to her but in sexual abstinence. The homoerotic pedophilia she claimed did not convince me; [it rather] reflected her own sexual wishful phantasies.
3 The particularity of this identification consists in her projecting the reproaches first and then reinternalizing them. The object serves merely as support for the superego projection. The ego in the defense does not identify with the reinternalized aggressions but fights them with a new introjection. In part III of this study, we will have occasion to take a closer look at this intricate process.

5 The diagnostic dilemma

Recall that *subjective disavowals* in particular stand in the way of elucidating the relationships between individual and society. We found these [disavowals] to be the consequence of a general prohibition on thought established by political dominion and economic profit to defend their interests. Our analysis had to make its way via the overcoming of this inhibition. We now turn to dreams and neurotic symptoms. We're discussing perverse phantasies, horror at the sight of the female vulva, castration anxiety, and incest wishes. Our work must prove itself in confronting the resistance against insight into *embarrassing intimacies*. The contrast between inside and outside is impressive, and we may look forward to finding out what synapses and mediation processes emerge from their combination.

As for masochism, the theories we have encountered so far have not put us in a position to understand even just the inner processes. Neither the thesis that masochism is the defense product of an originary sadism nor the thesis that masochism testifies to the effect of a general death drive is able to explain the very particular structure of *masochistic conflicts*. This much we have learned from the account of the three analysis fragments: for none of the patients, our usual psychoanalytic art of interpreting dreams was able to grant insight into what really moves them.[1] Meanwhile, we cannot but have the *impression* that, however different their phantasy worlds and however incomparable their sexual lives may be, these people are linked by a *shared structure of their conflicts*. We must suspect, though, that we are not confronting here the consequences of *the most general* human impulses, be it death drive, be it aggression inclination, but acute, particular conflicts that have been solved in a very peculiar way. I therefore propose to take a closer look at this *particular kind of conflict resolution*.

We know that Freud initially understood masochism to be the product of a defense: out of anxiety or under the pressures of conscience, sadistic pulsional impulses are turned back against the self. Later he conceived of the symptoms as indicating a structural conflict: the sadistic superego is directed against the ego that has become masochistic. Finally, Freud recognized in the striving for self-destruction and submission the effect of the death drive. This subordinated masochism to the power of the "Nirvana" principle, a tendency toward reducing tension in the psychical; the rules of the pleasure–unpleasure principle could no longer be seen to explain masochistic phenomena.[2] Henceforth, such phenomena counted as evidence that the death drive theory had a right to exist. Yet Freud was never entirely satisfied with this solution, since masochism assumed a theoretical position, it clinically did not deserve. To be sure, masochistic traits can be found in almost all neurotic constellations; so-called normal people, too, are not entirely strangers to the pleasure of subordinating themselves and receiving orders. Many "accidents" can be ascribed to an unconscious drive to injure oneself: the tendency would be unconscious and express itself in the form of parapraxes. In the analytic cure, too, we come across the "masochistic resistance," when patients hold on to their neurosis and seem to be willing to do anything except lose their tormenting symptoms. Masochistic tendencies, you'll find, often impose themselves against conscious positions such as defiance and independence and do indeed seem to be related to unchangeable foundations of the psychical.

I will, however, wait with my judgment. Perhaps some cases of "masochism" can be interpreted as consequences of a common *superego problem*. We know that no pulsional relinquishment is capable of appeasing the superego, that, on the contrary, conscience demands the submission of the ego all the more bluntly the more satisfactions fail to appear.[3] With regard to aggression in particular, the ego is in a hopeless position before the censoring agency—if it permits a physical satisfaction of the sadism, it is tormented by guilt; if it prevents the drives breaking through to action, it is guaranteed increased reproaches. Not because the relinquishment pushed it into phantasizing; the superego knows the content of the sadistic wishes long before the ego does and keeps them in check with punishments and threats. Yet ultimately, the aggressive pulsional quantities must be invested *somewhere* and make their way via the punishing agency to the ego. The sum of all violences in the ego remains equal, we might say. It makes sense that an ego thus plagued easily seems "masochistic." A simple defense, too, the so-called *reaction formation*, appears, insofar as the ego confronts aggressive tendencies with it, as submissiveness. Another defense, the *identification with the victim* of one's own hostility, forced on the ego by the superego on the logic of "As you do unto others, so I do unto you!" has consequences that look "masochistic." The more evil the ego willed for its "victim," the more sensitively conscience reacts, the more craving for submission and repentance emerges in the process. A further defense, the *identification with the aggressor*, can equally seem "masochistic" when it does not completely succeed; then the aggression is not turned back onto the attacker but operates only a partial introjection, which makes outer object and superego appear united in cruelty. *Undoing*, also a defense mechanism that makes use of animistic ideas, can amount to self-destruction and submissiveness; one thereby seeks to disavow the consequences of one's misdeeds. Finally, a *quantitative factor*, too, seems "masochistic"; when, compared to the capacity of the superego, the intensity of pulsional energies is too great, pulsional anxiety arises and paralyzes the ego. When pulsional quantity and the strictness of the superego are overpowering in comparison with the formation of ego structures, and the defense in particular, the I "suffers." In both cases, it becomes submissive, servile, and dependent.

How different, though, is the quality of masochism in the case of the suffering that gave the phenomenon its name! Leopold von Sacher-Masoch describes it in his novel, *Venus in Furs*:

> Here I am back again, soaked to the skin and burning with shame and fever. The servant girl has delivered my letter, I am condemned, lost, delivered into the hands of a heartless woman whom I have now insulted. She may even kill me; well, let her do so, for although I do not want to live any longer, I am unable to take my own life.
>
> I walk to the back of the house and see her on the terrace, leaning over the railing with her head in full sunlight and her green eyes gleaming.
>
> "Are you still alive?" she asks, without moving. I remain silent and hang my head.
>
> "Give me back my dagger," she says. "It is of no use to you, since you have not even the courage to kill yourself."
>
> "I have lost it," I reply, shivering with cold.
>
> She eyes me scornfully.
>
> "Did you lose it in the Arno?" she shrugged. "Ah, well. Why didn't you leave?"
>
> I murmur something which neither she nor I can understand. "Oh, you have no money," she exclaims. "Here!"
>
> And she tosses me her purse with a contemptuous gesture.
>
> I leave it on the ground. For a long time we are both silent. "So you do not want to go?"
>
> "I cannot."[4]

This pleasurable-tormenting climate is extremely different from the impression of helplessness and strictness the struggle between ego and superego leaves. We really have to wonder how the two could be mixed up. When a capable businesswoman, our "kitchen fairy," first, in her dream, makes me "pissed off" and then comes on time to her session, where she doesn't say a word about wishes that suggest themselves; when the "physicist" lets himself be plagued by his lover but feels no pleasure in his masturbation orgies; when the "acrobat" steps into an inner trap because she is unable to "juggle" her craving for revenge and her erotic wishes, we must not simply suspect problems of guilt. On the other hand, it is of course not the *sadomasochistic content* of their phantasies that deserves the title masochism but a *particular genetic development*[—a] psychosexual development, we now add, that leads to *masochistic conflicts* and to corresponding particular strategies for resolving them.

I thus want to propose to conceive of masochism from now on as a *nosological entity*. If it is to be a *neurosis* in its own right, though, then the task of our further work must be to furnish proof of the *masochistic psychosexual development*. The observation of the constitutional component, the fixation to a traumatic situation, conflicts that ensue, and the change in the pulsional vicissitude compared to other neurotic developments will have convinced us that the phenomenon of masochism finds a just place in theory when it is no longer judged according to its effect but studied based on the history of its genesis.

We thereby reverse the epistemic process Freud chose for himself.[5] We are looking for a theory whose suppositions compellingly lead from the hypothetical starting situation—as is the case for all other neuroses as well—to the symptoms we are presented with. We mustn't think, though, that merely a gap in neurosis theory or even Freud's intention to support the death drive with clinical vividness is responsible for the uncertainty in facing masochism. It is for good reason that psychoanalysis has little interest in diagnoses it can state—if at all—only post festum, after an analysis has ended. Yet it doesn't have a choice. It elaborates its judgment only as its activity unfolds.[6] The attribution of a neurosis to a diagnostic entity only emerges thanks to the development of the transference process and not thanks to the manifest symptoms. In every neurosis, we find components of different diagnostic categories. We derive no advantage from naming a syndrome one way or another but attach importance to exploring a psychical *conflict* that can be structured hysterically, phobically, or obsessional-neurotically.

We did see, however, how much effort it took Freud to locate masochism in the psychical apparatus at all. Now it was a form, now the motor of a defense; it was a pulsional derivative, character structure, perversion, and feminine position. Finally, it became a no longer reducible, autonomous drive.[7] In his late writings in particular, Freud called masochism merely a grave form of the resistance against the analytic cure. That is why we will content ourselves with having, for now, established a *dimension* of the phenomena. Yet if masochism does not stand for an individual pulsional demand but designates a whole neurosis, the greater share of our work of elucidation is yet to come.

Notes

1 Freud called the interpretation of dreams the *via regia* toward understanding the unconscious. In unclear circumstances, psychoanalysis indeed disposes of no other means than the interpretation of dreams, the observation of the emotional development, and the countertransference reactions.
2 See above, I.9.
3 Freud 1930, 128.
4 Sacher-Masoch (1869) 2006, 257. The concept presumably goes back to Krafft-Ebing [(1886) 2011, 89–152].
5 See above, I.9, #74–75.

6 Freud thinks that psychoanalytic diagnoses proceed in the manner of the king in Victor Hugo who claimed to know an infallible method to recognize a witch. He would cook her in a cauldron and then taste the soup; that way he would be able to say: yes, that was a witch, or: no, that wasn't a witch. [See Freud 1912a, 253.]
7 See above, I.9.

6 Two paths to masochism

One theoretical difficulty is that the existence of masochistic strivings seems to restrict the claim of the quest for pleasure to be the basic principle of all psychical processes. Yet the clinical observations proving that pleasure is taken in suffering cannot be doubted, nor can psychology (on the basis of innumerable other observations) do without the pleasure principle. This fact, among others, was what moved Freud to suppose the death drive. Masochistic tendencies henceforth counted as evidence for the operation of a genuinely self-destructive drive. Psychoanalytic experience has taught me that the hypothesis of the death drive is indispensable for elucidating a fundamental phenomenon in psychical life. I propose, however, to dissolve the unfruitful association of masochism and death drive again. Establishing masochistic tendencies has no need of the death drive, and the death drive can very well assert its existence without the evidence of masochism. By contrast, we should not rashly seek refuge with the pleasure principle and suppose that psychical and physical suffering do cause the masochist a kind of perverse pleasure after all.[1] There is no reason why in the case of masochism we shouldn't look for another, repressed content behind the manifest surface. Why must we deny masochistic symptoms what seems self-evident in the case hysterical ones, for instance? Masochism is the only exception in the psychical where what is manifest, the connection between pleasure and suffering, already counts as an *immediate* effect of unconscious forces. The neurotic symptom of hysteria by contrast is being understood as a multiply refracted compromise between pulsional expression and defense. We grant that every sign of hysterical illness has a development history; we seek out its genetic and economic components to resolve it; we believe that these components, once they are rendered lively again in the analytical transference situation, can be changed and that new and, we like to think, better conflict solutions can be created. It is hard to see why this path should remain blocked for masochistic symptoms. A lack of theoretical comprehension alone cannot be the reason.

We already suspected that in masochism, the psychical and the social are connected in a way that is yet unclear to us. A hysteric woman is a psychically conspicuous person in any social organization. In a machoistically oriented society, she might be particular apt at testifying to the unpredictability or on the contrary to the frigidity of women. But she does not lose the aura of the pathological, the effusive. In an administered society, an obsessional neurotic is a worker, a civil servant without blemish or blame, but no matter how useful he is, he is immediately identified as a neurotic, as a "strange bird."

It's different for masochists. We do not allow them the pathological significance we immediately grant depressives, schizophrenics, perverts, hysterics. In everyday life, their behavior is the object of sneering comments:[2] "I can see and hear that you're suffering. But I think that's nothing but a charade. Your suffering is meant to hush up the fact that you're enjoying your situation such as it is and don't want it any other way." Not only the aggressive and abrasive content of this "interpretation" draws attention but also the fact that the evidently perceived suffering of another does not trigger alarm or the impulse to help but a peculiar reproachful interpretation.

That cannot be a coincidence. If, as Freud says in *The Interpretation of Dreams*, the unconscious of one person understands the unconscious of another, then we must suppose that these reactions, on the one hand, are able to tell us something about the unconscious tendencies of masochism, and that they are also, on the other hand, suitable to drawing attention to a particular *social exploitation of masochism*. What I mean by this: a neurosis is indeed the success of specific individual-psychical conditions, yet it is equally—at least in its immediate effect, namely, in changing the inner and outer *subjective* reality—the site and the medium of social processes.

How neurotics deploy their neurosis in their life-conditions, *what* they thereby effect for themselves, and how they are thereby treated, is the visible trace of the struggle in which, step by step and apparently without external influence, a revolutionary process fails. This articulation designates neither the "secondary gain from illness" nor phenomena of countertransference[3]; what I have in mind, rather, is the fact that the neurotic conflict reinvigorates and must bring to an end not only the oedipal confrontation (the clash between pulsional demand and conscience) but also the struggle between individual and society. Individual suffering is the arena of a particular turmoil: acute inclinations emerging from a biography are being filled with pulsional energy and meet with fierce resistance from equally pulsionally charged forces, the inner prohibitions. In the process at issue, however, a struggle between individual and society takes place that goes far beyond the domestication of the subject for the benefit of a cultural norm.[4]

Neurosis is *revolutionary* because it begins with an insurrectionary impetus that—ignoring all threats—attempts a liberation from restriction and resignation. Neurotics, of course, do not want to shake off the commandments of culture in general but primarily the *additional burdens of a particular social organization* that *exceed* the *unavoidable pulsional restriction* imposed by the fact of living with others. And it is said to fail not because revolutionary failure is an axiom of psychology and history but because this names the usual outcome of subjective, of individual, and also of collective revolt against social dominion. For the subject, every rebellion leads not only to inner conflicts and an increased relinquishing of drives but, beyond the individual and the "interpersonal," to an anxiety [about] having attacked and harmed the established power. I thus emphasize the difference between subjective impulses, social relationships, and the *objective* power of a social dominion of politics, economy, or religion. We may have anxiety crises for attacking individual bearers of power; we can also foreshorten, in a subjective defense move, dominion as such to the individual measure of its representatives. Yet in truth, we find in [dominion] an opponent that functions according to other laws than the ones we suspect in ourselves. Misjudging the difference between the subjective exercise of power and the laws of objective dominion, on the one hand, and the consequences of individual morality combined with the obfuscation of the mechanisms of power, on the other hand, form the psychical coordinate system, all of whose vectors converge in assigning guilt to the individual.

In a relationship of dominion, the mere idea that life and the order of society could be thought differently is, for everyone, an aggressive act punished by feelings of guilt. This applies indiscriminately, albeit with different preconditions for the oppressed and the profiteers. A prohibition on thought bears down on everyone; any rebellion—even unconscious—inexorably leads to even more self-punishment, assimilation, and resignation. These processes seem common to us, perhaps even necessary to maintain a social order. We argue, politically, pedagogically, and psychologically, thinking to thereby establish a minimal, indispensable measure of restriction. In doing so, we all too gladly forget to take particular *conflicts of interest* into account. The revolutionary impetus in the individual fails—internally, as well—not because of resistances *in principle* but rather because of that *excess* of deformation and channeling of its pulsional forces that a *specific* social order obtains by force for its purposes. This surplus borne by a large share of people to the detriment of the individual and the benefit of dominion is *in no way a restriction of drives but a complex of promoting subjective impulses that are agreeable to power and inhibiting those that are useless for it.*

There is a point of contact between neurotic conflicts and political-revolutionary rebellion. At the beginning of both stands, the unwillingness to accept a demand by external reality to relinquish a drive. Hysterics refuse to relinquish their first love object and hold on to their oedipal wishes. Basarov and Gustav Landauer,[5] however, refuse power the very submission that the structure of their *inner* conflicts urgently *demands* of them. We do well to investigate the subjective roots of political engagement, and we will often find that alleged incoherences, tactically unwise actions, fit in very well with biographically anchored tendencies. In the social as well, people cannot but remobilize forces developed in the course of subjective history and strengthened in inner conflicts. It would be naive, however, to reduce the failure of revolutionary movements to the influence of psychical factors. If it were only about the struggle between pulsional restriction and pulsional liberation, no revolutionary movement would have to worry about succeeding; in the pulsional source of individuals, it would have an inexhaustible reserve of forces on its side.[6] Yet it is also not permissible to blame the failure of psychical revolts and social liberation on external misery and threats of violence. The examples that show an evident psychical compulsion rather than external inhibitions are too numerous. The third way, pointing to psychical defense mechanisms, we blocked ourselves. The identification with the aggressor often cited as the cause of failure presupposes a feeling of guilt that is subjectively founded in each case and serves to interpret the positions between individuals; it is unsuitable, though, to explaining socially effective phenomena. What, then, are we to think?

If it is still correct that for the individual judging social processes, subjective factors (memories, affects) are inseparably blended with the assessment of objective factors, then there are forces and laws at work in the social that do in fact seem to permit, even in their objectivized forms (the institutions of the state and the economy), a reciprocal conditioning of individual demands and "practical constraints," social "developments," and so on. Yet—compared with the influence of the objective laws and the effect of the instrumentalized will of a few powerful people—the share of individual strivings, even the share of the sum of individual strivings is so meager that we cannot speak of an association of subjective tendencies with already objectivized forms of human effort. The mystification of the individual as the subject of history overlooks that in the social, a qualitative leap takes place from what is going on between two or more individuals to the phenomena between society and individuals. [This leap] has primarily *quantitative* effects on already familiar axioms of ego analysis, mass psychology, and sociology. Multiplying individual strivings (the collective) just does not suffice to describe mass phenomena; in turn, we must not expect that in the social, rules apply that are entirely foreign to human psychology. In the transition from individual—unconscious—striving to social processes, we will thus prepare for three phenomena: the quantitative distortion of otherwise familiar principles; "parasitic" processes (when psychical and social forces reciprocally make themselves useful for their own purposes); and the appearance of new factors that are neither known to psychology nor provided for by the social sciences. I already cited an example of this third consequence: we saw that under particular circumstances, the aggression drive produces an objectified form of its demand, a form that neither is the intention of the individuals nor corresponds to a collective interest yet could also not be explained as the result of social laws.[7]

With regard to psychology, the stopgap of quantitative reflections comes as no surprise, since even in therapeutic technique, comparisons of magnitudes are essential. Time and again, we must reassess, for instance, the strength of the defense relative to the intensity of the pulsional energy. Neurosis theory, too, cannot make do without the observation of the quantitative preconditions of a state of affairs:

> The neuroses (unlike infectious diseases, for instance) have no specific determinants. It would be idle to seek in them for pathogenic excitants.

They shade off by easy transitions into what is described as the normal; and, on the other hand, there is scarcely any state recognized as normal in which indications of neurotic traits could not be pointed out. Neurotics have approximately the same innate dispositions as other people, they have the same experiences and they have the same tasks to perform. Why is it, then, that they live so much worse and with so much greater difficulty and, in the process, suffer more feelings of unpleasure, anxiety, and pain?

We need not be at a loss to find an answer to this question. *Quantitative* disharmonies are what must be held responsible for the inadequacy and sufferings of neurotics. The determining cause of all the forms taken by human mental life, is, indeed, to be sought in the reciprocal action between innate dispositions and accidental experiences. Now a particular instinct may be too strong or too weak innately, or a particular capacity may be stunted or insufficiently developed in life. On the other hand, external impressions and experiences may make demands of differing strength on different people; and what one person's constitution can deal with may prove an unmanageable task for another's. These *quantitative* differences will determine the variety of results.[8]

Although we acknowledge that a distortion in the quantitative relation of its factor will have the greatest consequence for a psychical process, we have trouble imagining how a social force gains influence in the innermost [world] of the human, the life of the drives, without taking refuge in subjective categories (identification, passivity wishes). And if what we suppose is correct, that masochism is an autonomous form of neurosis, then does it not follow that masochistic strivings are *pathological*? We might, to reassure ourselves, say that masochism has nothing to do with our everyday reality, and if it does, then it is an exaggeration of a common readiness for conflict. Perhaps we would have to settle for the observation that the difference between the neurotic illness and a military mentality of submission, between pathological self-sacrifice and the relinquishments demanded by a sadistic religion and crude methods of education is merely one of degree: too much masochism is neurotic, a little masochism is necessary. To recommend this view, we might cite the fact that for adapted, normal life in our culture, some *obsessional-neurotic* character traits are indispensable.[9] A popular formula, after all, says that modern society as a whole, and the forms of social intercourse in particular, are neurotic.

Both reflections, of course, are trivial. If the masochistic condition is a general condition, if moreover the degree of masochism demanded by the social dynamics is either proof of its own deformation or unavoidable (human "nature"), then there is no need for analysis. If, however, masochism is a neurosis, then the masochistic phenomena forced by the cultural ideology, too, must be considered the product of a pathological development; not just individual [but] sociogenic masochism, too, is thus treatable with therapy and accessible to a trained understanding.

For the continuation of this study, I choose a different approach. We note: masochism is an individual-psychological category, a neurosis; it emerges from conflicts in the life of the drives of which the individual is not conscious. Yet a particular ego structure, too, must be acknowledged as masochistic. This structure is not solely the achievement of changes in the id, it presupposes purposeful forces outside the individual that once more render the outcome of masochism unavoidable for the individual. I do not think, however, that social power is originally "sadistic" while the individual is moved by primarily masochistic strivings. It would also not go far enough to claim that an egotistical power promotes and exploits people's tendency to submit and then leaves it at that.[10] Instead, I suspect *that the individual as well society, each prompted by different causes, with different means, and with different intentions, produce the same symptoms.*

We will find that the characteristics of neurosis only seem to look like the socially generated syndrome.[11] Subjectively, both produce suffering, and only the analysis of their unequal lines of development and of the wholly divergent signs of decay will be able to make the case for a two-fold foundation of masochism. It is now up to us, step by step, to wrest the traces that lead toward masochism from an also two-fold resistance. The combination, for the purpose of further analysis, of social theory and psychology is opposed on the one hand by social amnesias (disavowals) and on the other hand by shame, which covers up secret satisfactions.

Notes

1 Morgenthaler (1984) 1988 and Holder and Dare 1982 equate masochism and sexual perversion. For Benjamin (1985) and Torok ([1964] 1985), masochism appears identical to "female submission"; see also Reik (1940) 1941.

2 At the end of his book, even the circumspect and well-equipped Theo Reik cannot help mocking masochists:

> The masochist, too, loses all battles, except the last. He knows—at least in the anticipating phantasy—that the prize beckons after he has experienced all defeats. He lets his opponent, sadism, taste all the pleasure for the hour—he even joins in the feast—but he patiently waits for the moment to bring the great turn. He tells himself in anticipation that one more such victory and the enemy will be defeated. Masochism is sadism in retreat, but with the inner expectancy of the ultimate push forward. It is characterized by unconscious defiance in defeat and by the secret foretaste and foreknowledge of coming conquest.
>
> This secret feeling of superiority draws its power from a phantasy that denies the laws of time and that keeps extending the suspense. If not in his lifetime, the masochistic character will assert himself after his death and gain the rights denied to him on this earth. Posterity will judge him better and will take revenge on his enemies ....
>
> In its pathological distortions and in its exuberance it endangers the progress of civilization because it imposes needless sacrifices and too great psych burdens on the ego and on communities. From a biological necessity suffering

grows into a psychic luxury. Time, to be sure, cures all wounds. Those, however, which we inflict on ourselves, are the most difficult to heal....

That is the grim tragicomedy of the martyr-attitude of modern man or at least of its essential characters. (Reik [1940] 1941, 430 and 433)

3 We speak of a "secondary gain from illness" when further advantages are added to the direct, unconscious satisfaction someone draws from their neurosis. A wish impulse not primarily involved in the disorder uses the symptoms to reach its own goals; this "overdetermines" neurotic symptoms, that is to say, multiple wish complexes participate in the same phenomenon. The countertransference names the analyst's unconscious emotional reaction to the patient's pulsional demands, which are stimulated in the course of the transference. The observation of countertransference reactions is one of the few instruments at the psychoanalyst's disposal. Using this tool is instilled in the "training analysis" and can only be *lege artis* [in keeping with the laws of the art] if this analysis was a therapeutic one, that is, if it has made the analyst conscious of their own conflictual issues.
4 See below, II.8 and II.9.
5 [The anarchist] Gustav Landauer was brutally murdered [by right-wing militias] on May 2, 1919, as a political prisoner (see Mühsam 1929). Basarov is the hero of Ivan Turgenyev's novel *Fathers and Sons*.
6 Marcuse, by contrast, holds that the relationships among people can be liberated by a re-eroticization without repression. The overthrow of "the sexual tyranny of the genitals" [Jay (1976) 1996, 110] and the return to the infantile structure of sexuality would put an end to alienated labor and to the reification of the body as well, which is founded on [this alienation] (Marcuse [1955] 1956, 234–37. According to Marcuse ([1964] 2002, 18), the "pacification of existence" can invoke the Nirvana principle for its justification.
7 See Part I above.
8 Freud 1938b, 183–84, Le Soldat's emphases.
9 Parin writes: "*Our* ego has undergone the most important formation for the vicissitude of the aggression in the anal phase" ([1973] 1978, 191 [Parin's emphasis]).
10 Fenichel pursues a similar train of thought when he discusses the connection between striving for possessions and pulsional impulses. "The instincts represent the general tendency, while matters of *money* and the desire to become wealthy represent a specific form which the general tendency can assume only in the presence of certain definite social conditions" (Fenichel [1934] 1953/1954, 101, Fenichel's emphasis).
11 The identity of phenomena in the case of different origins and economic bases is nothing new in either psychoanalysis or the social sciences. The overdetermination I postulate for psychical phenomena, indeed, also applies to the relationship between individual and society. Both sides can participate in the same symptom that becomes palpable in the individual vicissitude, both can have advanced [the symptom] with different degrees of force, both can have derived gain from it with diverging success.

7 Voluntary servitude

One of the first and to this day the most prominent proponent of the thesis that political dominion exploits people's masochistic inclinations for its own advantage is Étienne de La Boétie, who around 1550 published an essay with the title *Discours de la servitude volontaire*. To my knowledge, La Boétie is the first author to unequivocally and without restrictions engage with the *feasibility of human suffering*. He wonders

> how it happens that so many men, so many towns, so many cities, so many nations at times tolerate a single tyrant who has no other power than what they grant him, who has no other ability to harm them than inasmuch as they are willing to tolerate it, who could do ill to them only insofar as they would rather suffer it than oppose him.[1]

Of course, numerous thinkers before La Boétie pondered explanations for tyranny and servitude among humans, including Aristotle (to whose political theory La Boétie refers to multiple times, if not literally, then on the level of content), for whom servitude is conditioned by the nature of human beings, their habits, and [their] political institutions:

> All that we have said may be summed up under three heads, which answer to the three aims of the tyrant. These are, the humiliation of his subjects, for he knows that a mean-spirited man will not conspire against anybody: the creation of mistrust among them; for a tyrant is not overthrown until men begin to have confidence in one another; and this is the reason why tyrants are at war with the good; they are under the idea that their power is endangered by them, not only because they will not be ruled despotically, but also because they are loyal to one another, and to other men, and do not inform against one another or against other men: the tyrant desires that his subjects shall be incapable of action, for no one attempts what is impossible, and they will not attempt to overthrow a tyranny if they are powerless.[2]

Now, it is precisely these ostensibly reasonable explanations that do not make sense to La Boétie. Tactically retreating from force of weapons is one thing; the process, though, of people letting themselves, without need, be reduced to servitude and "voluntarily" turn themselves over to oppression seems incomprehensible to him. Playing love of freedom off against weakness and cowardice cannot yield satisfactory insight:

> one must feel more sorrow than amazement, to see a million men serving miserably, with their necks under the yoke, not compelled by force majeure but seemingly rather charmed and enchanted...
>
> If two, three, or four do not defend themselves against one, that is strange, but still possible—indeed, one can then say that it is for lack of courage. But if a hundred or a thousand tolerate one single man, can we not say that they do not want, not that they do not dare, to deal with him...?[3]

La Boétie recognizes immediately what others will understand only much later: while the lever of oppression is applied "outside" in the service of power, the compulsion could remain effective in the long run if it were not being met from the inside. The lust for power of some allies with them for the moment incomprehensible interests of many: "Where did he get so many eyes to spy on you, if you are not granting them to him? How does he have so many hands to strike you, if he does not get them from you?"[4]

People of course do not stop serving their oppressors. La Boétie notes that there is no need to fight for oneself actively revolutionarily; already the insight into one's own interest can help end the undignified situation. And he searches for reasons why not even that is happening. His first idea, which he mentions in passing and which neither he nor his commentators take up again, is surprisingly psychological. He thinks of a position toward power that repeats the infantile situation of the child before its parents:

> First of all, I believe it is beyond doubt that if we lived with the rights that Nature has granted us and teachings she imparts, we would be naturally obedient to our parents... Of the obedience that everyone has to his father and mother, with no other prompting than from his nature, all men bear witness, each for himself.[5]

If freedom is the natural state of human beings, then they must first have been defeated or *deceived* before they became servants. Through deception and cunning, people become dependent, get used to that condition, and forget that they once were responsible only to themselves: "It is unbelievable how people, once they are subjected, fall so quickly into such a deep forgetfulness of freedom that it is impossible for them to reawaken and regain it; they serve so freely and so willingly that you would say to see them that they had not lost their liberty but won their servitude."[6]

The first cause of servitude, then, is *habit*. Consciousness of freedom has been lost, servitude is handed down through the creation of legends: "People say they have always been subjected, that is how their forefathers lived. They think they are required to endure the ill, and convince themselves by examples."[7]

Yet all this cannot suffice to keep people in the state of subjects for centuries; they would rebel. Neither violence nor education nor habit can resist the urge for freedom if "bordellos" and "taverns," shallow "pastimes" did not seduce people.[8] Not compulsion, which only creates resistance, but their own pleasure is what beguiles people and makes them voluntarily forego any fight. The seduced become lonely and lose even the remainder of historical bonds. What four hundred years later, Leo Lowenthal describes as the *atomization* of the individual under terror, whose memory is actively being destroyed by power, in La Boétie appears as a kind of inner exile:

> In general, now, the good zeal and emotion of those who have retained their devotion to freedom in spite of time—though they may be numerous—has no effect, because they do not know each other. Under a tyrant they are deprived of their liberty to act, to speak, and almost to think.[9]

The final instrument of oppression to settle between the tyrant and the people is a hierarchy, "the source and secret of domination, the basis and foundation of tyranny." These are the collaborators of violence, "those marked by burning ambition and unusual greed."[10] They let themselves be hired as henchmen to satisfy their cruelty, to enrich themselves, and—just as importantly—to escape suffering and oppression themselves.[11] While La Boétie grants the victims a forgotten but not entirely lost consciousness of themselves, he sees in the instrumentalized servants of power people estranged from themselves. Precisely those who—truly voluntarily now—consciously and intentionally enter the service of dominion are destroyed as subjects; they have no life of their own anymore, they are merely "accomplices."[12]

La Boétie's explanations are obvious, and it seems incomprehensible that no others before him, his friend Montaigne for example, had the idea of studying the *psychological* causes of servitude. The idea is indeed irresistible: if tyranny is not only dominion by violence, maintained by external hardship, then we must suppose that people are servants *voluntarily*. The oppressed will have their reasons for *letting* themselves be dominated.

Francis Bacon, Spinoza, Montesquieu, Tolstoy, Gustav Landauer, and many others shared La Boétie's view. Yet the general history of the reception of his *Discours* is very much an example of societal forgetting. Indeed, it seems as if people do not *want* to know about their possible liberation. The insight is guarded in libraries as an academic treasure; there is no need to trouble oneself with physical destruction, the interests of dominion are already served by *disavowals* that deprive the theses of their political context and render them emotionally "neutral." Yet the *Discours* can only be understood as a beacon of revolution, and power has never treated it as anything else. Those who have dominion felt recognized; La Boétie's thoughts were dangerous and had to be eliminated. For if the theory of voluntariness proved to be right, if it were taken seriously, it would be in the oppressed own's hands to liberate themselves once more. The "voluntary" submission, however, does good work already in preventing its own consciousness. Despite multiple translations (into German for the first time in 1593) and repeated new editions, the study has remained as good as unknown.

It cannot be denied that La Boétie's theses are seductively persuasive: Recognize the mechanisms of dominion and be free! If you really want it, independence will succeed! The idea that we bear the meaning and purpose of our oppression within ourselves is invigorating already because it raises the prospect of a relief for which we are solely responsible. I do not, meanwhile, conceal that I find La Boétie's idea misleading. It does indeed *seem* as if people did not even want enlightenment, never mind liberation. They disavow the information that is meant to make them conscious of their situation and remind them of [their] sovereignty, and instead hold on to the notion that they are defeated by *external violence*. This prompts the judgment that people are not only idle and sluggish but also subject to an unconscious compulsion to repeat that, once subjected, makes them subservient forever.

Notes

1 La Boétie (1574) 2012, 2.
2 [Aristotle 1984, 5, §11, 1314a: 122–23. An appendix to the German translation of La Boétie Le Soldat used (La Boétie [1574] 1980) includes this passage from the *Politics* on pages 100–1.—Trans.]
3 La Boétie (1574) 2012, 4.
4 La Boétie (1574) 2012, 7.
5 La Boétie (1574) 2012, 8.
6 La Boétie (1574) 2012, 13.
7 La Boétie (1574) 2012, 17.
8 [La Boétie (1574) 2012, 22.]
9 La Boétie (1574) 2012, 18.
10 La Boétie (1574) 2012, 30 and 31. [What the English renders as "domination," the German renders as *Herrschaft*.]
11 "[A]s if they could earn anything that belonged to them, since they cannot say that they belong to themselves" (La Boétie (1574) 2012, 33).
12 La Boétie (1574) 2012, 36.

8 The search for the "subjective factor"

In 1977, two Argentinian psychoanalysts, Horatio Amigorena and Marcel Vignar, published a study entitled "The Tyrannical Agency," in which they study the psychical consequences of a military dictatorship; they reach conclusions that resemble La Boétie. The "tyrannical agency" is the superego, which becomes the accomplice of external dominion. The authors describe the changes in the inner structures under the influence of open violence:

> For totalitarian power, it is not enough to exercise repression in an outside that organizes and prescribes the norms of the life of each member of the community in great detail. Totalitarian power must impose itself violently on the inside, like an internal system of controls, hierarchies, and surveillance, and thus become the agency that structures the subject itself.
>
> This is perhaps the most archaic and most disguised form of power. It inscribes itself in an interiority that conceals it, it takes on the air of a tyrannical agency, and it acts without any apparent scandal.[1]

When power has established itself in the inner world, people are caught in a trap from which there is no escape. Open rebellion leads to death, and submission in hopes of evading the henchmen ("I submit officially to avoid having to humble myself") proves to be illusory. The psychoanalysts recognize that in a dictatorship, submission, and rebellion are no longer opposites.

In 1945, Leo Lowenthal described different means employed by a terror regime to break individuals psychically. He explains that the "interruption of the causal relation between what a person does and what happens to him" is the goal of modern tyranny. The "breakdown of memory and experience," the transformation of human beings into "raw materials" amounts to a cynical triumph of dominion. "Can one imagine a greater triumph for any system than this adoption of its values and behavior by its powerless victims?"[2]

Time and again, insight obtains the same result: through open violence, people enter into dependency, and are defeated by physical distress and by active, silent measures of dominion. Their submission is cemented by a

The search for the "subjective factor" 163

psychical mechanism: the identification with the aggressor. With the interests and goals of the rulers internalized, dependents cannot but serve a cause set on destroying them. It makes little difference whether individuals identify to protect themselves or whether the submission takes place "voluntarily" to satisfy repressed wishes. The fact is that power and terror encounter no absolute contradiction in the powerless but covert complicity.

This observation violates our sense of justice, and it is difficult to believe in the genuine existence of a psychical process that drives individuals to psychical and physical ruin. If there is a death drive, it should apply to *everyone*—except if the application of power had managed to employ for its purposes not just individual people but the psychosomatic drive as well. It apparently profits from the inclination to self-destruction while the individual is only subject to this inclination.

Psychology and history search for the "subjective factor" that is to explain what reason cannot grasp. If we do not want to believe in the eternal return of the same "coincidence" that protects dominion (for example in the notorious assassination attempts that "narrowly" fail to attain a dictator), we hope to find advice coming from psychological insights. When none can be found in the outside world anymore, looking for inner inhibitions does indeed suggest itself. While it presents itself as farsighted, the inclination to suspect "associations" between subjective and objective factors merely assumes the standpoint of dominion once more and indulges in the illusion that there might be an *interdependence* between the powerless individuals and the power potential that politics and the economy have at their disposal. The thought, however, that power after all arises from none other but the will of an individual that many follow, or from the democratic decision of many, and thus is very much a consequence of *subjective motives* and can therefore be interpreted psychologically once more, deserves notice. While it denies the qualitative leap power experiences the moment it objectivizes, it does point out that dominion is willed and made by people and can thus also be changed by people. When in the "Marginalia to Theory and Praxis" of 1969, Adorno says that "without psychology... it is impossible to understand" how "the objective constraints are continually internalized anew," "how people passively accept a state of unchanging destructive irrationality and, moreover, how they integrate themselves into movements that stand in rather obvious contradiction to their own interests,"[3] he assigns psychology a task it willingly accepts. It remembers passive longings, inclinations toward self-devaluation, the consequences of unconscious feelings of guilt, and agrees with social critique: in the long run, the persistence of inhuman dominion cannot be explained otherwise than by "subjective" factors.

There is no denying that a pulsional readiness for aggression and pulsional passive strivings shape people's inner misery. Given the dilemma of observing cruelty and passivity in comparison with the objective deployment of power that acts back on the subjects, most will bring themselves to acknowledge the insignificance of subjective factors for social development. The *psychological* insight, precisely, into the *objective* conditions teaches us that, the sovereignty of pulsional forces in the inner [world] notwithstanding, the crushing triviality of subjective efforts in historical processes and the return of the drive in an objectified form benefiting political power demand being judged by another standard than the psychological one. Those, meanwhile, who think they can reduce objective power to the lust for power and the greed of those who exercise it must soon confront a difficulty. They find themselves in the embarrassing situation of having the sadism of those who have dominion be joined by just as weighty a motive on the part of the subaltern: masochism is not just to facilitate the application of the means of power, it is to make that application seem desirable for many. I will leave aside for the moment that in such reflections, subjective and objective categories blend, pulsional wishes appear on the same level as social principles. Let's say that genuine inner forces, particularly the work of pulsional defense, introjection, and identification, first come to meet the foreign interest in hopes of a satisfaction, then include it as motives in the subjective events. Let's say, further, that the subject does not want to relinquish pleasure infantilely enjoyed and therefore now operates a transference to dominion rather than to the parents. We can even admit that the ego is unable to distinguish between the pressure coming from the drives and the seductions offered by power; indeed, it becomes manipulable in the first place because power demands something from it that its pulsional tendency has long wanted. Yet how come that in the long run, the individual does not notice the effective absence of physical satisfaction and no contradiction opens up between their wishes and reality? And how are we to understand that the ego does not at least perceive the agency of the foreign intention in its domain?

La Boétie thought of the power of seduction; Leo Lowenthal observed active, goal-oriented influence being exerted; psychoanalysis speaks of unconscious processes that repress internalization. All these notions share the idea that social power pushes something on individuals, imposes itself on them, subjects make foreign interests their own, and so on. I consider this tendency to postulate a movement that *does something to* the subject to be a wish-fulfilling illusion. In truth, rather, it is the other way around: external dominion *robs* individuals. We will see later that it diverts and exploits their *pulsional energies* unnoticed; for now, we can claim that no contradiction *can* arise in the inner world because power does not *push* anything on the subject, no foreign interest *ensconces* itself in the subject. The subject, rather, loses a piece of its inner life. It would have to discover in itself, not something foreign but something lacking, detect a leak as it were in its psychical apparatus or a defect in its emotional processes. That it does not want this, precisely, and rather holds on to the illusion that it is being given something, that something is being pushed onto it, has largely psychical causes that are founded on the repression of sexual phantasies (castration). When, therefore, it seems voluntarily to extend its hand to its submission, this happens because the subject, *artificially impoverished in pulsional intensity*, interprets the lack psychologically ("I masturbated too much" and the like), whereas dominion is capable of transforming the diverted energies into objectivized forms to supports its power. The trust and devotion a religion inspires in its followers, for instance, translate into objective power for the religion. The pleasurable illusion it offers could not be maintained if there had not been a qualitative leap from the projection of the individuals to the institution "religion." People seek a justification for the diminishing of the pulsional energy and receive from faith the hope for recompense. They attach wishes to an idea and have occasion to satisfy themselves in its name, primarily aggressively. When the idea attains objective forms, codex, tradition, and so on, it will also be able to exist without followers. Yet it has no *power* unless it is able to turn back onto the subject. What it deliberately demands from subjects is submission. It imposes itself through its representatives; not because of a decision by the latter but because it is already driven by an autonomous dynamic. The *psychical energy*, extracted from people in their engagement with reproaches and unfulfillable expectations, does not simply fizzle out "into space" but *step by step is given to religion as power*. Only this process taking place at the synapsis between the psychical and the social creates the imperceptible but *constant shift of forces* that finally appears as "voluntary" servitude.

It is paradoxical but undeniable that the very search for the "subjective factor," the search dedicated to the interest of the subject, amounts to collaborating with its oppression. It legitimizes the psychical exploitation by shedding light on one side of the coin, namely, the unconscious sources of the dependence, but leaving the other side, the invisible but energetic *objective* strategies, in the dark. Here, increase in power; there, unfulfilled hopes, increased pressure from conscience, depletion of pulsional energies, and in addition the reproach of submitting "voluntarily"—the disparity gives a sense of why it is so difficult to gain insight into these matters. It is not just shame about admitting embarrassing illusions to oneself that must be overcome, it is above all inhibitions of thought, which the objective forces, fearing for their advantages, oppose to their becoming conscious. The prohibitions on thinking, to be sure, in turn, make use of subjective conflicts, but they arise under the dominion of an external force that thereby defends the source of its energy.

Notes

1 Amigorena and Vignar 1977, 790.
2 Lowenthal 1946, 2, 3, 4, and 6.
3 Adorno (1969) 2005b, 271.

9 A little parapraxis

In the course of this study, a peculiar parapraxis caused confusion for me concerning the performances of ego and superego. In my notes, I found the following quote from Freud's *The Ego and the Id*: "Whereas the super-ego is essentially the representative of the external world, of reality, the ego stands in contrast to it as the representative of the internal world, of the id." The quote is obviously wrong, ego and superego are swapped, and their functions placed inversely.[1] The correct quote, of course, is: "Whereas the ego is essentially the representative of the external world, of reality, the super-ego stands in contrast to it as the representative of the internal world, of the id."[2] Yet the confusion is not entirely unfounded since there was a time in our lives when the superego did indeed represent *one* part of the external world, namely, shortly after its emergence, the internalized prohibitions of the oedipal rival. The *function* of the superego later remains unchanged in the restriction of the drives and thus resembles the effect of the reality opposing the pulsional wishes. What I forgot, however, is the not insignificant fact that the *contents* of the superego, too, largely remain unchanged in the course of development. The internal reality of the superego therefore cannot be identical with the—external—reality the ego is familiar with. In adulthood, too, the agency of conscience largely follows the commandments that formed it in the early stages of its emergence. Yet characteristically, the reality of the ego in the course of development acquires two dimensions: it separates into an internal reality filled with memories, phantasies, and wishes, and a second reality that stems from the perceptions of the external world. In the ego, internal and external confront each other as equals at best. The ego is able to distinguish emotional impulses and thought-images from influences of external reality. We might say that the ego makes use of internal reality to interpret the external world and to make predictions, which it needs in order to create the best conditions possible for the satisfaction of wish demands. In short, the two realities in the ego are necessary for the functioning of the psychical apparatus.

The superego by contrast only ever knows one reality, that of the infantile, oedipal conditions.[3] It reacts as if the infantile conflict situation continued to exist unchanged, and it is not even wrong about that; the infantile demands are tenaciously maintained, albeit in repressed form. The existence of the agency of conscience is internally justified only by the *continued existence of the incestuous wishes and the murder impulses*, which conscience must prevent from making contact with reality by means of countercathexis (repression energy). It thus comes no more as a surprise that the return of the reality of the superego is ardently wished for than the observation does that this reality must be distorted by anxiety. At the time of the Oedipus conflict, one has not yet had to abandon hope for one day reaching the aim of the strivings, winning the mother for oneself and depriving the paternal rival of power, [though] in turn one had to endure the daily torments of anxiety. The motive of oedipal submission is the special form of this anxiety, the idea of castration. The oedipal relinquishing of the drive takes place only under the moving impression of the difference between the sexes. This [difference] also comes to drive the separation between oedipal and postoedipal reality. The infantile conflict sets the conditions for a later choice of object and becomes the criterion for whether one will in the future acknowledge the difference between the sexes that the unconscious up to this point denies.

The superego thus has reasons enough to insist on the childhood reality. Yet what can prompt the adult ego to operate a swap? It will want to exploit a function of the superego *to gain access to areas of the inner world under a taboo*. Conscience, itself earlier a part of the ego,[4] emerged from a compromise between pulsional wish and anxiety. While it now represents the refusal, it has preserved a direct access to the repressed. As long as it denies its current conditions, the ego can participate unhindered in the superego's pleasurable wish world. If the superego can keep its strongest weapon, the threat of castration (e.g., when phantasy assumes that women, too, possess a phallus that is taken away from them again as a punishment), then the ego can refuse to believe in the difference between the sexes once more. Since for the reality of the superego, the oedipal struggles have not been finally decided either, the ego will in addition be able to deny both the defeat before the rival and the mourning the forced relinquishing of the love object has caused.

Of course, the ego has to pay a price for all these advantages. It cannot acknowledge simultaneously a former and a current reality except if it considerably restricts one of its functions, reality testing. On an earlier occasion, I pointed to the failure of reality testing in distinguishing between external and internal world. This failure was part of the intention of a coalition between pulsional wish and reality. The new diminishment of reality testing serves the ego. The *pleasure principle* demands compensation for the oedipal slights, yet the *reality principle* is not bypassed but only deceived a little; nothing is "invented," one reality merely replaces another. The pleasure principle makes use of the fact that for the ego, *the* reality has at least six dimensions. The ego is familiar with an internal and an external reality, it also distinguishes the world of wishes and phantasy from the censorship aimed at the inside, and it confronts both with the reality of internal reason. The ego must be able to judge whether an anxiety affect has the status of an emotional reaction or whether it ought to count as a warning signal from the superego.

In the external world, the ego recognizes further features; it decides whether its perceptions are qualified as "objectively real" or "apparently real," made real by particular interests.

I thus must not hesitate to admit the motive of my parapraxis. It was the wish to conjure up the past once more and to deny bothersome facts related to the establishment of the superego. Let's dwell for a moment on the superego; for our topic, knowledge of the details of its constitution is essential.

The agency of the superego emerges at the age of four or five, at the end of the oedipal conflict. The infantile wishes are repressed with regard to castration anxiety, and the internal structure, too, that operates the repression and will maintain it in the future as well, owes its existence to a defense, to introjection. The cathectical energies of the pulsional demands are withdrawn from the external world and redistributed in the inner, bound to different structures. The libidinous forces gather in the repressed phantasies and in the ego, whereas the aggressive impulses form the core of the superego.[5] The more intense the child's pulsional demand was, the stronger the subsequent narcissistic charge will be; the greater the child's hostility toward its rival was, the more pulsional charged and aggressive the superego will be. The strictness or tolerance of the "real" father can promote or inhibit this tendency only to a very limited extent. Conscience precisely does not represent the parental prohibitions but is the *internalization of one's own hostile impulses*, which evolved in the struggle with demands to relinquish and with threats. The superego thus acquires the character of one's own aggression. It also sublates in itself the form and the quality of the former conflict. The defense mechanism for alleviating castration anxiety, the identification with the aggressor, distinguishes only a part of the process.[6] With the identification, one bypasses the sense of guilt—one does not deserve punishment, has not done anything wrong, instead the father is in the wrong, and so on.

The two-fold mechanism the superego requires for its emergence is, first, the projection of one's own aggressiveness onto the rival and, second, the internalization or re-introjection of the hostile impulses. These subsequently turn against the ego as reproaches. It would of course be naive to believe the internalization of aggression to have captured the entire amount of pulsional energy. Cruelty, meanwhile, will not be content with attacking the ego with feelings of guilt. Whereas *prior* to the institution of conscience the pulsional demand was primarily directed at external objects, it is turned inward by the superego and yet in phantasy remains attached to the objects of the external world.

The superego is not in and for itself hostile to the drives. It is not simply a refusing agency but acts on the pulsional wishes like a filter: certain satisfactions remain excluded from realization, others are reshaped, shifted, put on new paths, others again urgently promoted. Among us, it is primarily aggressions directed against in the widest sense *paternal authority* that are unwelcome. Other kinds of aggressive satisfaction, anal-sadistic modalities, for instance, are not only permitted but belong to the normal equipment of our wellbeing. Aggressive impulses that do not bother authoritarian institutions but rather let themselves be roped in by them are tolerated by the superego as well. A child cursing God will be punished; a child looking down on followers of a different faith will be admonished, to be sure, but if it identifies emotionally with the religion, it will nonetheless regard those of a different faith as barbarians.

The superego forms as a reaction against aggressive strivings that at one point in the development posed a threat to the ego.[7] It subsequently becomes both a barrier to and a channel for aggressiveness. It uses up pulsional energy itself, is sadistic with the inner world, but allows satisfactions that are not directed against the parental authority or its substitute objects.

Properly considered, the institution of the superego has not succeeded in, or never had as its goal, taming the human's pulsional inclination toward aggressiveness. The main achievement of th[is] psychical agency concerns an *inhibition of aggression toward older rivals.*

I already mentioned the dilemma of the sense of guilt earlier. For conscience, it is a matter of indifference whether one transgresses a prohibition in phantasy or in the act, since the superego does not punish the execution but the disapproved impulse. The conscientious thus become entangled in all the more conflicts the more they spare the external world from their sadism. The internal result of the development consists merely in converting the infantile anxiety into the later guilt affect. Yet when we inquire into the *cui bono?* Of the process, the beneficiary is unequivocally the external authority. To protect itself, the resolution of the oedipal crisis has set up a taboo. Yet is that not a paltry, and moreover a cynical end? Are we to believe that by the very constellation of their psychical setup, human beings are destined to be subjects, destined to servitude?

If the superego does not achieve a diminishing of the aggression, merely the sparing of previously hated and now idealized objects,[8] then it cannot a forteriori impose a *relinquishing of the libidinous drive.* The child in no case "relinquishes" its wishes, but it deprives them of the quality of consciousness, it represses them. It neither abandons the claim to the object nor is it ready to change the physical (genital) aim of its wishes. The threats of the superego, though, effect a loosening of the *connection* between pulsional aim and pulsional object.[9] In the unconscious phantasies, the combination of incestuous object and sexual wish continues to exist. The internal redistribution of forces, moreover, makes use of the ambivalence of the drives and allows large shares of the libidinous strivings to go to the rival. The pulsional forces now opportunistically seek aims and satisfactions where they offer themselves. The unsatisfied forces that no longer manage to link up with the oedipal wishes thus come together in a sexual dependence on the former enemy. The defense works with the same aim; for the defense, the wishes' turning to passivity is the lesser evil over against active aggression. Finally, the external world, too, welcomes the increase in docile devotion. All of a sudden, pulsional impulse, defense, and reality agree, while the observer pondering the consequences will, on the whole, be in favor of the tender commitment to the opponent but, in the individual case, will follow it with skepticism.

Notes

1 To my surprise, other authors, too, fall prey to this tendency to confuse the functions of superego and ego. Such is the case, for instance, of Fenichel, who in discussing the "vicissitudes of the superego" cites Freud's "Introduction to *Psycho-Analysis and the War Neuroses*" and swaps superego and ego (Fenichel [1945] 1996, 109). Even Freud himself must admit, in a footnote in 1923, when he introduces the ego as "the representative in the mind of the real external world": "Except that I seem to have been mistaken in *ascribing the function of 'reality-testing' to this super-ego*—a point which needs correction" (Freud 1923b, 28 and 28n2, Le Soldat's emphasis).
2 Freud 1923b, 36.
3 For a diverging view, see Lincke 1970.
4 In 1923, Freud calls the superego "a grade [*Stufe*] in the ego" [Freud 1923b, 28].
5 At this point, I would like to draw attention to the interesting distinction Maria Torok makes between introjection and incorporation: introjection of the drives and incorporation of the object are two mechanisms that "truly operate against each other." The incorporated object marks the place, date, and circumstances under which a pulsional wish was excluded from the introjection (Torok 1968, 722). Torok here makes use of Ferenczi's much too little appreciated concept of introjection (see also above, #14n7).
6 See the discussion below, Part III.
7 Generally, we can associate castration anxiety with prohibited genital wishes. What is prohibited, however, is not the genital satisfaction in itself but the phantasies connected with it, which mainly pursue incestuous aims. When we look at the quality of the pulsional energy, we see that hysteria develops a genital anxiety from the consequences of the drive's *intensity*, whereas in masochism, the same threat arises from the *aggressive* cathexis of the genital. Castration anxiety is culturally promoted and maintained. By contrast, education transforms another fear, that of the anal-sadistic phase of development, into an anxiety pleasure. This takes the form of ideas about something being crushed inside the body or the entire contents of the body liquifying, of leaking, as it were. Through the use of the unconscious equation feces = money, both the accumulation of possessions and the defense against the fear of having to hand over something valuable can become pleasurable. The structure of the pleasure, however, is decided not by the genuine pulsional quantity but by the objective social status. The larger share of the pulsional energies opportunistically flows toward that outcome where it encounters the least resistance.
8 In analyses, we time and again observe hatred, anger, and resentment arise when such idealizations fall apart. Otherwise idealizations that are given up leave mourning behind.
9 Freud warned against conceiving of the connection between a drive and its object in too narrow terms, for example in Freud 1905a, 146–48, or in Freud 1915a, 122: "The object [*Objekt*] of an instinct is the thing in regard to which or through which the instinct is able to achieve its aim. It is what is most variable about an instinct and is not originally connected with it, but becomes assigned to it only in consequence of being peculiarly fitted to make satisfaction possible."

10 On the utilization of pulsional energy

Stephanie had to cope with a superego that demanded absolute submission from her. It mockingly attacked her for even the smallest pleasure impulse. She was unable to afford a new dress or to contradict me during a session without being plagued by severe inner reproaches. She had developed a few defense strategies that amounted to a compromise between punishment and wish fulfillment. At the time of her regression, when she could no longer train, she combined urge to masturbate and need to control by walking through town for hours on end wearing pants that were too tight and shoes that were too small. Later, the drugs helped her obey the prohibition; for weeks, she lay in bed weakened and immobile. Her wish to present herself seductively had been paralyzed by the objection of the superego. Stephanie's mother was a cold, domineering woman. She terrorized the family with various suicide attempts, was herself addicted to pills for a while, then neglected children and husband but demanded love and leniency for herself. The hypothesis that Stephanie identified with her mother is evident. Her masochism accordingly would consist in having transformed the hatred of the egotistical mother into identification with her, the murder phantasies against the oedipal rival into unconditional submission.

From the family history, Stephanie knows that she was an unwanted child. Her parents had to marry because of her. Her father was still a student, and immediately after the birth, she was given to a woman who cared for her for about a year. At the age of 14 or 16 months, the mother took her in but often left her by herself because she had to continue to work. She remembers the calming sound of the ticking clock as she was waiting in her bed for her mother to return. Another lively memory from childhood concerns a scene in the toilet, where she believes herself overpowered by the mother who is pulling a tapeworm from her anus. Associated with this is a suspicion of regularly, in early adolescence, having been genitally examined on a pretext by the mother's brother.

For the analyst, such allusions are unequivocal. In the unconscious, there are no murderous impulses directed at the mother at all, on the contrary, sexual excitation (the "ticking of the clock"), the wish to receive a penis (tapeworm) from her, and exhibitionist phantasies are being associated with her. There can be no doubt that she did not identify with the mother out of submission but out of *mourning* the loss of the ardently desired love object. (In the first case, the superego would be marked by the identification, in the second, by contrast, the ego.)

Shortly before the dream with the drum, two events took place. Stephanie had let her father invite her to dinner. He still owed her a birthday present. She had asked him for a special postage stamp, and he had succeeded in finding it. On the day of the meeting, Stephanie was very excited. She found herself of little beauty, then began putting on makeup and had the idea of painting a mask on her face, the way people in this region do for carnival. We can imagine the result: the father was horrified and ashamed to go to the restaurant with her. She was dumbfounded but accepted the rejection in mocking triumph. A few days later, the father got in touch again. He offered to mount a bookshelf in her apartment. Stephanie agreed. And this time, too, she succeeded in putting the father to flight. She managed to do her acrobatic exercises, half-naked, in his presence, such that the old man took to his heels, bewildered and excited. Stephanie thus had developed a technique for fighting her male rivals; she excited them sexually and then left them hanging. She mocked the men's narrow-minded, nonsensual attitude and thus took revenge for the defeat she had had to accept as a child. She had to prove to herself that the penis she was sorely missing in herself did not procure the father any satisfaction either.

The second event before the dream concerned a colleague at school with whom she had fallen in love. For a while, she downright courted him although he did not seem to think much of her. She chased him with letters and calls, and he remained cool and dismissive. Not with shame, as in confessing her sexual practices, but with annoyance she reported that she hardly ever feels *greater satisfaction* than when he turns her away and remains unshaken by her begging and pleading.

We need a small excursus to understand the quality and the causes of this satisfaction. Freud's thesis on masochism (prior to death drive theory) says that the masochistic superego is particularly strict and implacable. The original object of sadistic wishes has been given up and replaced by one's own ego. We would think, then, that Stephanie projected her superego onto her colleague. The satisfaction of being treated badly by him would then be nothing but relief from internal reproaches.

I would like to point out a few things in relation to these ideas. The thesis that aggressive pulsional forces can be defended against, that is, kept away from consciousness, be prevented from cathecting an action, and be invested intrastructurally (i.e., *between* ego and superego), is tenable only if two preconditions are admitted. First, the forces needed for the defense (countercathexes) and the aggressive potential invested between ego and superego must *quantitatively* correspond to the pulsional energies to be defended against or have developed a regulatory mechanism that enables a lesser force to vanquish a greater quantity. Otherwise, a quantitative pulsional surplus arises, and it will not be possible after all to prevent the disapproved breakthrough into consciousness and to the object. Second, the aggression is not simply re-introjected and turned against the ego but split into an externalized idealization (to bind the residual aggression) and a share that initially goes to the ego. Only in the subsequent defense process does the superego, through its communication with the id, gain in aggressive energies that it deploys as guilt-feeling potential. The turn against the ego takes place only when feelings of guilt and idealization of the former aggression object combine and the ego sees no possibility for insight into the originary connection between pulsional wish and reaction of the superego.

Pulsional forces stem from the id and via the ego functions push for actions on one's own body and in the external world. When they are inhibited, postponed, and kept away from consciousness, they can in the best of cases be qualitatively changed, neutralized, sublimated, and desexualized (in smaller affect-cathexes, they can also enter the ego).[1] A large amount continues to push toward reality. If this were indeed turned against the ego, the ego structure would likely be permanently damaged by an inundation with energy.[2] Even if we consider that additionally, pulsional energies are diverted to maintain the ego's own defense (countercathexes), a huge amount, compared with the forces bound in the phantasies, of pulsional energy supplied by the unsatisfied pulsional source remains. What happens with it?

In Stephanie's analysis, it is precisely this cathectic energy that she directs at me in the transference. She has positioned herself toward me as she did toward her colleague. She lets herself be rejected by me; she tries to seduce me and enjoys the frustration as "greatest satisfaction." In the unconscious, of course, it is the other way round. There, the analyst becomes the representative of the vindictively watched and hated father. In secret, she must sexually excite me and delight in my powerlessness. In the dream, however, she wishes I might satisfy her like the beloved mother. This is how she splits libidinous demands that are repressed from aggressive demands that are projected. The former experience a pleasurable hallucinatory satisfaction in the nightly phantasy, while the sadism remains largely frustrated. What does usually, that is to say, not within an analytic transference, happen with this amount of unsatisfied energy? Pulsional energy in the long run cannot remain unbound. It invests wishes in the unconscious and thereby commits itself to certain kinds of satisfaction and objects. Depending on whether the wishes are loosely or closely related to areas of conflict, the cathexis is prevented from progressing to consciousness and action.[3] The idea here is that the libidinous energies almost completely transform into pulsional wishes, whereas aggressive energies, on the one hand, also form contentual wishes but, on the other hand, build up defense structures that turn against the original aims of the drives and keep them in check. The pulsional forces, one might say, strive from the id via the cathexis of contentual wishes to the physical senses and to action.

The defense, in turn maintained by pulsional energies, represents a structural barrier that modifies and channels the pulsional flow. Psychoanalysis is familiar with a number of such barriers: pulsional postponement, cathexis defense, repression, and so on, that can intervene at different critical points of a pulsional process. One site of the pulsional defense, on the boundary between the unconscious and consciousness, may be the most spectacular—this is where a large number of the neurotic symptoms we know of form.[4] Consider, though, that the possibilities of psychical conflict are not limited to the antagonism drive versus defense. I am of the opinion that the pulsional energy itself, even before it forms contentual wishes and long before it encounters the defense, might be changed and disturbed in itself. The consequence of this would not only be very special drive processes that would have to arrange themselves with unusual kinds of strivings or excitations; the defense, too, would display peculiarities vis-à-vis the habitual, since it, too, is maintained by pulsional energy.

When we take the balance of power between id and ego into account, we will not assume that a diverted strand of pulsional energy opposing the majority of forces is able to stop and tame them. Even if we take modern regulation techniques as a model of the ideas; even if we admit that the defense occupies strategically important positions, for example, that it shields the access to conscience; even if defense mechanisms claim for themselves the advantage of affect signals (anxiety, guild, unpleasure, etc.) in the ego, they are nonetheless unable to control all the pulsional wishes rushing up simultaneously. The pulsional energies have a habit of gathering, of forming "complexes"—in therapy, we speak of the overdetermination of conflict-contents. We might admit that the defense only needs to concentrate on these conflicts and could leave other, "harmless" wishes alone. (I'll set aside for the moment my objection that there are no harmless wishes. The id will know to invest itself in all phantasies just as the superego will suspect opportunistic pulsional cathexes in every impulse.) Yet in comparison with the energies the *defense* has at its disposal, the *pulsional potential of the id* is to be considered *incomparably greater*. Panic-like states of anxiety as soon as the defense fails just a little bit, repeated pulsional breakthroughs when a pulsional wish is able to make use of the defense-energy as well, leave no doubt as to the *magnitudes*. The psychical apparatus is able to impose pulsional postponement, the superego can force repressions via the threat of castration, but *the majority of the pulsional energies that are not bound, not invested in the defense, unsatisfied, is ready to be socially utilized*. It becomes the prey of those forces outside the subject that know how to appropriate and exploit it. In a system of dominion, the *individual-psychical energy joins the means of production capital, land, and labor on equal footing*.

This fourth category is the *secret source* power draws on without subjects becoming aware. In addition to the cumulation of the other means of production, the *exploitation of the psychical resource* proves to be the most important contribution to its existence, and it is the basis of social "influence." The word "influence," of course, with obfuscating intention reverses the direction of the action. It is not the dominating that effect something in the dominated [, the dominated] are not being "influenced"; on the contrary, the dominated have their energies diverted and used up to move interests foreign to their own. In so doing, dominion makes use of the *conversion of psychical pulsional energy into the objective power of ideologies and social laws.*

I will say it again: the pulsional energy that is not satisfied and not bound by the defense, and this is the quantitatively greatest share, is confiscated without subjective intention, that is, not on the path of object cathexes and not through projection, by social dominion as a source of energy lying fallow. [Social dominion] confiscates the conversion of subjective impulses into objective power, that is to say, *the shifting in the balance of power* that appears as "voluntary" submission, yet it definitively *binds* the energy to itself by bringing the objectified forms of power, its institutions and instruments, into its possession. It is understandable that this process must take place in secret, protected from the consciousness of subjects, and that its consequences are presented apologetically, in an inverted causality.

Notes

1 It is only with skepticism that I can agree with the theory of neutralized energies and autonomous ego functions (Hartmann [1955] 1964). Insofar as pulsional energies can be "desexualized" at all, they will most certainly remember their origins and rejoin their "pulsional armada" the moment a conflict arises in the ego. Truly "neutralized" energies solidly tied to the ego, it seems, can be supposed only for the emergency functions.

2 This of course applies not only to aggressive energies; the libido, too, can turn against the ego. The ego thereby becomes a "love object" for the id (see Freud 1923b, 46).

3 Eissler remarks that pulsional wishes come with a "label," a kind of mark of origin that makes them unmistakable. He thereby alludes to Freud's phrase from the study on "Negation": judgment is an intellectual substitute of repression, its "no" a "hall-mark" of the disapproved unconscious, "a certificate of origin—like, let us say, 'Made in Germany'" (Freud 1925a, 236 [Le Soldat probably took the quote from Eissler 1962]).

4 This defense barrier is where the psychoanalytic work usually takes place. Our senses do not reach much further than the border area between ego and id. It would be more correct theoretically to count this domain as part of the preconscious, for we can only speculate about what is going on in the id. Identifying what is unconscious with the id leads to a very imprecise conception of the psychical apparatus. Broad swaths of the superego and the ego are unconscious as well, and while what is defended against—which is dynamically rendered unconscious by a countercathexis—does enter into the economic sphere of influence of the id, it cannot be considered a part of it.

11 Aggression, the difference between the sexes, and infantile neurosis

One might think that reality testing could be left to rational judgment. Reason should be able to separate the outer from the inner world, feelings from perceptions. We saw, however, to what extent the reliability of reality testing depends on the success of the oedipal conflict resolution. If the repression is insufficient and the loosening of the connection between sexual drive and object insufficient, then reality testing, too, can be corrupted. Mistaking inner and outer reality is the consequence of psychical mechanisms like identification and projection; yet it is *the condition* for foreign influences to make it into the inner world unhindered without being recognized as intruders. Insofar as the error serves the pleasure principle, reality testing fails when it comes to elucidating the origin of a perception. Reality testing is only exceptionally at the disposal of the *reality principle* such that social exploitation of the psychical energies can set in at this point.[1] Authority must first succeed in abolishing the subjective differences between inside and outside. It cannot accomplish this task with threats and manipulations, it must in every case secure the cooperation of the ego. Yet the parapraxis I described above proves just how easily the ego is ready to misinterpret reality as soon as there seems to be even the slightest chance to fulfill an unsatisfied and unconscious wish after all. Psychically, promises and seductions are much more effective than threats; they put the subject in the position of poor "Hans in Luck," who chases a pleasure and in so doing gets entangled ever more in internal guilt and dominated by foreign power.[2] Heinz Hartmann makes these connections clear. He writes in an essay on schizophrenia:

> Every neurosis adulterates insight into inner reality; and reality testing of the inside is never perfect even in the normal person (with the exception, maybe, of the ideal case of a "fully analyzed" person—if there is such a human being). In schematically contrasting what a neurotic and a psychotic would do in a given situation, Freud says: the neurotic represses the instinctual demand, while the psychotic denies outer reality. In this case, we could say that in the neurotic testing of inner reality, and in the psychotic testing of outer reality, is interfered with.[3]

To socially critical psychoanalysis, Hartmann's statement must seem extremely optimistic (if this symptom applied only to schizophrenia) or as extremely prescient: in his sense, we are all socially produced psychotics. Yet even an extensive disruption of reality testing cannot explain the masochistic symptoms. Neither the misjudging of reality nor the strictness of the superego can be held responsible for the special *conflict* from which masochists suffer. The socially relevant submission, too, is not an act that pulsional wishes or the superego demands by allying with the external power. In my view, this [submission] is rather the consequence of an unsuspected, secret energy surplus in people that, without their participation, is diverted and consumed by power. The later declaration of this process as masochism merely serves as a disguise and to reassign guilt to the victims.

What, then, is masochism?

Analytic experience teaches me that in patients who later develop a *masochistic neurosis*, we are justified in supposing that aggressive energies invaded the early ego.[4] This must have been a sudden, massive pulsional invasion with irreversible consequences that confronts the ego with the irresolvable task of finding, in no time, ways of satisfying a surplus of aggressive forces. The pulsional demand cannot be refused because the ego has no appropriate defense mechanisms at its disposal. In the cases I encountered, the invasion is to be dated to the period between the tenth/twelfth and around the sixteenth/eighteenth month, the phase that in psychoanalysis is called (following Donald Winnicott) the time of transitional objects or (following Margaret Mahler) the early practicing phase. I explicitly do not speak of a traumatic event because in this early phase of life, the structure of the triggering external situation seems unimportant to me, besides being impossible to ascertain sufficiently.

Around the age of one, to be sure, Stephanie had to cope with the switch from the foster mother to her biological mother, who then probably took less care of her. In my other analysands, however, there was no evidence of any drastic external events such as the birth of siblings, illness, object loss, and the like. What remains undoubted is the fact of a sudden and irreversible aggressive inundation in early childhood. For our purposes, it does not matter whether we posit a congenital amplification of the aggression, as Freud did in his 1919 study, "A Child is Being Beaten," or whether instead we lean toward supposing increased frustration aggressions (weaning, birth of siblings, incompatibilities with the mother, etc.). What is important is a *relative amplification, over a longer period of time, of the aggression pressure that permanently changes the relationship between libido and aggression in the ego.*

We may imagine this process in the inner world to be dramatic. The child stands at the threshold between the oral and the anal phase. The oral-sadistic impulses threaten the introjects being formed. The internal images it seeks to create when it is anxious or hungry are as it were "eaten up" by the aggressive surge. The tender bonds it was to develop in the symbiosis with the mother are loosened by a constant unease without physical causes. All newly emerging structures subsist on primarily aggressive energies. The ego becomes uncooperative and unyielding, the preautonomous superego, a preliminary stage of what will later become conscience, is vicious and full of hatred. The delicate relationship of libido and aggression in the fusion of the drives, what will later be called ambivalence, threatens to fall apart. The two pulsional strands, which usually support each other in the quest for pleasure, stand in each other's way: aggressive cathexes snatch any possibility for satisfaction from the libido, and the libido defends itself by scaling down its development and remaining passive. The ego, however, is overburdened because it is forced, without being equipped for it, to provide the energies rushing at it with space, with means of binding and of satisfaction.

For the businesswoman I have been calling "kitchen fairy," the peak of the anal-sadistic phase coincided with two unpleasant events. The family moved into a new home in the country, shortly after the mother had given birth to a boy. While in the city, the "kitchen fairy" had shared the parents' bedroom, she now got a room of her own. The little brother attracted all of the parents' attention because he was sickly and much too thin. The "kitchen fairy" consoled herself by playing in the garden with water and stones, building sand figures, and tenaciously digging in the earth for grubs, which she collected and kept hidden under her bed. It was possible to link a later acrophobia with the childhood play. Usually a good driver, she was unable to drive on roads leading across high bridges; on hikes, too, she could not cross any water, climb any observation towers. In such instances, a bodily phantasy appeared in her unconscious in colossal magnification: "down" there, where the water's flowing (the urine comes out), something terrible has happened, I don't want to look! The discovery of the difference between the sexes had fused with hatred for the little brother, with rage about the mother's unfaithfulness, and with the anal ideas acute in this phase of development. She could not explain to herself the way her sex looked other than with an idea that seems logical according to the logic of someone that age: the missing penis has fallen into the toilet bowl like a stick of stool into the water! The phantasy is not anxiogenic but on the contrary consoling, for if the missing member was lost this way, then, like stool, it could be reproduced at will; all it took was to stuff one's face. The little girl ate and ate and became *fat*. She had to learn, though, that her resolution led nowhere. The mother's pregnancy gave her two new ideas. She indulged in the idea that the shared bedroom arrangement was dissolved to punish *her* for the nightly excitations she felt listening to the parental intercourse. The loneliness in the new room seemed to her to say that it only served her right to be excluded, [since] she did not come to her mother's aid in the father's attacks. The girl now interprets the pregnancy, the mother's "fat" belly, in keeping with the sadistic idea of coitus. The father has hurt the mother, he beat her, and he stuffed something inside her that rises like the yeast dough in the kitchen. In the girl's eyes, the mother's growing girth became a source of mocking reproaches. It was as if the mother constantly confronted her: Look what the father could do to me,

Aggression, the difference between the sexes, and infantile neurosis 179

and you couldn't. Yet shame and self-reproaches were joined once more by hope. If the mother ridiculed her, became unfaithful to her, and now great changes in her body were happening, then there could only be one cause for it: the mother is in the same situation as she, also chases the lost sex, and has finally found a way to regrow one in the bile. The birth of the brother, though, taught the girl differently; neither the mother nor she had gained anything. In turn, she had to discover on the new arrival the very body part that drew all her attention. The distinction between the sexes is particularly apt at attracting aggressive energies. The phantasies about how it is that some individuals have a penis and others do not bind sadistic ideational contents and affects like shame, guilt, mockery, and ridicule. Anxiety about losing the penis, envy, and anger that arise from the thought that one might never come into the possession of a member that others obtained seemingly without effort, consume aggressive cathectic energy. All efforts to evade castration anxiety (in boys) or to compensate the lack (in girls) use up quotas of aggression. In the case postulated here that a significant surplus of free aggression must be dealt with, conflicts of this kind, which usually come to play a role only later, are treated preferentially and intensively.

The young "kitchen fairy" worked out a two-fold strategy. She increased her efforts at putting an end to the difficult situation and plotted revenge. This notwithstanding, she started denying the difference. She thought to herself that the penis is merely a bag of urine turned inside out, a kind of bladder. She herself did not have something like that because, a good girl, she always went to the toilet *in good time*. If she held back the urge to urinate, a "little sack" would quickly form on her as well. Boys, she thought soothingly, are nothing but "fat girls." She took revenge on the mother by refusing food ("I'm not accepting anything from you, even if you now tried to push it on me"). She easily outdid her brother in school and was not stingy with demonstrations of her intellectual advantages. She became independent, cheeky, bright, and distrustful.

Lying alone in her bed at night, however, the work for her really began. She had now become convinced that the missing genital was concealed *in* her body and that it was up to her to find it. She developed various tactics to pull it from nose, ears, mouth, and navel, and kept her phantasy busy with the questions of the how and the why of the current hiding place. Finally, the cathexis of the genital area with libido led to the supposition that the penis must be concealed in her vagina. She tried to liberate it by scratching and drilling, by applying various tools. It was not easy post facto to judge whether these manipulations and the injuries she sustained were invested with pleasure or instead promoted her tension. In any event, the hopelessness of her efforts must have moved her to take a regressive step. She turned to a masturbation technique she maintained almost unchanged into adulthood. She imagined she is being put on a table, naked, her hands and feet tied to the table's four legs. She is then gently pushed underneath a huge pendulum hanging from the ceiling. While the pendulum is swinging slowly back and forth above her and is lowered millimeter by millimeter, a wild animal (wolf, lion, and the like) appears at the lower end of the table, between the legs, tearing at its chain to attack her. The animal, too, is coming ever closer since every move further loosens the anchoring of the chain. She reaches orgasm at the last moment of distress by tensing all her muscles to the utmost without touching herself with her hands. (As a child she had deployed, instead of this phantasy, which recalls literary models, her being bound to the edges of her bed and, as her counterpart, the family doctor or one of her cousins.) *One* intention of this scene is easy to guess. The regression has led her back to anal modalities. The penis was to be pressed with force from the vagina, like the stick of stool from the anus. This was to be her revenge for all the defeats and the humiliation done to her. This resolution and the blend of excitation, hope, and defiance took full possession of her. While she did continue to complete school with superior casualness, she used every occasion to tense her muscles, something she did with such vehemence that for a time, it was feared she suffered from epileptic fits.

Another source of the idea suggests itself. When the girl doubts the mother's love and takes the birth of the brother to be proof of her faithlessness, then the pressing and pushing on a table is to be seen as a representation of the labor pains. The "kitchen fairy" has identified with the lost love object, the mother. By taking over the mother's pains, she tries to get her to return. Her hurtful rebellion against the mother helps her deny the mourning. She finds a late substitute for the identification when as an adult, although she does not want to become a mother, she takes care of home and kitchen like a matchless mother. This is to be seen as a compromise: she proves to herself that she succeeds in everything she sets out to do, that in her hands, everything flourishes and thrives—and must be aware every day that the one thing she really cares about is spoilt forever. The shame she feels looking at her genitals reminds her that it was she who mutilated herself. One by one, she holds her father, mother, and brother responsible for her anatomy; at bottom, though, she is convinced that she herself broke off and lost her penis during her first masturbatory manipulations. The energetic connection between the sustained aggressive cathexis of the genital wishes and the sadistic contents that characterize her masturbation phantasies makes this turn against the self-easier. The superego involves the forces available in shame and reproaches once the majority of aggression energy is used in the masturbation. This is how the adult can be seen, despite the aggressive pulsional surplus, as a friendly, sociable person.

How does it happen that she reaches orgasm not with the help of repeated, rhythmic stimulation of the genitals but by a *linear intensification of the motoric tonus of the whole body*? Did she really not touch herself with her hands only because she feared a repetition of the grave mishap? And what are we to make of each of the sadistic ideational elements? What does she need the pendulum for, and what is the "wild animal"?

One might be right to think that the "kitchen fairy" recounts only the terrible part of the masturbation phantasy and keeps the pleasurable end to herself. It might also be the case that the pleasurable share is repressed and that she could not say anything about it. Perhaps she prefers an expected punishment, in order to then enjoy the pleasure all the more unhindered.[5] Up to now, our interpretation assumes that the masochistic is not so much about relationship problems than about the consequences of the early invasion of aggression with regard to processing the difference between the sexes. What then are we to do with the information that the woman had established a warm and close connection with the analyst and was capable of creating a comfortable mood around her, something of which someone who displays *early* psychical disruptions is hardly capable? The "wild animal" must put us on the scent. At one point, the patient casually remarked that for a long time she wet her bed. This symptom, however, and the intention to be satisfied sexually "all stretched out" are to be interpreted as the return of the repressed. The aggression had become predominant on almost all levels in her life. She had become sadistic in her phantasies, compulsive and coarse in her sexual practices, the way she conducted her business was just but often harsher than necessary, yet the real *sexual wish*, the way in which she imagined genital satisfaction, was *passive*. All urgent aggressiveness notwithstanding, she had reserved for herself, in the sexual, a passive position. By necessity, one might say, for is passivity not the natural expression of the female anatomy? How is she supposed to be active when she is missing the very thing that makes sexual activity possible? We are not talking here about passive and active behavior, though, but about *genital* activity. It is not a matter of course that even in phantasy, in the sexual wish, and in the physical need, she stuck with the idea that something had to happen to her. (This tendency was already apparent in the dream reported at the beginning, where she expects *me* to be angry *at her*.) She could for example have developed a rescue phantasy, like the little girl who wants to "murder" her mother.[6] We should not hastily assign the fact to the defense or to genuinely passive strivings. Even if we found in her aggressive wishes throughout, there is nothing speaking in favor of supposing her sexual passivity to result from the aggressiveness being reversed. Insofar as it is the superego that demands the defense against the pulsional impulses, the passivity of the *sexual wish* will not simply arise from this. On the other hand, one might claim that it is an originary passivity of the *pulsional aim* that is imposing itself. Finally, there is the question of the gain in pleasure. It is not evident at first sight at which point of the pulsional process and through which phantasies the pleasure is attained. The patient cannot say anything on this point: for her consciousness, the pleasure is physical and equated with the orgasm. Yet of course her contentedness and pleasure gain are doubtful, or else she would not have gone into psychoanalytic treatment. Is it the extent of the pleasure that seems insufficient to her, or is it the means that bother her? Is it a different kind of pleasure she wishes for? Possibly she can maintain

182   *Voluntary Servitude. Masochism and Morality*

the current level only by making great internal efforts and fears for the further reliability of her forces.

Let's return once more to her masturbation phantasy. What could the "wild animal" be that threatens her between the legs? It is first a symbol of her genital wishes. The pulsional cathexis of the genital seems to her "like a wild animal," it demands, it is greedy, and it can be neither tamed nor satisfied. Let's not forget that for the patient, there is an immediate causality between her sadistic wishes and ideas and the external form of her genitals. For her, it is clear that—because of her aggressive raging in the infantile masturbation—responsibility for the loss of the penis lies with her. Now a pleasurable reversal results: Not *I* am an "animal" and have lost, due to lack of self-control, the valuable member, but *it* was evil, has bolted, it serves it right to be tied up and having to struggle to return to me, *to its original place!*

The pleasure here is supplied by different sources. The guilt defense refers to the idea that the penis is alive and has made off; not she but it itself has caused the "hole" it has left behind. We must not be surprised by the strange logic of this explanation; it is no more absurd than the idea that she had damaged herself. The train of thought is close to infantile animism, which provides all things and body parts with a will of their own. And we know that the superego will raise no objections against such justifications since it expresses its own reproaches according to an archaic logic as well. Beside the advantage of the guilt defense, there is the confirmation of the hope to once more become "complete" after all and, last but not least, the aggressive satisfaction. She is evil toward the penis, leaves it hanging, and torments it. It must endure what she is suffering from: helplessness and frustration in looking at the genital. The orgasm arises in the moment in which the lost member finds its way *back* to her. In the unconscious, the moment that seems terrible to consciousness because the "wild animal" attacks her is the fulfillment of her narcissistic penis wish. The pendulum swinging above her is a three-fold condensation: it stands for the projection of the threat of conscience, for the memory of the index finger's movement back and forth during masturbation, and equally for the familiar gesture of "wagging one's finger" at little children. It must moreover represent the rhythm of the sexual excitation that is no longer part of the physical tension.

We find that the masochistic patient who seems so dependent on external care, on the love of her boyfriend, cares exclusively about the rehabilitation of her genitals. We already observed this fixation in Stephanie, who gave the impression of being willing to die for a little love and "help." She seemed submissively to beg for love from the colleague and the analyst, and yet her dependence was not aimed at any person (no "object" in the psychoanalytic sense) but indicated her entanglement in a conflict about the constitution of her genitals. The "physicist," too, was concerned with being safe from punishment and with punishing his *fucking dog*, that is, the phallus. Whether the object dependence that is the first thing we recognize in all masochists is

Aggression, the difference between the sexes, and infantile neurosis 183

regularly to be interpreted in a similar way is something we cannot yet decide at this point.

Unwittingly, we got ourselves into a confusion of physical and psychical tension. We speak of the rhythm of excitation and call it irreconcilable with a simple linear amplification. We usually imagine the rhythmic, repeated stimulation of an erogenous zone to be pleasurable, not the maximum of a muscular tension.[7] Yet in building up *pulsional tension*, different laws apply. Since we already left the question of activity and passivity open earlier, there are a number of theoretical considerations to be supplemented here.

In the psychosexual development, aggression energies, to the extent that they are not already bound to pulsional wishes, serve to fashion and maintain the defense structures in the ego. Within the psychical apparatus, aggression has the effect of an "activity potential." The sexual drive is of course "active" as well, but the *physical aim* of unfused sexuality can be considered the innervation and excitation of the mucosa at various points on the body (erogenous zones). In this sense, the sexual aim is originally "passive." Nonetheless, even for the earliest oral stage, a libidinous satisfaction without activity is very hard to imagine. The breast-fed child must perform active sucking motions. By contrast, aggressive satisfactions without libidinous participation, such as crying or kicking are everyday [activities]. Infants' biting their lips and fingers as well as their licking their lips would be an early example of a pulsional fusion.

The *pulsional fusion* of aggressive and libidinous energies, the *normal pulsional ambivalence* is a *condition* of the pleasure principle we take for granted of course. A sudden and excessive increase of the aggression pressure has unforeseen consequences especially in the *alloying of energies*. As a first characteristic of the disorder, we can note that, where the *libido's saturation point for aggressive energies* has been exceeded, the cathexes of the libidinous object tend to split into its component parts, into "good" and "bad" objects.[8]

In the transition from passive satisfactions to active modalities (more precisely, from largely *sensorial activity* during the oral-receptive phase to also *motoric* activities during the oral-aggressive and anal phase), an excess of aggressions should have unfavorable effects as well. This is because the aggressions are preferentially invested in active satisfactions. An aggressive surplus will increasingly promote activity, while passive shares in the gain of pleasure attract no libidinous interest (no cathexis). Passive pulsional aims will be able to participate in the general pulsional vicissitude only to a diminished extent. Now, what are active and passive *pulsional aims*?

Pulsional forces that we suppose to exist separately in the id as libido and aggression *fuse* as soon as they become effective in the ego. Although they cannot deny their *original quality*, [and although] they are always ready to defuse once again, they suffer a vicissitude dictated by these conditions in the ego. The ambivalence of the drives is one of the trickiest and yet unquestioningly accepted conditions of the life of the drives.

When we speak of pulsional vicissitudes, the term "pulsional aims" keeps insinuating itself without it being clear what exactly is meant by it in each case. In the genetic development, the pulsional forces, as partial drives, successively and telescopically cathect different wishful phantasies that we call *pulsional wishes*. We thereby designate general pulsional aims of an oral, anal, phallic, and genital kind that consist in sensorial and motoric activities. We say that the libido cathects a wishful phantasy. The pulsional forces, however, also conquer *physical targets* of satisfaction, so-called erogenous zones.[9] These are initially bound to the modalities of the partial drive, later they move freely—a genital satisfaction, for example, may very well fulfill an oral pulsional wish.

The attributes "active" and "passive" in theoretical usage become "aims," which makes them prone to misunderstandings because they are better suited to designating paths of the excitation process, namely, the sensorial and motoric shares of the (wished-for) *excitation*. These paths become pulsional aims insofar as they imperatively show the wishful phantasy the way. The wishful phantasy is then described, as an abbreviation, by the wished-for course of the excitation. We speak of active and passive pulsional wishes. *Yet no "passive" pulsional wish exists: this expression labels an aggressively or libidinously cathected wishful phantasy whose physical satisfaction can be obtained only on the path of a sensorial excitation.*

Finally, the drives have *personal aims*: the self and the objects. Yet Freud rightly emphasizes that the connection of the pulsional wishes with their objects is a loose, possibly a culturally promoted one.[10] Much confusion—especially in the context of masochism—has been caused by conceiving of the connection to the objects onto which a wishful phantasy is projected as an intimate libidinous dependence. The situation is further complicated by the kind of *energy quality*: free, unbound, neutralized, defused. The kind of *investment of cathexes* is again something else. Pulsional energies can be invested narcissistically or be deployed objectally; they can be tied into structures or attached to pulsional wishes. A pulsional wish can be *conscious or dynamically unconscious*, that is, repressed. The introduction of the defense once more makes the general structure of the drives, what I call *pulsional tectonics*, several degrees more complex. Energy qualities are thus internally refracted, pulsional aims, erogenous zones, and the objects are shifted, exchanged, and condensed.

The *gain in pleasure*, finally, is composed of the qualitative excitation and the cathectic quantity of the pulsional wish, which are measured by [the qualitative excitation and the cathectic quantity] of the de facto satisfaction. The gain in pleasure is not linear[11] but defined by the perceptual identity with earlier wish fulfillments. The *pleasure principle*, of course, already accepts the excitation (that is, the actualization or hypercathexis) of a phantasy without the corresponding action; in this case, though, we will always be able to count on the psychical innervation of the erogenous zone that, as pleasurable tension, satisfies *physically*. The *pleasure affect* arises at every point of the *pulsional process* insofar as an association with conscious shares of the ego can be obtained. The affect itself most often remains *preconscious*, that is to say, descriptively unconscious.

Repressed contents and affects, everything that once was conscious but was then, in an act of defense due to the objections of the superego, withdrawn from the ego, are *dynamically unconscious*.[12] It takes a constant *defense function* to keep the repression intact against the will of the drives to impose themselves in the ego, a defense that becomes visible as countercathexis in the therapeutic resistance. The structures, the effect of the defense, the somatic pulsional sources, psychical principles, and so on, by contrast, are *definitely unconscious*. The *vicissitude of the drive* is usually determined by the repression, but the pulsional tectonics that emerged from the dynamic influence of the repression becomes itself a condition of the further development as well.

Insofar as the quality of the drives and the forces of the defense continue to harmonize, we have no reason to address anything but the *contentual conflicts*. At issue in the analytic cure are the object relations and the dynamic between pulsional demand and defense. For many neurotic developments, investigating the vicissitudes is enough, and *studying the pulsional quality* rightly seems superfluous. The consistency of the cathectic energy, the fusion of drives and its being bound to certain erogenous zones are presupposed as given and confirmed by experience. Yet how are we to establish a connection in the coincidence, in the case of masochism, of aggressive pulsional wishes with passive pulsional aims?

The early ego has certain possibilities for postponing drives, techniques of disavowal, and avoidance against internal and external dangers. Defense mechanisms properly speaking are developed only later. In the first year of life, it is most often the mother who, as an "auxiliary ego" (Anna Freud), performs the defense function and relieves the pulsional tension by means of physical satisfactions. Aggressive satisfactions are facilitated as much as libidinous ones, for example by means of biting rags, pacifiers, and toys that can be taken into the hand and into the mouth and squeezed. The dependence on objects, which is normal at this time, does not lead to anxiety but to reactions of anger when satisfactions fail to materialize. The ego learns very quickly that the anxiogenic needs come from the inner world, while satisfactions in and on the body, for the moment, take place only in the presence of an object. The anxiety affects (anxiety concerning loss of objects, later loss of love, and so on) are consequences and results of the defense (projection) against the *always primary pulsional anxiety*. This latter arises when a pulsional tension is not relaxed in time or [relaxed] inadequately. What a pulsional anxiety really is, however, what threat from the inner awaits the ego, that we do not know.

In *The Ego and the Id*, Freud points out that we do not have access to the threat that the ego seems to know: "What it is that the ego fears from the external and from the libidinal danger cannot be specified; we know that the fear is of being overwhelmed or annihilated, but it cannot be grasped analytically."[13] In "Inhibitions, Symptoms and Anxiety," he voices the suspicion that it is "excessive amounts of excitation," "economic conditions," changes of a quantitative kind that induce neurotic developments.[14] Later, in 1938, he stresses his view that quantitative differences (quantitative disharmonies in the psychical) lie at the basis of neurotic conflicts.[15] If we maintain the supposition that in masochism, the ego at the threshold between the oral and the anal phase is exposed to a *suddenly occurring and sustained aggression pressure*, then this *economic* change—*prior to* all contentual conflicts—has far-reaching consequences. With the defensive capacities remaining the same, the rising pulsional tension first prompts an increase of pulsional anxiety, which, unless additional possibilities for satisfaction are available, is immediately projected. At this point in time, it takes the form of anxiety about losing the object and of dependence on the object. The infantile split between a "pleasure ego" and the unpleasure projected into the external world, which usually makes waiting for the next satisfaction possible, is disrupted. When the external world must be charged aggressively, it can no longer be idealized; what can be expected from it is mostly unpleasure and pain. The child, however, simply cannot relinquish it because its objects must be available for the projection of the aggression. The consequence of the psychical loss of object, insofar as the object is no longer available in reality or the aggression pressure invalidates the defense, is the repetition of the trauma. The renewed absence of the satisfaction ends in anxiety about being helplessly exposed to the desires rushing in. Since the psychical site of anxiety is the ego, the early phase-appropriate dependence on the object is opposed by the wish for aggressive satisfaction. The object, however, is not the *aim* of the pulsional demands but is needed as a helper, as the *assistant of the satisfaction*. The idea that aggression must always be directed *against* someone, and be it one's own self, is something I consider to be wrong.

The excitation of aggressive phantasies is not especially satisfying because of the contents; contentual, sadistic, and libidinous-sexual wishes can barely be told apart. What distinguishes aggression is a particular kind of *cathectic energy* as well as *special aggressive-erogenous zones*. The stimulation of these body parts, among which we count the vocal cords, the hand, and the anal orifice, combined with corresponding pleasurable memories, yields an *aggressive satisfaction*. The share of the objects is secondary and becomes significant only through the connection between the physical excitation and an event in the external world. The orientation of the drive toward the objects, in which some would like to recognize the destructive intention, must not interfere with the judgment that the *aggressive gain in pleasure* consists in the excitation and satisfaction of a particular physical tension. We will have to grant aggression, similar to the libidinous development, its own modalities on the different genetic levels of maturation. In the oral, we must name as aggressive possibilities of satisfaction biting, crying, and licking. The oral mucosa, by contrast, which is stimulated by lingual movements, experiences a libidinal cathexis.

The hypothesis that libido and aggression in the course of infantile development enter into a connection belongs to the foundations of psychoanalytic thought. Freud speaks of an "alloying" of the [two] kinds of drives, whose modification entails "the most tangible results."[16] The concept of *ambivalence tension* addresses the admixture ratio of the drives within the alloy. Ambivalence is conceived as a measure for the diverging intentions, in each case, of libido and aggression. The causes of the ambivalence are usually not investigated. If there is enough evidence for the existence of ambivalent wishes, which by itself is not surprising, pointing to the contradictoriness of the life of the drives suffices. Yet it is of some interest whether the ambivalence rests on a fusion of the drives that *have not been operated* at all or is instead to be imputed to *too great an intensity* of the individual components that do not come together in a compromise. If a part of the ambivalence is repressed, the ego has not "endured" the tension. It is unclear, however, whether the discrepancy is in itself unpleasurable or whether perhaps it is contentual categories that trigger the defense. Even if the two reasons work together, the question remains unanswered why the alloying is more successful for smaller pulsional quantities and why the tension rises with the intensity of the demand. We might imagine just as well that the fusion of the drives becomes all the more reliable the greater the energetic "thrust" effected by the id is. Loving and hating someone simultaneously not only puts us at odds with ourselves, it significantly increases the emotional connection with the person concerned.

I found it useful to proceed in my reflections on ambivalence according to the following idea. Libido is to be able to connect with a quantity of aggression only within certain limits; whatever available pulsional energy does not enter into the alloy remains "unbound." The libido is granted a limited absorption capacity, a *saturation* with aggressive energy. The unbound, surplus aggression quantities, however, are to turn back on the alloy and break up the fusion relationship to the very extent to which they themselves found no use there. When the pulsional alloy reaches a certain tolerance value, when the libido's saturation capacity is exceeded, then even the ambivalence tolerated up to that point disintegrates into its component parts. Only this process allows the defense to repress one of the two pulsional components. The common pulsional ambivalence that can be demonstrated in every psychical process is thus a characteristic of the just as regular saturation of the libido with aggression. With these suppositions, we escape the dilemma of on the one hand considering the alloying of pulsional forces to be an axiom of theory but on the other hand understanding "*ordinary* ambivalence" to be the consequence of "an instinctual *fusion that has not been completed.*"[17] Only an *additional* measure of aggression results in that movement in the saturation ratio that appears as unpleasurable ambivalence tension. A burden of labor, caused by the liberated energies, is assessed as unpleasure. These energies must be bound to new wishes, repressed, or satisfied. Perhaps the turbulence in the cathexes, the process of splitting in itself, is already unpleasurable.

Finally, the unpleasure might come from what we notice first in the symptoms: the *contentual* incompatibility of the wishes. While the repression of a wish by the superego, which bases its judgment on contentual criteria, is the most consequential part of the inner movement and one that is relatively easy for understanding to access, it is likely not even a necessary condition of the unpleasure.

The degree of saturation with aggression that can be endured without decomposition seems to be a congenital variable. Not so for the degree of ambivalence tolerated by a culture, that is, endured by a conformist ego, without setting the defense into motion. The repression of a share of the emotional ambivalence, which our cultural education regards as an accomplishment, is not psychologically necessary, nor should we mistake this "achievement" for the decomposition that comes about under great internal aggression pressure. The cultural commandment is a defense process and leaves behind the tendency of the repressed to return; the defusion of drives, however, is an alarm signal for the ego.

In contrast to the dramatic processes in the inner world, the external appearance of infantile masochistic neurosis is inconspicuous. While I hold on to my thesis that in early childhood, an *irreversible shift of pulsional energies from libido to aggressiveness* takes place, it is possible to interpret the outsize aggressive pulsional tension as phase-appropriate, the withdrawal of cathexes as defiance, forced autonomous functions even as maturity, intelligence, and so on. Where the signs are more urgent, especially where the regression to orality is more pronounced, we will speak of an infantile depression.

The first problem of masochism consists in coping with the aggression quantities. When the defense cannot absorb everything, the early ego has an opportunity, not without risk and danger, to use freely floating aggressions for itself. In using unmixed aggressive energy here, instead of the usual "neutralized" energy, to build up the ego functions (for the "autonomous functions"), it forces these to develop prematurely. We might say that it appoints the mercenary army of pulsional energies as civil servants in the administration.[18] The result won't be long in coming. The aggressions promote and deal with the task of structure formation as if it were a pulsional satisfaction, and the superego will rightly suspect cunning pulsional forces to participate in the ego's pleasurable functioning and react accordingly. Part of masochists' passivity can be explained by this. What for others is association with the "pleasure of functioning" remains suspicious in masochism because pulsional aggressions are at work unabated even in the activities of the ego. The trademark "Made in Id" that all artistic productions, wanderlust, and so on bear points time and again to sadistic impulses, revenge, and combativeness.[19] Otherwise, unsuspected endeavors immobilize under the pressure of conscience. In masochism, ego functions that in other neurotic constellations are appropriated by sexual libido are the instrument of a sadistic satisfaction that is pleasurable and thus worthy of repression. The loss of activity and joy of life that masochists experience in the course of the oedipal conflict can be traced to the newly emerging difficulties. The superego first opposes the pulsional cathexis of the ego functions and deprives these of their energetic basis. Yet it was precisely this *aggressive cathexis of the ego* that largely compensated for the disruption in early childhood. We owe it to the binding of aggression in the ego, that is, to the fact that it makes those disposed toward masochism seem bright and carefree, that despite the early point in time at which the trauma occurs, the infantile neurosis unfolds without pathological symptoms.

Notes

1 See Lowenthal 1946. Freud repeatedly pointed to the task of reality testing, which by no means corresponds to a simple rational judgment function. Its position vis-à-vis the "reality principle" is like that of a ship's compass to the current of the water. "The reproduction of a perception as a presentation is not always a faithful one; it may be modified by omissions, or changed by the merging of various elements. In that case, reality-testing has to ascertain how far such distortions go. But it is evident that a precondition for the setting up of reality-testing is that objects shall have been lost which once brought real satisfaction" (Freud 1925a, 238). "Since memory-traces can become conscious just as perceptions do, especially through their association with residues of speech, the possibility arises of a confusion which would lead to a mistaking of reality. The ego guards itself against this possibility by the institution of reality-testing, which is allowed to fall into abeyance in dreams on account of the conditions prevailing in the state of sleep" (Freud 1938b, 199).

2 [See Grimm (1812) 1983.] Lu Xun (pen name Zhou Shuren) has his famous sad hero of the tragedy of the 1911 revolution in China fool himself and transform every humiliation into a "moral victory": "And yet within ten seconds, Ah-Q had set jubilantly off on his own way. He was now the top self-abaser in China, and once you'd discarded the inconvenient 'self-abaser,' you were left with 'top'" (Lu [1921] 2009, 86).

3 Hartmann (1953) 1964, 201. [The reference is to Freud 1924b.]

4 Freud's original theory went toward understanding masochism as a defense product of sadism [see above, I.9, esp. #67]. All authors (Theo Reik, Wilhelm Reich, Ludwig Eidelberg, Wilhelm Stekel, Kurt R. Eissler, Fritz Morgenthaler) agree that in one way or another, masochists are caught up in an aggression problem.

5 Such is the obvious thesis of Theo Reik in *Masochism in Modern Man*: "The shifting of the psychic accent from the original instinctual aim to the threatened punishment solves this riddle... . No! He does not enjoy pain, but what is bought with pain! He does not strive for discomfort, but for lust that must be paid for with discomfort" (Reik [1940] 1941, 191).

6 See above, Chapter II.2.

7 This seems to be so "natural" that I cannot find in the literature any reference to our distinction. *Erotic beating and whipping*, too, happens rhythmically; a single stroke is not felt to be pleasurable. Some masochistic practices (strangulation, compression), however, indicate just this preferred *linear* increase of a tension.

[Today's sexology confirms Le Soldat's observation on the different forms of increasing physical excitation as much as it does the differentiation of physical excitation and psychical experience of pleasure. The linear increase of excitation by tensing the muscles corresponds to the earliest mode of excitation available to the baby for regulating states of tension. See, for example, Bischof 2008, 1–2.]

8 According to Spitz 1962.

190 *Voluntary Servitude. Masochism and Morality*

9. I do not agree with the view advocated by Hartmann, Kris, and Loewenstein that aggressive satisfaction does take place in specific zones (1947, 33). Starting from an experiment Eissler conducted, I think that in the course of [psychosexual] development, aggression, too, cathects preferred body areas, namely the mouth, later the hands, the feet, then the entire muscle apparatus (see Eissler 1938). Traces of these aggressively cathected zones of the body reappear in preferred kinds of suicide: poisoning, shooting, jumping to one's death, and so on.
10. Freud writes in a footnote in *Three Essays on the Theory of Sexuality*: "The ancients glorified the instinct and were prepared on its account to honour even an inferior object; while we despise the instinctual activity in itself, and find excuses for it only in the merits of the object" (Freud 1905a, 149n1).
11. [A summary of the results can be found in] Moser and Zeppelin 1973.
12. Eissler (1974) holds that under specific conditions, direct communication is possible between the repressed id and consciousness. Kris ([1950] 2000) on the contrary thinks that what is unconscious "can reach consciousness directly only by a pathological detour" (Eissler 1962, 26n26). Freud says, on the "Question of Lay Analysis," that "if the ego is in possession of its whole organization and efficiency, ... it has access to all parts of the id ... For there is no natural opposition between ego and id; they belong together, and under healthy conditions cannot in practice be distinguished from each other" (Freud 1926b, 201).
13. Freud 1923b, 57.
14. Freud 1926a, 130.
15. [Freud 1938b, 183–84; see the quotation in this volume, #114.]
16. Freud 1915a, 122–23, 1920, 53–55, 1923b, 42, 1933, 104–5; the quotations are from Freud 1933, GW 15, 111 [the English translation elides the word *Legierungen*, "alloys"—Trans.] and Freud 1938b, 149.
17. "The question also arises whether ordinary ambivalence, which is so often unusually strong in the constitutional disposition to neurosis, should not be regarded as the product of defusion; ambivalence, however, is such a fundamental phenomenon that it more probably represents an instinctual fusion that has not been completed" (Freud 1923b, 42).
18. The designation "mercenary army" comes from Freud. [It is unclear which passage Le Soldat has in mind here. As Le Soldat herself does earlier (#), however, Paul Parin compares aggression to a mercenary army; see Parin [1973] 1978, 191 (Le Soldat quotes a different part of this passage above, #).]
19. See below, note #284n56.

12 The principle of the death drive

Between two and four years of age, the "physicist" underwent a mild infantile depression.[1] The causes could not be found. He refused to eat and grew very thin. His mother, then a very youthful, cheery woman, called him "listless." She had married a second time, an older man, set back by a bankruptcy and a car accident but striking for his beauty. The patient was the only child from this union but had to share the mother with three siblings from the first marriage. The woman did not find happiness. She tenderly dedicated herself to raising the children and took care of herself and the home with devotion, but when the "physicist" was thirteen years old, she left the family. Before that, she had been writing poems and tried to make a living that way; when that failed, she urged the patient to engage in literary production. He, however, was only interested in physics. He wanted to know "how substances belong together and react with one another," "why a plane can stand still in the air," and "whether it isn't possible after all to calculate the area of a circle with complete precision." He was a cheeky, curious, and intelligent child with a phantastic capacity for immersing himself in a problem. School gave him no trouble, but when he should have taken up university studies, ambition, and curiosity suddenly left him. He muddled through the exams and abandoned his studies before the doctoral examination. He found employment in a lab and vehemently fell in love with one of the barely sixteen-year-old apprentices. Already as a child and in adolescence, he had felt attracted exclusively to men. He had fallen in love countless times and then dissolved the relations in exhausting scenes of reconciliation and renewed conflict. By the time of his first "great love" for the young man working on a project with him, though, he had become suspicious and fearful. The former curiosity was alive only as a jealousy with which he tormented his lover. He drank a lot. He squandered his money and accused the friend of stealing from him. At this point, he was living with his mother again. From this time, he reports a masturbation technique. He had practiced it already as a child and later changed it only a little. He took panties from his mother and sat down at the desk to work. He wrapped his penis first in the panties, then in a piece of paper, finally he put a plastic bag over it and masturbated with the left hand while with the right hand, he wrote down physical calculations. As a child, he asserted, he was

DOI: 10.4324/9781032666273-29

having no phantasies doing this. Later he was thinking of accidents, plane crashes, natural disasters, and the like. He let a later lover force him into marrying the lover's sister. The boyfriend threatened to leave him otherwise. The mother welcomed the marriage for "religious" reasons although she knew about her son's homosexuality. The father did not attend the ceremony. A few months after the wedding, the mother suffered a cerebral hemorrhage and died. The patient held the father responsible for her death—he did not take care of her and had her taken to the hospital too late.

The "champagne dream"[2] was followed by memories of the death of the mother. She died, [he said,] lonely *as a dog*. He would like to abuse the father like the guy in the dream, everything is the father's fault, he took his mother from him. Why is she dead and not he? I for my part, though, interpreted the dream not as fulfillment of death wishes but as conditioned by the anxious idea that he could lose his penis and that the analyst would reproach him for his constant sexual excitation. I saw the dream's wish fulfillment in the exhibitionist bragging. But I now understand that this phallic triumph is blocked by the identification with the mother, whom the analyst/father treats "like a dog." The ambiguity of the allusion is quite justified, since the "physicist" loved his dog more than anything and was with him day and night.

The "physicist's" masochistic symptom is to be interpreted not as submission and not as dependence on an *object*. The young guys, from whom he puts up with everything, are projections of his penis. When these withdraw from his love and he, if he really wanted, could make them stay, he is struggling against his acute castration anxiety. In his phantasy, both father and mother were closely related to castration: the father as perpetrator, the mother because she put up with "that" coming from the father. (The reproach that the father killed the mother appears as the displacement substitute, which can become conscious, of the idea that the father castrated the mother.) Since both parents are "contaminated" by the thought of castration, they cannot serve as love objects. The "physicist" can only love himself, more precisely: he can be concerned only about the intactness of his most important body part.[3]

The manifold associations of the "physicist" on the subject of death provide us with one more occasion to appreciate the link Freud established between masochism and death drive. Perhaps there really is a more direct path to masochism than the one we have discovered. Freud once even speaks of "people who are complete masochists without being neurotic."[4]

The claim made here that masochism is a neurotic disorder contradicts Freud's thesis that masochism is a direct derivative of the death drive and a genuine, regular, and unavoidable motif in the psychical. I consider the death drive theory to be a necessary consequence of psychoanalytic reflections. The theory of the drives and the concept of the unconscious, thanks to which psychoanalysis can rightly claim to have contributed to elucidating the conditions of human life in the first place, do not work without death drive theory. I thus have no choice but either revising my view that masochism is a neurotic development or proposing to liberate masochism from the burden of having to serve as evidence of the death drive.

The linking of masochism and death drive emerged not from clinical insight but in the course of a theoretical reflection. Freud in *Beyond the Pleasure Principle* did not want to present his theory as a "speculation." In a young science, speculation is only reluctantly tolerated, even if it means nothing but a doctrine's theoretical consequence that, although evident, cannot be proven. The supposition of the process we call primary, too, is a speculation. Yet it is so familiar to us that we would not think of seeing it as a *theoretical* construction; without its help, we would hardly be able to work therapeutically.[5]

I will show later that the effect of the death drive, too, can be made evident clinically without having to depend on masochistic symptoms. In my view, the association of aggression and death drive is dubitable as well. In the current form of theory, the origin of aggression is to be sought in the death drive; aggression appears as a derivative of the death drive. However, although death factually *entails* the destruction and annihilation of the living, the *metapsychological* articulation of death in any other form than as the *abatement of pulsional energies in the id, followed by the collapse of the ego structures*, is a romantic idea that hypostasizes the anxiety about our own destruction. Death appears to the subject, for itself or in observing others, as destruction: a life is annihilated, relationships broken off, works, and ideas ruined. Under the influence of anxiety and pain, we project aggressive impulses onto the end. The *phantasies* surrounding death are undoubtedly destructive and sadistic ones. But the *process* in itself can be called neither pleasurable nor painful. Subjectively, death is not a destruction but the ceasing of the life-functions. In assessing this banal fact, psychoanalysis should not be deceived by projections.

Death drive theory arose as the negation of an illusion. Freud turned against the anxiety-sparing idea that death is foreign to life itself and [that] when we die, we yield to an external compulsion. He says, "the aim of all life is death," and because the lifeless preexisted the living, the drive that is seen as "an urge... to restore an earlier state of things" must be a death *drive*.[6] This, however, is inherent to life and emerged *ab ovo* in the coming to life of the inorganic.[7] If we are willing to accept the psychoanalytic axioms, we will have to admit this consequence as well. In the psychical, just as in the physical, there is a *development toward death*. Sexuality, pulsional satisfaction, and the pleasure principle, too, ultimately serve the death drives; in *Beyond the Pleasure Principle* and in *The Ego and the Id*, Freud awards them the right to rule over the Eros. The quest for pleasure must impose itself against the death drive and wrest from it its share from the energies gathered in the id.[8]

So far, there will be little doubt about Freud's insights. However, it is far from obvious why the death drives should express themselves in the form of destructiveness. Of course, the *subjective assessment* of death is largely one of a hostile process, yet to the extent that we refrain from evaluation, the *subjective moment* of death must already be considered to be the extinguishing of the life-functions. I therefore propose defining *psychical death* as the abatement of the pulsional forces in the id. The death drive hypothesis thus postulates an impulse in the id that reverses the direction of the drives, pulling them back from the ego and the external world into the id. As a result of this tendency, a counterimpulse to increase the formation of structures in the ego initially forms, *but ultimately the abatement of the pulsional energies effects the collapse of the psychical structures*.

Likewise, aggression is to be liberated from its being bound to the death drive, the destructive and sadistic strivings are to join the sexual libido. Aggression and sexuality are the pulsional types whose appearance and effect *obey* psychical principles. Pleasure principle and reality principle are the two basic rules all psychical processes must follow. I think we understand Freud's death drive theory better and avoid a number of contradictions with other parts of metapsychology when we conceive of the *death drive not as a pulsional force but as a principle of psychical processes*.[9]

Death drive, pleasure principle, and reality principle are thus three *restrictions* with which the action of the pulsional forces, sexual libido, and aggression must comply. Where the psychical is concerned, the presupposition of the pleasure principle is uncontested; the necessity of orienting the inner processes by the conditions external reality posits leaves no room for choice either. Insofar as the death drive opposes the libido (the "Eros") and not the pleasure principle, the *theoretical* consequence is the coincidence of death drives and destructiveness. This conclusion is promoted by the projection that death is a destructive process. Yet if the death drive expresses itself in the pulsional forces slackening and ultimately faltering, then it cannot simultaneously pursue the aggressive satisfaction of its own destruction wishes. If destructiveness is a pure pulsional pleasure, then new, previously unknown, or unnoticed indications of the death drive's action must be found.[10]

The *principle* of the death drive is justified by yet another fact. Neither in the material nor in the psychical can we conceive of a force whose effect would not be limited by a counterforce. In every dynamic process, antagonists prevent the process from quickly converging in a stable point. The intention, it seems, never was to *suppose* the destructiveness of pleasure principle and reality principle, yet for theory, the assumption of an antagonism between pleasure principle and death drive makes death drive and pulsional *defense* coincide. That is a consequence we can in no case approve of.

In what follows, I'll undertake a small excursus and for that purpose assume the standpoint that the "ego" is not merely a psychical agency or structure but that the term also designates an *economic ensemble* or an energetic system. The totality of forces effective in the ego at a given point maintains a relationship with the economy of the superego (which I'll neglect here) as well as with the energy "reservoir" in the id.[11] The theory conceives of the pulsional forces as a demand to work from the id to the ego. It sees the energy quantities flow from id to the ego. It thus assumes a dynamic in which the id sets the conditions and the ego must process the consequences. This model is reinforced by the genetic development insofar as at birth, the ego is only a disposition and must wrest its forces, form, and orientation from the id. I have already proposed elsewhere, however, to conceive of the dynamic relationship between ego and id in the sense of a mutual *gravitation*. There is nothing we can say for the moment of the effect of the ego's gravitational force on the id. The gravitational effect of the id on the ego, by contrast, appears as *pulsional tension* and as the *tendency to form structures*.[12] While the pulsional tension in the ego can be understood as resulting from the attraction the greater source of force in the id directs at it, the phenomenon in the ego to establish and extend structures throughout its entire life must be attributed to another impulse. For the psychical, psychoanalysis assumes a fundamental *tendency toward integration*. Although Freud in a short note from 1938 ("Splitting of the Ego in the Process of Defence") shed doubt both on the constant inclination of the ego and on its capacity for integration, clinical practice today assumes that *under all circumstances*, the ego tries to mediate between divergent strivings, operates condensations, and works toward compromise solutions. We acknowledge this tendency in the ego and count it among its gravitational forces. A compromise solution for an internal conflict indicates that the ego has been able to assert its position over against the id. When the ego actualizes the defense forces—and it does so in every pulsional process as long as no traumatic situation arises—it opposes the pulsional demand with an inversely polarized impulse; when the ego combines divergent strivings, that is, when it condenses simultaneous pulsional wishes, adjusts superego prohibitions and ideal prescriptions, and considers conditions of reality, this activity requires an impulse in the ego that runs counter to that of the pulsional energy—even if the ego makes use of pulsional energies to carry out its work. In both cases, it can rely on its own gravitational force. Yet insofar as the ego initiates a satisfaction, its impulse will go in the same direction as that of the id; id and ego as it were offer the pulsional forces a *channel*. Although this appears to the observer solely as the result of the intention of the id, centrifugal forces of the ego participate in the wish fulfillment. The ego here gets rid of its energy, it transforms ego forces into so-called hypercathexes. We normally notice nothing of this contribution to satisfaction; only once the death drive temporally stretches the processes in the ego or the quality of the pulsional energy changes for masochism does it become clear in the more frequently occurring *divergent tendencies* that we previously did not pay enough attention to one part of the causality.

The centrifugal impulses in the ego ensure that the ego can keep itself alive economically without suffocating in structures. In every pulsional process and in every single perception, including inner perceptions, the ego is not only forced to take up new structures, but it also binds these to itself thanks to the effect of its own gravitation. The periodic slackening of its force of attraction, or rather already the rhythm of the forces in the id (the "death drive") makes it such that the ego can operate introjections, dissolve structures, and promote aggressive hypercathexes in the first place. The cathectic displacements or pulsional defusions occurring in this context must not be misunderstood as a defense in the service of a satisfaction. They are themselves pleasurable wish-fulfilling processes of phantasy. The internal situation in this peculiar satisfaction, which arose via divergence and must yet be ascribed to the gravitational effect, can in no way—excepting its genesis—be distinguished from the one that goes back to an immediate impulse of the id: the phantasies relating to a conflict receive a hypercathexis, and the ego can get rid of an unpleasurable tension without this giving rise to anxiety. After this process, though, the pulsional energy appears not as an addition to the repressed, nor as repression energy or in the object cathexis, but bound to the ego as "narcissism."

Assuming gravitation between the agencies thus leads to the claim that there are forces at work that are opposed to the drive. This *centrifugal* effect ensures that the ego does not from the outset drown in the disproportionately larger source of the id. If the pulsional tension in the ego is the direct effect of the id attraction, then the centrifugal force of the ego is to consist in the pulsional *satisfaction*. While the drives themselves do urge their fulfillment, we must postulate a tendency in the ego that not only effects the postponement (defense) of the pulsional demand but shows [the pulsional demand] ways and means of relief. The tendency to establish structures, in turn, especially of the superego, which thus counts as part of the ego's energetic domain, is due to the direct effect of *ego gravitation* as well. In building and consolidating its structures, the ego protects itself from being appropriated by the id.

Let's look at the situation in detail. We might still accept that formations of structure testify to the effect of general ego energies, but it seems improbable that *pulsional satisfaction*, too, should be the consequence of a force anchored in the ego. This objection is easily countered. The task the drive poses the ego is of a psychical, not a physical kind. The aim of the drives, by contrast, is always physical satisfaction. The psychical stands between the origin of the drives, a physical longing, and their aim, a satisfaction in and on the body; the psychical is initially suitable to securing the physical satisfaction and to obtaining repetitions of pleasurable stimuli, but very soon—to the extent to which the ego forms—it becomes the site of psychical gains in pleasure. The pulsional tension demands as far-reaching a cathexis as possible of the *phantasies* with pulsional energy. We recognize the result of this invasion in the "pulsional wishes," energy-charged complexes of shares of memory, cognitive, and hallucinatory contributions. We must not be deceived, however, by the fact that physical satisfaction, too, is categorically and "pulsionally" demanded. To observation, it appears as if the drive itself dictated the fulfillment of the wishes; meanwhile, we overlook that the suspected effect of a greater force covers over the *direct consequence* of a lesser function. It is always the ego that demands, imposes, and implements the *physical* fulfillment; it thereby seeks to evade the invasion of the inner world by the pulsional energies. Every pulsional satisfaction leads the psychosexual energy back to where it comes from: the somatic. When the physical satisfaction of a pulsional wish appears as the intention of both forces, of the id gravitation

The principle of the death drive 197

as well as of the centrifugal ego tendency, responsibility for leading judgment astray lies with a coincidence of something effected with a genuine force. The id gravitation, that is, the drive, *expresses itself in the ego* not as an impulse in the direction of the id but as an urge that strives away from the psychical toward relaxation in the body. Engaging more closely with the problems of delineating ego and id, we will see in the criterion of the preconscious in particular that the energy flow is not unambivalent. The apparent direction of the drives results from a *countermovement* in the ego that absorbs the impulse, that is to say, the energy of the id gravitation. This [countermovement], however, comes with an orientation of the centrifugal force of the ego and covers it up because its energy quantity is several times greater.

We now understand better why the drive cannot be contented with a physical satisfaction of whatever kind. It is bound to the body only by its origin (the id) and of necessity by the *content* of the phantasies. But it is an exclusively psychical factor and thus knows only psychical fulfillment. The pulsional aim in the narrow sense thus consists in the unhindered cathexis of the inner world with pulsional energy. The cathectic economy of the ego by contrast demands the discharge of the energies via the abolishment of a physical displeasure. Pulsional satisfaction, of course, does not succeed directly here either but via the relaxation of the somatic pulsional source, which in turn prompts the psychical pulsional pressure to subside for a brief moment. In the psychical, however, a satisfaction is recorded in no other way than through the pleasure affect and the subsequent reaction of the prohibiting agency; the pulsional tension continues unchanged because no relief has occurred at its origin, the id gravitation.

Let's now risk taking a further step in this speculation. If we believe the ego is capable of centrifugal impulses, then similar forces for the id won't be long in coming. It was possible to expect the understanding to recognize the ego's gravitational effect in structure formation, that of the id in pulsional energy, yet the *centrifugal forces in the id* put our imagination to a hard test. That is because they are perceptible to the ego not thanks to a decrease of the pulsional pressure but on the contrary thanks to an increase in the id's demand [that the ego] work. How does this come about? In our elaborations so far, we have left aside an important factor: time. Neither the ego nor the id is temporally unlimited configurations; they have a beginning (in intrauterine development) and dissolve at the moment of death. If the ego fulfills its function by forming structures, that is to say, constant units of energy bound to a purpose, then it will in the course of development reach a degree of saturation of possible structure formation. We cannot believe that the possibilities for the continued formation of the ego, which is ultimately a *biological* entity, are limitless. And just as the ego succeeds to some degree in setting up a structure, after which this setup ossifies and falls apart again, so the id, too, will have to endure changes in old age. (The timelessness of the id *contentually* stands in a different context, and "death wishes," too, are not characteristics of the aging of the id.) We must imagine the processes in the id that correspond to the collapse of the ego structures as a kind of implosion: *the pulsional forces collapse and withdraw into the id, and finally withdraw from the psychical as such*. This effect can in no case be attributed to the gravitational forces. For if the id were to cave in under the pressure of its own force, the drives, then this would be observable in the ego being inundated by drives and subsequently in a dissolution of the boundaries between ego and id. Only once we assume a process in which the id gets rid of its own forces, that is to say, on the condition of a *centrifugal impulse* can we expect the sought-for effect, the subsiding of the pulsional pressure. The abatement of the pulsional energies appears to the ego as a reversal of the pulsional direction and leads to the dissolution of the structures that have become useless.

Now, here, too, we should not let ourselves be guided by the wishful thinking that likes to shift phenomena of decay to the end of life. Destruction and death in that case seem to belong together. Our train of thought, meanwhile, suggests, first, that *the destruction of ego structures and the fluctuation of the pulsional pressure are everyday phenomena that are intensified and extended at the moment of biological death by the cessation of the somatic pulsional source* and, second, that *psychical death cannot be considered the consequence of aggressive pulsional strivings*.

When in 1920, Freud constructs the urge toward death as a drive and not as a principle of the psychical, he considerably mitigates the difficulty of his idea that life, psychical life as well, carries the motor of its own annihilation within itself had imposed. Death is represented again as an aim of the life of the drives, a nasty aim, but still something *striven for*. Our reason defends against such an absurd, unpleasurable striving, yet at least death stands before us as the object of the life of the drives and does not *dispose of us*. Activity is delegated to the unconscious drives that cannot be controlled by the ego, but it is still situated in the psychical. Dependence is what humans seem to endure the worst, and always and everywhere they look for possibilities to disavow it. Freud repeats, albeit at a higher level, as negation of the negation, the wish inversion that seven years earlier, in "The Theme of the Three Caskets," he had so brilliantly interpreted.

In this [earlier] work, Freud spells out why the motif of a possible choice between three sisters, three questions, three caskets, keeps returning in myths and in dreams. He explains that the choice is never a "free choice, for it must necessarily fall on the third if every kind of evil is not to come about, as it does in *King Lear*." Freud continues: "Lear carries Cordelia's dead body on to the stage. Cordelia is Death. If we reverse the situation, it becomes intelligible and familiar to us. She is the Death-goddess who, like the Valkyrie in German mythology, carries away the dead hero from the battlefield." In granting the aged and dying man a choice, a wishful reversal takes place. "Choice stands in the place of necessity, of destiny. In this way man overcomes death, which he has recognized intellectually."[13]

We find ourselves at the end of our excursus with a burden and with a theoretical relief. Psychoanalytic insight is unable to change anything about helplessness in facing biological death. No death drive and no destructiveness can promote our own death unless they name biographically conditioned, contentual wishes. On the other hand, we have acknowledged the *principle of the death drive* in the psychical; we see in it the *condition of an everyday quality of pulsional processes: the fluctuation of pulsional pressure*. (We will have occasion in part III to place what our theoretical speculation here has yielded in a context that is closer to experience.) At least we succeeded in liberating masochism from a heavy and foreign duty. For if aggression has nothing to contribute to the functioning of the death drive, then masochism is exonerated as its crown witness.

Notes

1 See above, II.3.
2 [See above, #98.]
3 By object choice according to the "narcissistic" type, we understand love for persons that in the unconscious phantasies represent the subject itself, its earlier or wished-for self, or parts of it, in particular, in masochism, the idealized genital spared by castration anxiety.
4 Freud 1928, 179.
5 In the theory of science, speculation is very much acknowledged as a necessary and fruitful step in the process of insight (see "Spekulation" in Klaus and Buhr, eds., (1964) 1972, vol. 3, 1027–28; Kuhn [1962] 2012).
6 Freud 1920, [38 and 36]: "It seems, then, that an instinct is an urge inherent in organic life to restore an earlier state of things which the living entity has been obliged to abandon under the pressure of external disturbing forces; that is, it is a kind of organic elasticity, or, to put it another way, the expression of the inertia inherent in organic life."
7 "Eros, which seeks to force together and hold together the portions of living substance. What are commonly called the sexual instincts are looked upon by us as the part of Eros which is directed towards objects. Our speculations have suggested that Eros operates from the beginning of life and appears as a 'life instinct' in opposition to the 'death instinct' which was brought into being by the coming to life of inorganic substance" (Freud 1920, 60–61n1). Natural science is unlikely to embrace the notion that death prompts a transformation into the inorganic. After death, the organism decays into carbon compounds as well.
8 Freud 1920, 62–64; Freud 1923b, 42–46.
9 The *principle* of the death drive is not identical with the "Nirvana principle" Freud adopted from Barbara Low, which aims "to reduce, to keep constant or to remove internal tension" (Freud 1920, 55–56).
10 See below, III.1.
11 Freud 1938b, 150–51.
12 "Pulsional tension" names an economic process. The tendency to form structures, by contrast, is a function of the energetic relationship between ego and id. The economy of the drives as I understand it here is concerned with the quality and the vicissitudes of the psychical cathexes (pulsional energy quantities), while the postulated gravitational forces describe the tensions between the structures.
13 Freud 1913b, 300, 301, and 299.

13 Masturbation technique and anxiety signal

The peculiarities of masturbation in adulthood are variations, developments, and repetitions of the technique pleasurably practiced in childhood. The way in which one masturbates is defined by wishful phantasies; yet since these must be considered compromise formations of pulsional wish and defense, the fastest way to understanding the unconscious demands is to interpret the technique, that is to say, the physical action, the way we interpret a neurotic symptom. The masturbation technique contains all impulses of the original wishes in condensed form; every detail of the physical manipulation must lead, via associative links, to the central conflict. That is the reason for the particular interest we have taken in the intimate practices of the "kitchen fairy," the "physicist," and the "acrobat." If neither the theory, nor, accordingly, clinical observation allows us to make headway on the question of masochism, then we must keep to the obvious, to the transference process. "Transference" refers to the relationship that arises in the course of a psychoanalysis between analyst and patient. This relationship develops a peculiar dynamic: it repeats the infantile conflict. We have had to realize that despite the warm atmosphere masochists know how to generate around them, the projections are not of an objectal kind but always concern the genitals alone. The *curiosity* about the genesis of one's genitals, about the difference between the sexes, and about the anatomical constitution of the analyst dictates the entire course of the transference. The analyst, too, is swept up by the curiosity and must guard against getting into the kind of excited search for the "lost member" from which their patient suffers. On the other hand, they can make use of this same actualized sexual curiosity to track down the scheming neurotic conflict. The details of the masturbation practices reveal themselves in therapy only after years of meticulous work on the resistance. Patients conceal their intimate actions like a secret treasure, and we are quick to show consideration for shame and discretion. Yet the following teaches us how right masochists are to protect their sexual practices as a *valuable* secret.

Early infantile masturbation allows the maturing ego to postpone the fulfillment of the pulsional wishes. When the satisfaction is opposed by external obstacles or the wish internally induces anxiety, the pulsional quantities are shifted to phantasy, and a satisfaction-like action is performed on the body.

Infants lick their lips or suck at their pacifiers, excite the anal zone with their fingers, and so on. The cathexis defense, an early protective mechanism in the ego, is the psychical counterpart to infantile masturbation; together, they free consciousness from the bothersome pulsional energy. Unlike later defense movements, the cathexis defense is not directed at demands with reprehensible contents but merely at an excitation quantity felt to be overpowering. While it does become visible in the object cathexes, which diminish proportionally, it is not directed against them but rather at the *intensity* of the internal excitation.

We have postulated an invasion of aggressive pulsional quantities, more precisely, a shift in the admixture ratio of the drives due to surplus aggression at the end of the first year of life. We have further claimed that a masochistic development arises only if the increased aggression pressure and thus the disparity between the two kinds of drives endures. Yet what happens with the surplus of aggressive energy that cannot become ambivalent [by fusing with libidinal energy]? A part, we suspected, will be used in the construction of the defense. The cathexis defense, too, is contaminated by the aggression. It is charged with pulsional energy and ready at any time to detach from the union of the ego. It would thereby give up its defense function and would rejoin the pulsional forces striving for satisfaction. In that case, however, the ego's first weapon against the supremacy of the drives has become unreliable.

In the infantile masturbation of the anal and early phallic phase in masochism, the ego is forced to defend against the pleasurable sadistic phantasies. There is no reason to suspect the psychical system of defending against *everything sexual*. In masochism, the hostile strivings at this time are subject to greater defense than libidinous [strivings] not because they would be more embarrassing or more prohibited but solely because of their *greater quantity and intensity*. In the preoedipal period, then, an equilibrium emerges in the ego in which defense formations and unconscious phantasies are aggressively charged. The ego fears not so much the particular content of the phantasies as it does the repetition of the traumatic situation: the aggressivization of the pulsional energies and the loss of the possibility of pulsional alloying.

We understand that the pulsional strength could be the first cause of the anxiety; too great an intensity annihilates the ego structures established for the defense and renders the ego helpless. Yet the qualitative change in the drive (concerning its capacity for alloying), too, leaves a powerless ego behind—powerless, this time, not before the id but over against the external world—because the libido that aggression has left withdraws sexual satisfaction from the ego's influence and exposes it to the whims of the objects. Usually, that is to say, in other neurotic formations, aggression serves the defense against embarrassing libidinous wishes, or a part of the aggression is used to defend against another part that is bound to a disliked wish. Censorship in that case takes offense at the wishes' reprehensible content. For masochism, however, we recognized the primary pulsional danger to be the *quantity of the energies*. This quantity is experienced in the ego as pulsional intensity and remains a threat, no matter whether it attaches to impulses with a harmless content or to prohibited ones.

We must, of course, ask why an aggressive pulsional invasion would be such a terrible thing. After all, although we make use of metaphors from physics and energetics to describe the psychical and have no other way of expressing the relationships between ego, id, and superego beside dramatic concepts,[1] it is not the case that the ego is literally "inundated" and disempowered, washed away by the pulsional forces. What, then, are we to make of the *anxiety*? Why does the anxiety affect have such an effect not only on the ego but on the entire psychical apparatus?

We have no justification for our view of pulsional inundation as unpleasurable and anxiogenic other than a habit of thinking. In truth, an aggression invasion would mean at most that the ego would have to unconditionally place itself in the service of the pulsional satisfaction. Even if from our conscious vantagepoint we are used to attributing a striving for freedom and an urge for independence to the ego, with which we like to identify, doing so does not go without saying. The ego, precisely, does stand in the service of pulsional satisfaction. Nor is the pleasure principle an option for explaining the effect of the anxiety because the pulsional *satisfaction* would in itself be pleasurable. Reality at this point in time cannot have any serious inhibiting effect yet, [since] at [this] early stage of development, reality testing is still controlled too much by the pulsional wishes themselves. We must thus suppose that *the prospect alone of a pulsional satisfaction of the most intensive kind has an anxiogenic effect*. Why, we cannot say.[2]

Possibly, this phenomenon has to do with the earliest experiences, when pulsional energies were indeed capable of ruining young, still unstable ego structures. Perhaps quantitative factors play a role as well. We would then have to attribute to the pulsional forces a capacity for amplifying and replacing each other in a kind of chain reaction once the bounds of defense have been crossed unhindered.[3] It also appears evident to us that a pulsional storm cannot take place without temporal limits. Every observable pulsional breakthrough (think, for example, of anorexics' binge eating) is exhausted in timespans we measure in minutes, half an hour at the most. But who says that the ego has the ability to estimate a temporal process of this magnitude?[4] Our rationally acquired ability to deal with the dimension of time can of course be no model for the automatic functions in the ego. The *anxiety signal* that occurs when rejected, embarrassing contents storm back into consciousness, by contrast, is clearer. It would indicate an unpleasure to be expected, warn against the reaction of the superego, and thereby protect the ego.

We must admit we're groping around in the dark here. The ego seeks to avoid anxiety and unpleasure and therefore stands in the way of an *intensive* pulsional satisfaction. It does so "voluntarily," that is to say, without being compelled to refrain [from satisfaction] by either external force or the objections of the superego. The only motive of the self-restraint seems to be the anxiety affect. The unpleasure that thus arises can obviously not be conjured in any way. *When* a pulsional demand is judged to be too intense presumably depends on congenital factors. The anxiety that controls the automatic functions in the ego is measured by temporal variables, by an *expected rhythm of the variations of the pulsional tension*, that are unknown to us. We do not know whether the ego is afraid of too long a period of helplessness or instead of the endlessness of the pleasure. We can only, *post festum* as it were, confirm that the aggression invasion in early childhood was anxiogenic. As "natural" as this fact may seem to us, we have no explanation for it. Let me emphasize once more, though, that the anxiety can in no case be traced back to the quality of the pulsional energy (the aggression). The *automatic anxiety* does not give preferential treatment to the aggressive pulsional component; as a quantity, [the aggressive] counts as much as the libidinous component. The superego's assessment of the content as well as the subsequent *anxiety signal* concern the phantasies cathected by the pulsional energies and are thus completely different from the affect of being overpowered by the drives.

The problem of self-destruction needs only brief treatment, since the aggression is not "directed" *against* the ego but demands satisfaction *from* the ego. The fulfillment of aggressive wishes in phantasy, however, is by no means destructive but rather—for the structures to which the energy is bound—neutral. It is recognized as pulsional and therefore as dangerous only in the *interpretation* by the superego or in reality testing. From the psychical point of view, the *physical satisfaction* of the aggression cannot simply be seen as threatening since it merely consists in the stimulation of special erogenous zones. [What can count as threatening] for real anxiety is the perception of the reaction triggered by the wish fulfillment in the external world and in the objects, while for automatic anxiety it is the destruction of ego structures, which, however, is caused not by the aggression but by a great quantity of pulsional energy, whatever its quality.

The structural binding of the aggression, which we must stipulate for masochists in the second and third year of life, relieves the ego and cannot be recognized as a symptom. The cases I am familiar with, to the contrary, are characterized by unusual precociousness. The children quickly learned to talk and to walk and had no bigger problems in toilet training. The pedagogical success is an effect of the pulsional force invested in the ego functions. The children appear independent, autonomous, and bright. Yet behind the manifest surface, a neurotic development is making headway. Its first *hidden characteristic* is that in every pulsional process in the ego, libidinous and aggressive strands separate such that the *ambivalence seems to decrease but in reality increases.*

The ambivalence perceptible in object relations or the narcissistic cathexis of the self-derives from the admixture ratio of the pulsional components. We experience an impulse as ambivalent when libidinous and aggressive intentions can be pursued simultaneously with it. Usually, the ambivalence generates a tension. Ego and superego cannot endure or tolerate the simultaneity of love and hatred. A share of the pulsional striving is repressed.

In the unconscious, though, it remains intact as an element of the original wishful impulse, makes its demands, and is always ready to advance toward consciousness and the motor system. When one pulsional component is defended against, the decrease of the ambivalence will rightly be considered deceptive. The repression, however, leaves a clear symptom behind: *the ambivalence tension*. Yet this, precisely, is lacking in masochism. There, the disentangling of the drives is an automatic process and does not come about under the influence of the superego. As soon as there is a constant excess, that is to say, as soon as the admixture ratio of the pulsional component has shifted in favor of aggression, every new pulsional demand must express itself in that form as well: in the cathexis of a wishful phantasy—which is always a *hypercathexis* in addition to already existing energy—the aggressive component is no longer able to join the *saturated admixture ratio*. Yet neither is it able to remain free, and it will try to detach the energies already bound from each other.[5] As the result of an economic chain reaction, *polarized cathectic quantities* arise *that attach to one and the same wish without fusion*.

The ambivalence tension is usually founded on the difference between consciousness and unconscious. The repression-intention and the tendency of the originally alloyed pulsional components to reunify collide. This presupposes the axiom of pulsional fusion. It remains in force unchanged in masochism but, secondarily, due to the saturation tolerance, [the fusion] is broken up. The superego does not respond to the intention to alloy (which [albeit intact] no longer [constitutes] an economic automatism) with repression; it saves itself the laborious defense and takes recourse to *isolation*. The tension thus appears not between consciousness and the repressed but between two parts of the same wishful impulse. Instead of, for example, the erotic component of masturbation being conscious while the sadistic is repressed, both remain intact but are associated each with different pulsional aims and erogenous zones. Thus, the perception of the genital is cathected libidinously, that of the hand aggressively, or the other way around. Nor does the masochistic superego tolerate any simultaneity of love and hatred. Its effect thus amounts to a *definitive prohibition on masturbation*.

When the "physicist" came into analysis, he was already the father of two children. He had not given up his homosexual ties, he depended more than ever on the favor of his young lovers and beside that lovingly cared for his two sons, Roy and Elmar. He regarded his wife, whom he had married under constraint, as a "sister and companion," and it was obvious that in his unconscious phantasies she had taken the place of his deceased mother.

But he was much more fascinated by his children and by the chase for his young friends' reluctant love. Roy, his elder son, was dreamy and passive, Elmar, the younger son, was a bold, bright, cheeky little kid. The patient insisted on imposing his own notions of his children's inclinations. Thus, Roy was to do sports and attend children's groups, while Elmar was to draw and make music. In this tendency, the "physicist" identified himself with his mother, who had once planned for him a career as a poet. We find a predilection for conducting experiments with people, for working out long-term life projects for others, while remaining "altruistically" waiting and passive oneself, a kind of "sacrificial attitude," in every masochistic constellation. It is usually suspected to be a reaction formation against egotistical strivings, that is to say, an identification with the victim of one's own aggression. Here, however, the situation was different. The prospect of Roy getting a raw deal in life, of being taken advantage of by others, filled him with rage. He also imagined the danger, though, of Elmar becoming a good-for-nothing and enjoying only empty amusements. He managed to arrange his time with the children in such a way that he never saw Roy and Elmar together. The sight of the two children together triggered in him a feeling of embarrassing annoyance. He tried to explain this impulse to himself and concluded himself to be the culprit. He was cheating on the children, on the one with the other and on both through his love for Z., the lover; he was convinced his sons were jealous of each other and each for himself angry with him. He therefore began setting the children against each other and wanted to find out which of the two was more attached to him. The patient had constructed in his object relations a complete arena for projecting his internal battles. He tried to observe the irreconcilability of the psychical forces and was on the lookout for possibilities for rescue. Yet all that ever took place was a repetition of the original conflict. The mother and Z. belonged together; his wife, the sister of his first boyfriend, had an (incestuous) family claim as well as, thanks to her anatomical "lack," a prerogative over the boyfriend's virility. Because of the oedipal taboo, he had to stand between the two. Since for him, the boyfriend is the incarnation of his penis and the wife attracts the former feelings for the mother, he must simultaneously try to bring the two together. He cannot endure the woman's penislessness, which reminds him of the prospect of castration; he wants her to have a "boyfriend" the way he does. Only as a "phallic woman," that is, as a person who is a woman and a mother and nonetheless possesses a penis, could she be a love object for him. Yet his oedipal longing to defeat the father has won out over his castration anxiety. Probably amplified by the aggressive charge of the life of the drives I postulated, the triumph over the rival had greater weight. With the marriage and the existence of the children, the corpus delicti of the tabooed sexual relationship, he was exposed again to castration anxiety; the superego was raging internally and had to find an external object: the analyst. He subsequently shows her that the disavowal of the death of the mother, passing over death and oedipal taboos fills him with satisfaction and pleasure, that under no circumstances he is willing to relinquish it, but that he demands from the analyst/father/superego to stop, once and for all, threatening him with castration. To that end, the "physicist" had already come up with a kind of deal.

He began moving away from his older son and devoted himself exclusively to the little Elmar. He forced the child to take piano lessons, bombarded him with philosophical problems, and had fits of rage when he showed little interest. He thereby provoked in the boy anxiety attacks and dramatic revolts.

206 *Voluntary Servitude. Masochism and Morality*

In the analysis, he had positioned himself toward me as passive and submissive. As a "good boy," he wanted to gain my sympathy and avoided any allusion to the fact that I am a woman. In this situation, he reported a second dream:

> A wastewater treatment plant, a kind of fish farm. Elmar has drowned. I must rescue him. I jump into the lake, the water is dark and slimy. But I get him out. He is still alive and breathes softly. ... Then I hear voices mocking me, Elmar is dead or not yet there (not yet born?); they say I exaggerate.

His strategy was easy to see through. The "wastewater treatment plant" is, of course, the analysis; it is simultaneously to be a "fish farm." In the manifest dream, he wants to save his son Elmar from drowning. Since we are already familiar with the unconscious equation rescue = kill, we can try the hypothesis that the "physicist" wants, in reversing the oedipal intention, say, murder his son. Yet there is no evidence for such a tendency. A connection with the "acrobat's" rescue phantasy only leads to the supposition that the patient wants to have sexual intercourse with his own son, for which there is no basis either. We remember, however, the peculiar "games" he played with his children: now he wanted on no account to see them both simultaneously; now again he set them against each other; finally, he kept Elmar for himself and plagued him with excessive care. The children served him to project his ambivalence. Thanks to his passivity, Roy, the older son, was particularly suited to personify for the unconscious the intense sadistic impulses, whereas little Elmar was to protect the erotic sexual strivings. That the two could not peacefully get by is only too understandable. But not enough with this. Just as in his masturbation technique, the aggressively cathected hand is denied direct contact with the stimulated penis, so Roy, the representative of the aggression, is not to meet with Elmar, the *projection of his member cathected with passive libido*. The consequence would not be, in analogy with the feminine phantasy, a self-castration but the *resuscitation of aggressive phallic impulses*.

When in the dream, the patient suggests to the analyst pulling "Elmar" from the water, to *"farm [züchten] fish,"* he is trying to provoke her into taking over the function of the "aggressive hand" and to "discipline [züchtigen]" him, that is to say, to *masturbate him*. The castration he fears from the analyst/father would thus be transformed into a violent-pleasurable satisfaction. He has in mind here not only the sexual gain in pleasure, but he also creates at least two additional advantages for himself. The masturbation rids him of the embarrassment of having to deal with the sex of the analyst: did her "Elmar" "drown" in the wet, slimy milieu of the genital? Just the theoretical possibility of a missing penis inspires him with panic. On the other hand, the prospect of her/him being equipped anatomically the way the father once appeared to the little boy is rejected as impossible ("exaggerated, it can't be that way"). Knowledge of the true state of affairs finally wins when he threatens the analyst with scorn and mockery ("they're mocking me") should she want nothing to do with the demanded satisfaction. The second advantage consists in a ruse. If the analyst accepts to watch over "Elmar," the *passive genital*, here in the form of *the dream*, then he becomes free to indulge in the pleasure of satisfying his *aggressively cathected penis* in duplicate, on himself and projected in the person of his lover, and at the same time of having insured it against the threat of castration.

In masochism, the overpowering aggressive quantities prompt the sexual cathexes to become passive and conquer important parts of memory and of phantasy for themselves. That is why the contentual conflicts are defined less by the relationships of external reality versus psychosexual strivings conditioned by maturation than, rather, by the opposition between the pulsional wishes appropriate to the phase of development and the energetic situation, which can no longer be corrected. The little girl accuses herself of having destroyed her genital with the intensity of her sadistic wishes, the boy fears that the aggressive cathexis of his body, especially his hand, renders the impending *self-castration* unavoidable. Both can neither relinquish the masturbation nor escape the onslaught of aggressions. Beside the disentanglement of sexuality and aggression, a new divergence arises between *aggressive phallic wishes* that must be projected and are *idealized* in the object, and the *passive sexual wishes* bound in one's own body. The latter are the target of the remainder of aggression that cannot be projected and takes the form of *debasement and mockery*. The defense measures, however, are exposed to attacks from three sides. The defense is invalidated when the pulsional pressure increases further (through somatic changes); external obstacles, for example, the revocation of habitual possibilities for satisfaction, shift the balance back in favor of unbound energies. Finally, we must address the question of the gain in pleasure. So far, and for good reason, we have omitted the examination of the *pleasure quality under the conditions of masochism*. We will no longer be able to avoid that task. How are we to conceive of a psychical gain in pleasure that arises on the condition that aggressive pulsional forces conquer the sexual wishes for themselves and largely abandon, not the sexual aims, but the libido, to repression?[6]

Before we can begin this work in Part III, we still have some way to go in clearing up technical details. We have spoken of the disentangling of the two kinds of drives and in so doing overlooked that the split-apart pulsional strands display a strong tendency to reunite. What naturally enters into a reliable alloy does not like being split again by an excess of one of the components; in the masochistic constellation, too, aggression and libido strive for unification. Yet by pulsional economic necessity, masochists are condemned to *actively*, via the defense, get this split-up of their wish cathexes going again, which once had traumatically initiated their neurosis. The constant excess of aggressive pulsional energy threatens the already scarce bonds of sexual libido with the wishes. To preserve a certain quality of the pleasure, masochists must prevent this by all means available. Whenever his ambivalent impulses come together, the "physicist" increasingly deploys projections. He takes a new sadistic lover, signs up for analysis, to assert his phallic integrity, or devotes himself to his son Elmar, to succor his libido, which has become powerless. Yet what looks like the *defense* against an ambivalence of sadism and passive inclinations that has become unbearable is the goal of the defense. Masochists' ambivalence tension, in other words, is not the cause but the wished-for consequence of the labor of defense.

Such a thesis must astonish and require further justification. To that end, I will draw once more on the discussion of masturbation. Normally, that is to say, in other neuroses, the masturbation phantasy fulfills ambivalent wishes. The impulses usually revolve around the oedipal conflict, simultaneously enjoying sexual pleasure and celebrating the aggressive triumph over the rival in condensed form and via compromise solutions. The superego is given its due by having final say in the fashioning of the ideas and by always settling the process with elements of punishment and unpleasurable affects. Yet the cathexis of the erogenous zones of the body, too, is ambivalent; the penis is the target of equally aggressive and libidinous energies, and the vagina bears active and passive cathectic shares. For masochists, however, both the phantasies and the body-cathexis split into their constitutive parts. Passive pulsional aims associate with the *sensory erogenous zones* (the mucous membranes in mouth, genital, and anus, as well as the entire surface of the skin), while aggressive impulses pursuing active aims cathect the *motoric erogenous zones* (tongue, eye, hand, penis). The phantasies follow the diverging body-cathexis, where persons—and sometimes fetish-like objects, too—must represent individual energy quantities or the body parts these have conquered. While we might initially be inclined to think of a regression of the pulsional modality—there was indeed an early phase in life where such a sharing out of the body among the kinds of drives was nothing unusual—we quickly learn that this is not about shielding a pleasure from the objection of conscience by disassembling it into its constituent parts. On the contrary, masochists build up the pleasure by once more bringing together in phantasy those body parts that, thanks to the cathectic situation in this very medium, had become *untouchable* for each other. The pleasure thus generated is purely *psychical*, and we will have occasion later to address the *cessation of physical satisfaction* in masochism.

The ambivalence conflict and the curiosity mentioned earlier have a common denominator: shame. Hysterics accuse themselves, compulsive neurotics expect punishment, and masochists are ashamed. They do so obviously and ego-syntonically or are contraphobically cheeky and ostentatiously impertinent. *Shame* always arises as an unpleasurable affect in the ego, not when phase-appropriate phallic wishes are frustrated (which would trigger anger and anxiety) but when the *exhibitionist cathexes split apart into their constituent parts*. Shame is the anxiety signal of the phallic phase. It functions as a connection between polarized ego shares that here are cathected libidinous-narcissistically, they absorb sadistic energies. For the wish fulfillment, shame is the signal that sets the defense into motion. In that regard, it is a predecessor of the later guilt affect.

We might also say that shame is a form of unbound aggression that appears in the ego of the phallic phase; it appears intrastructurally and is thus a by-product of pulsional satisfactions whose gain in pleasure prompted (because of the cathectic energy's saturation tolerance) pulsional defusions. In the preoedipal period, the signal effect of the unpleasurable affects anxiety and shame develops an ego function that is no longer merely a limit for the drives and not yet entirely conscience. (Thus, when in masochism primarily shame or anxiety instead of guilt become visible, this is the consequence of a complex economic process and not the symptom of an extensive "regression.")[7]

For quite some time during difficult phases of the analysis, the "acrobat" would come to the sessions wrapped in scarves and wearing dark sunglasses. One day during summer, she showed up in a pretty, very low-cut dress. Content with the progress of our work, I let myself be carried away and remarked that I found the dress pretty and that it suited her very well. The effect of the compliment was devastating. Drowning in tears, she told me that just before the session a woman in the street had called her a whore. She had not expected that I too would insult her. Annoyed and angry, she left me.

What had happened? The transference had reversed. When she felt neglected and ugly, when she let herself be rejected by her boyfriend while she idealized the analyst, she operated a split and tripartition of her sexual wish in a manner similar to the "physicist." The aggressive impulse was projected onto the man, the analyst was to administer the intact and unattainable phallus, and she herself was identified with the debased vagina and the genital strivings that had become passive. The projections, on the one hand, made her helplessly dependent; on the other hand, they reliably protected her from anxiety and shame and became guarantors of the hope that, by conquering the analyst, she may yet come to possess the member she had lost through her own fault. For months, the supreme goal of all her efforts had been to seduce the analyst by any means, through eroticization, with reproaches, via pity, and so on. On that day, then, she had attempted a *recathexis*. This attempt aimed at once more internalizing her phallic-exhibitionist wishes, which she sought to trade in for the projection of shame. Therapeutically, the cathexis displacement was very welcome and had been prepared by binding the shame to the analytic process. She thus wanted nothing further than to be looked at and admired by me. The feared aggression, too, seemed to be conjured for a moment, absorbed before the session by the scolding stranger. My clumsy remark brought the whole thing down. Because I did not silently endure the demonstration of her ability to endure a pulsional tension, it seemed to her as if my intervention was an expression of envy, irony, and schadenfreude. Immediately, she once more transfers sadistic impulses onto me, and the surge of shame and mortification indicates the renewed breakdown of the ambivalence, this time provoked by me. The pulsional strands separate again and are projected onto different people. I become untouchable for her, she is angry "as hell" and starts taking pills again. Through the regression, she defends against the mortification I caused with my sober remark—instead of a ravishing declaration of love—but she takes the opportunity to distribute the cathexes anew. Up to then, the analyst was the representative and bearer of the idealized penis; she is now deprived of power and turned into the projection of the angry and helpless ego. In the transitional act of a short fit of addiction, she brings the physically impossible together: she takes her genital in her mouth. For her, the sickly sweet pink pills that "poison" her are associated with the wish that the analyst genitally satisfy her with her tongue. Her memory of having been licked in childhood by a kitten, of course, appears as a mystification of the past. The shame in recounting does not concern the real, erotic content but what is thereby repressed and obscured: the perception of her vagina as a hungry cat of prey that immediately devours everything that comes near it. This idea of castration goes back to the aggressive-sadistic cathexis of the vagina that as it were "devoured itself"; because of its greed, it immediately annihilated the budding phallus. The repression was initiated by the superego, which does not tolerate embarrassing objectal wishes. The shame, however, arises from the insight that a *constant aggressive cathexis of the female genital cannot succeed.*

My remark that she made herself pretty for me is understood by her as phallic boasting. That I point her tendency to seduce out to her while she was ready to internalize the idealized aggressiveness once more is something she can only understand as a scornful reference to her greedy, albeit passive, sexuality. For her, who above all believes her superego, her sexuality has become passive because, through her sexual greed, she has mutilated herself. Her inner censorship insists on the association of sadistic phantasies, aggressive cathexis of the genital, and castration. In truth, though, the aggressive cathexis of the vagina is unstable only because *the alliance with the motor system preferred by the aggression finds no physical correlate.* Women's labia only have limited movement, the vagina none at all. At the phallic stage of development, the constant aggressive cathexis of the male member, too, is fragile because activity focuses on the erection, a process not subject to voluntary movement. *Male phallic shame* therefore does not attach to the *lack* of a body part but to insufficient *virility and erectile function.*

I mentioned in a different context that a *memory trace* is required to form a wish in the psychical. A pleasurable wish fulfillment can succeed only insofar as a *perceptual identity* with earlier satisfactions is produced. The ultimate goal of all internal movements and redistributions is to open up access for the pulsional energies to the erogenous zones and to reinvigorate perceptual identities. Yet what is to happen with those pulsional forces that from the outset find no or only a very inadequate erogenous zone to satisfy their demands? No one will seriously claim that *anatomy* and not the *id* is what determines the drives' original quality. Such a thesis would amount to the statement, first, that women and men have genuinely different pulsional constitutions and, second, that the somatic pulsional source, that is, the origin of the id, depends on the external form of the genitals and is not conditioned by the connection between the psychical and the body in general.

It is thus not possible to hold anatomy responsible for the quality of the pulsional wishes, yet a seemingly "natural" female inclination toward *genital passivity* cannot be denied. How are we to explain this contradiction? Of course, there are difficult conditions for other pulsional qualities and body relations as well; in the anal phase of development, for example, activity finds its physical correlate in the muscles of the entire body and of the abdomen in particular, while the libido cathects the sensory mucous membrane of the anus. Pleasurable perceptual identities (defiance, negativism) arise when in phantasy, the two kinds of cathexis meet again. But for the genital phase, that is, the post-oedipal period, theory supposes a gathering of all pulsional components for cathecting the genital. To gain clarity in what follows, we must also mention that it is not a *region of the body* as such that is cathected but the *psychical perception* (representatives) of it. Basically, any given perception could be cathected with any kind of drive, yet the bond of the energy soon disintegrates when there is no corresponding perceptual identity following up. (The cathecting of a *wish* by contrast requires no pleasurable physical perception.) As far as the male genital is concerned, its psychical perception lends itself to being cathected with both kinds of drives: in masturbation, it binds passive energy components, through its erectile function, active demands. Male genital wishes form on the basis of constant cathexes of the corresponding perceptions; in this case, pleasure is hindered merely by contentual criteria, that is, when the superego erases the association of a cathexis with the perception again. (The repression, to be precise, does not eliminate the relationship itself but detaches it by means of an energetic operation, the countercathexis, from the preconscious phantasy compound.) In the "phallic" phase of development, the pulsional excitations for both sexes strive toward the genital but they encounter a different anatomical situation. The particular situation we find in masturbation affords a rather good opportunity to study the genesis of the phenomena of *penis envy and castration anxiety* that are unavoidable in the life of the mind.

When at the age of about four, little girls seek to invest their aggressive energies in genital wishes, the condition of their vaginas, insufficient for this purpose, confronts them with a difficult problem. To a limited extent, the labia and the clitoris can be cathected aggressively; for the corresponding binding of sadistic energies to the perception of the vagina, they must regress to anal or oral modalities. We observed in the "acrobat" how she sought to accommodate her genital aggressiveness successively in a defiant charging-up of the body's muscles, combined with anal sexual phantasies, and the idea of "vagina dentata" (the "cat of prey"). The perception of the surface of the skin, especially of the mucosa, refuses to be cathected aggressively. The members, sense organs, and muscles in turn are constant targets of aggression. There is a particular reason why the regression to orality can be cathected aggressively although the oral cavity has nothing to offer beside mucosa. The *oral erogenous zone* comprises the inner surface of the oral cavity but also the lips, the tongue, the vocal cords, and the budding teeth. The *current* perception of the vagina refuses the aggression, while the *regression* permits the sadistic cathexis of the tongue or the teeth that take the place of the penis being missed. In this way, a perception hallucination emerges, a "phantom member" *in* the vagina that is able to absorb the hostile impulses as long as the regressive pulsional change is maintained. Aggression finds a similar way out in turning back to anal modalities: the content of the intestines (the stick of stool) is identified with the penis and takes over the aggressive cathectic quantity.

Yet what we know as "penis envy" is the consequence of a further defense-movement. The absence of the physical correlate for the phallic cathexis has triggered anxiety. The pulsional energies that up to this point have always found a *physical target* for [their] satisfaction are now unable to discover a perceptual identity suitable for binding. Earlier, unpleasure and anxiety stemmed from the intensity of the drives or the absence of satisfaction. Now two new kinds of unpleasure set in: fear of the superego (guilt affects) and the existence of "free" aggression that cannot be bound permanently. In the economy of masochism, the *quantitative* burden especially plays a role. If "penis envy" consists in the defense against free genital aggression, then this effort must be particularly hard for women masochists who already suffer from an aggressive excess. The defense movements we summarize in the concept "penis envy" succeed only half-heartedly and remain unreliable. The sublimation, the distribution of the genital aggression across the entire body ("beauty"), attempts at restitution in the choice of object, and acting on one's body (disease, pregnancy, etc.) are unable to deploy the free cathexes to increase the gain in pleasure. While the female masochistic character forms around the problem of genital aggression, masturbation techniques and phantasy bring out efforts at compensating for the physical lack. In the case of the "masochistic character," the ego forms according to the conditions of the particular pulsional vicissitude and becomes itself a neurotic symptom; in masturbation, by contrast, penis envy is the means by which the conflict is to be spared a neurotic development.

For male children, the process is no less precarious. The observation of the difference between the sexes awakens ideas about how and why one might lose the penis. The shock caused by the sight of the "castrated" woman, of course, is not a sufficient cause for establishing an anxiety that won't diminish for the rest of one's life. The economic conditions of the phallic phase and the oedipal conflict, however, also converge in a state of genital anxiety that the perception of the other sex has helped to prepare. For more information, we once more turn to the pulsional economy in masochism, since the displaced emphases within the libido promise a plastic picture of the process. The common ambivalent cathexis of the genital does not allow the castration anxiety to become virulent until the oedipal age. When, in keeping with their degree of maturity, children polarize their objectal wishes, directing the predominately libidinous shares at the mother and the sadistic ones at the father while most of their attention focuses on the genital body zone, two effects ensue. First, a strand detaches from the genital pulsional aim that signals the demand to be masturbated by the mother and to penetrate her genitally; beside this, the wish arises to assail the father, too, with the penis, with the intention of killing him (to pierce through him, beat him to death). Both aims, however, unite to form *castration anxiety*. The idea of the penisless mother recalls the possibility of one's own castration, and the phallic attack on the father demands revenge according to an archaic principle: the phallus wanted to kill him, the phallus must go. There is no way to escape the dilemma for little male masochists either; they, however, must struggle with an additional difficulty. The cathexis of their genitals is predominantly aggressive: in opposition to girls, they have no trouble finding the physical correlate for the genital aggression; we must suspect, rather, that the unbound energies left behind by the preoedipal development now tend to cathect perceptions of the penis. The particular kind of the aggression, however, entails that the physical satisfaction does not amount to a relaxation. I have already taken a stance on the relationship satisfaction on the body versus pulsional satisfaction and can thus be brief. Both as regards the pulsional tension and as regards physical excitation, the aggression takes a peculiar course. After the satisfaction, the libido is silent for a short time, pulsional tension and physical excitation need a noticeable amount of time to reestablish themselves. The aggression tension, meanwhile, recovers immediately after the satisfaction. Under the conditions of normal ambivalence, such phenomena are not observed. The course the tension of the libido takes seems uniform, and there is no reason to search the sexual excitation for two kinds of rhythm. Masochists' unsuccessful and obsessive masturbation, however, suggests that the *aggressive satisfaction of the body* is a near-impossible task to accomplish, that, in any case, the sadistic excitation regenerates much more quickly and enduringly than the erotic. Normal masturbation has a different quality, it primarily serves the gain in pleasure—as does masochistic masturbation—but is deployed to *defend against* castration anxiety. To that end, the perception of the genital is increasingly associated with passive aims, the oedipal submission, and the libidinous-passive attachment to the rival are prepared. The danger masochists seek to evade through masturbation, by contrast, is castration *and* pulsional anxiety.[8] The latter consists in the fear of being overwhelmed by pulsional forces without any possibility of physical satisfaction and of having to face the disintegration of the ego structure. In keeping with the genital orientation, this anxiety takes the form of ruining the penis through the intensity of the drives. In girls we understood that this idea appears as a consequence of castration anxiety; they thereby try to explain [the anxiety] and to defend against it. In boys, castration anxiety occurs as the reproach of mutilating oneself through excessive aggressive masturbation of the genital. Male castration anxiety thus usually has two sources: one's own aggressive pulsional pleasure, which returns as the archaic revenge of the father, as well as a share of originary pulsional anxiety.

Notes

1. On the use of metaphors in science, see Demandt 1978.
2. See Freud 1923b, 57; see also II.11 above.
3. This idea corresponds to the "vortex theory" of the drives (see Hermann 1935 [a summary in English can be found in Willard 1939]).
4. We have some knowledge of the temporal dimensions that *consciousness* can comprehend and assess, and we also say that the *unconscious* knows of no temporal boundaries. We do not, however, have any conception of the *ego*'s possibilities to comprehend periods of time. At most, the rhythmical pulsional tension gives the ego some clues—which are not capable of entering consciousness. Perhaps the anxiety of the ego, as soon as the effect of the death drive sets in, is also prompted by the loss of a "timer" in the drives.
5. See above, II.11, #148–49.
6. "We are without a term analogous to 'libido' for describing the energy of the destructive instinct" (Freud 1938b, 150).
7. Masochism, for all that, cannot be called a "preoedipal" neurosis. The course transferences take in analyses leaves no doubt that the patients have attained a *structured and definitive oedipal position*. An emotional relationship is established easily. Yet what initially appears to be an inversion—passive pulsional aims paired with aggressively cathected wishes—at closer scrutiny turns out to be *the neurotic symptom*. While this symptom is essentially determined by anal and phallic, that is to say, preoedipal ideas of castration, it is shaped into a resilient psychical formation ("symptom") only by the tensions of the oedipal crisis.
8. The diagnostic difficulty consists above all in recognizing the defensive nature of the oedipal castration anxiety. For the [male] masochist, the phantasy of being genitally mutilated *as a punishment* is still easier to endure than the reproach of doing the same thing *to herself* is for the girl or the prospect of doing so is for the boy.

III
Masochistic pleasure

1 A contribution to decreasing tension

We have learned that masochism cannot be founded solely on either unconscious feelings of guilt or the "sadomasochistic" content of secret wishes. The thesis that masochists are more exposed to the effects of the death drive than others could not fully convince us either. We did observe a peculiarity in the life of the drives, but this concerned the *aggression vicissitude*. We conceived of the consequences of a change early in the development of the relationship between the pulsional components of the libido and of particular conflict solutions as *neuroses*. Castration anxiety and penis envy, which are more intense here than in other neuroses, an urgency to address the difference between the sexes, the absence of ambivalence tension even as the ambivalence remains, as well as a peculiar dampening of the gain in pleasure that cannot be blamed on the superego, seemed to us to be characteristics of the masochistic etiology. We have to admit that this is not exactly a lot. However, we still have to examine the *oedipal conflict*. Until the relationship of a psychical process with the childhood crisis, which is the vanishing point of all further development, has been cleared up, any judgment on it is by necessity fragmentary.

From here on out, we will take for granted that the form of the Oedipus complex, its course, and the way in which it is resolved is decisive for each individual. In masochism, the problem of aggression is at the center of the conflict; all other phenomena can be related causally to the particular pulsional vicissitude of sadism.[1] Usually, the oedipal child turns toward one parent with its love demands and harbors murderous intentions toward the other parent. If the supposition of an originary pulsional entanglement is justified, then such a *polarization* can take place only because of a repression (which is oriented differently for each object) or a regressive pulsional defusion. The latter is out of the question in a conflict conditioned by maturation, such that the common oedipal ambivalence must be considered the effect of a repression-like inhibition. The effective defense, the repression, will only later be the effect of the superego, yet the superego itself will emerge at the end of infantile development as the result of an unavoidable—unavoidable in our culture—solution of the conflict, of aggression internalization. Once the agency of conscience has been established in the psychical, the ambivalence is subject to a countercathexis, that is, defended against, and constantly associated with an *ambivalence tension*. This tension is explained by the struggle between the censoring forces and the pulsional impulses that insist on both wishes being satisfied simultaneously in the same object.

In looking at three cases of masochism, we have become convinced that ambivalent wish cathexes exist in juxtaposition without a corresponding tension being evident. In masochists, the impression of great ambivalence is generated only by the absence of repression. Opposing pulsional impulses impose themselves suddenly and without consideration for each other, without raising suspicions in the superego. Yet if the pulsional fusion is not only the regular result of psychosexual development but a general cultural phenomenon, then it is one more masochistic "riddle." Neither conscience nor our reason permits love and hatred toward the same person at the same time, yet in masochism, we find sadistic wishes beside passive goals that do *not* provoke a defense. No one will seriously suppose that masochists do not develop a conscience. A weakness of repression, too, is unlikely, since repression more than sufficiently proves its capability in other contexts. We must therefore suspect that the *masochistic superego* has obtained a very particular position toward ambivalence. How this is to have happened, of course, is obscure. Only children display a comparable tolerance for ambivalence, or it appears, in our cultural sphere, in massive psychical disorders. Yet masochism can be attributed neither infantility nor regression to psychotic states.

The psychoanalytic conception presupposes the drive as "the psychical representative of an endosomatic, continuously flowing source of stimulation," and pulsional energy is "regarded as a measure of the demand made upon the mind for work," as a kind of energy "that in itself… is without quality."[2] The notion that the id is a "great reservoir of libido"[3] does not heed the separation of pulsional energy that has become important to us. Libido and aggression appear to be "mixed" or "alloyed," and there is no reason to look into the processes of cathexis displacement in more detail.[4] I have attempted to present a thesis that, by assuming a "degree of saturation" of pulsional energy with aggressive quantities, explains the phenomenon of pulsional defusion without having to claim a constitutive predisposition toward ambivalence in the sense of an alloying *not operated*.[5] When we take this idea further and suppose that unbound aggressive forces attach to the remaining pulsional fusion and—precisely in their intention to attach to it—break it up, a new reflection will appear correct to us. If the relationship between the kinds of drives among themselves develops a dynamic that otherwise can only be the result of the defense, if, that is, this pulsional disentanglement does not come about because of a contentual conflict but is a process conditioned by the particular quality of the admixture ratio, then the effect for the ego will be beyond doubt. The ambivalence tension does not apply and with it a large share of the *gain in pleasure*. The pleasure measured in other pulsional satisfactions by the amount of libido excited, but also by the co-excited anxiety, is in this case diminished by that part that usually emerges from the overcoming of the resistance of the superego.[6] The wishes, to be sure, still bear the mark of the id, and their contents are bound to emotionally important memories the censorship is suspicious of, they are not able to become conscious, and yet they have lost the dynamic intensity of the repressed. Such wishes, we might say, "escaped" the censoring agency; yet in that case, we will need to explain why they are nonetheless unconscious and what process, if it is not the prohibition of the superego, blocks their access to consciousness. Second, the question arises why the pleasure principle does not come to bear, which after all does not permit any diminishing of the gain in pleasure unless it must. The pulsional impulses would have to urge being fulfilled, at least in separation, to make up for the loss. What we observe, however, is that the superego is concerned with something else entirely than the ambivalence problem and that despite physical satisfaction, the gain in pleasure is diminished.[7]

At this point, I will forego a discussion of whether this phenomenon, as an effect, is to be attributed to the death drive and its tendency toward psychical entropy [or] at most to the struggle between pleasure principle and destructiveness. I will postpone the investigation of the psychical causes, in any case, until we have understood a contribution of a different kind to the decrease in tension. I have pointed to the fact that ambivalence can be a consequence of pulsional defusion as much as of repression. I must now add a peculiar coincidence. What appears to us as pulsional defusion without the repression that usually comes with it, that is, the ambivalence without unpleasure tension, coincides symptomatically with the phenomenon that at the beginning of this study I called the *disentanglement of aggression and sexuality*, which is driven forward by *social forces*. This coincidence is all the more astonishing as we are used to unambiguous frontlines. There are indeed societies that allow consciousness to direct hatred and love simultaneously at an idol or an authority.[8] But our conception excludes something like that. We cannot reasonably say: I admire you more than anything, expect you to rescue me, and will now kill you. Instead, if and when we feel such impulses, part of the ambivalence is defended against. What remains, as symptom, is the one pulsional component as well as the unpleasurable tension that urges the return of the other. When we looked at the social disentanglement of the drives, we saw no signs of any repression. Rather, we thought we noticed that aggressive and libidinous strivings coexist without abolishing each other. The consciousness of individuals is not bothered by this, provided two conditions are met. First, a cathexis displacement must have taken place such that the libido appears low in energy, while the aggression in turn seems sexualized; second, this pulsional composition—which is the normal one in object relations—is taboo in the relations with the objective form of power. We may think of this as similar to, for example, the custom to interact with gods in a different language than with one's neighbors. This process, though, would be the negative of what ethnopsychological research postulates for some African and Asian cultures; there the ambivalence either applies generally or is required precisely in relations with authority. Now, what are we to make of the observations, what forces may we suspect behind the "*coincidence* ['*Zufall' der Koinzidenz*]," which [forces] condition the social taboo? The last question seems more easily answered. If we're willing to accept the theses presented so far, we will not remain doubtful about the *intended purpose of the pulsional disentanglement* for long. We said that a social dominion makes use of the energy displacement between subjective pulsional wishes and objective power (the "voluntary" servitude) to channel off subjects' unbound and unsatisfied pulsional forces. The conversion of psychical energy into objective power, whose institutions belong to dominion, turns individuals' unconscious wishes into a convenient and inexhaustible reservoir of force for dominion. The source, of course, does not bring to light useful things alone. Libidinous energies that cathect sexual wishes and for their satisfaction demand merely one's own phantasy and sensorial physical stimuli are of no interest to power. Sexual wishes are the slag in the ore mine, and they are pointed to with all the more verve the more and the more secretly aggressive forces are being mined. The mendacity and strictness of the rules of abstinence in a society's conscious sexual morality then always parallel the sexualization of the aggression. And the cathexis displacement is being promoted because erotic satisfaction must appear as a "waste of energy" to the social beneficiaries of the ambivalence. The interests of dominion require the pure gold of sexualized aggression. Only this energy can be aligned and deployed as belligerence, as economic rivalry, regressively as obsessive consumption, religious dependence, and political enthusiasm. Yet how does an external force achieve the psychical manipulation? It does not intervene in psychical life but merely conditions a process whose result—as already in the energy conversion—it makes use of for itself. Dominion here does not take power over the objective forms of pulsional energy but profits from a psychical chain reaction initiated [just] once. For, the aggression *cannot* be directed against the objective power because, even *before* it cathects wishes, that is to say, perceptual identities, it is largely channeled off. What remains is objectively insignificant, yet subjectively of sufficient virulence to get caught up in conflicts and to produce that surplus of confrontation that once more joins the energy stock of power. This also explains that, while the representatives of power are attacked and subjective aggression conflicts are unavoidable, the taboo on hostility toward the authority is reaffirmed time and again.

We have not yet said how the channeling off of the energy takes place; but at least we can now assert that the *intention of the social disentanglement of the drives* consists in *endowing the psychical forces extracted from the subjects with a desired quality*. The subjective energies are thus exploited not *in globo* but selectively, and the libido, diminished in its intensity and become passive, contributes to the perpetuation of the taboo insofar as it in turn expects aid and rescue from the authority once the loss of energy has spoiled the intimate satisfaction. We named one mechanism of channeling off energy in the *displacement and qualitative transformation* from subjective to objective force. We also realized that this process is not without danger.

A contribution to decreasing tension 221

When unconscious energy translates into objective power, and if in the process the aggression freed from the libido forms not only ideology and agency but once more an objectified form of itself, then this [form] accumulates a power that evades even the grasp of the dominion in whose service it yet stands. Another mechanism is banal but, under the circumstances, it has unsuspected consequences. I am talking about *seduction*. The drives' opportunistic inclination to satisfy themselves wherever and whenever an occasion offers itself opposes no resistance to the sexualization of the aggression. Everyday reality simply needs to promise opportunities for aggressive satisfaction often enough and simultaneously discredit the erotic ones, and a majority of cathexes will attach to wishes that have thus been excited. These, of course, are still disapproved and unconscious wishes—we are, after all, not talking about rational adjustments for the purposes of the ego but about economic processes of transforming and distributing pulsional energy. When we speak of seductions, then, this *characterizes a contradiction that arises between superego and reality when reality secretly allows for hope for an action that conscience, in phantasy, has already sanctioned with strict penalties*. Yet the more sadistic aims seem in fact attainable to people, and the more conscience relents in its opposition, the more passive and listless people become. This is incomprehensible because fulfillment must be preempted either by internal censorship or by external necessity; the drive does not relinquish by itself. If the opportunity does not correspond to the wishes, a lesser gain in pleasure will be clinched rather than none. We have, however, let a little something go unnoticed so far. The social power that promotes individuals' aggressiveness usually has no intention of satisfying it. While it baits the pulsional forces time and again with new aims, its own existence requires not the psychosexual energies as such but the *ensemble of an entire pulsional process without physical satisfaction*. (Only the wish cathexes, the superego prohibitions, the self-accusations, in short, the psychical investment in the entire conflict complex—minus those quantities that go into the work of defense—are available for the conversion.)[9] A physical satisfaction converts a majority of the cathexis into pleasure. And the gain in pleasure is merely a subjective sensation, the final aim of its striving for the individual but completely inconsequential for power. Aggression, meanwhile, once more accommodates this intention because, for unknown reasons, it can do without physical activity for much longer than the sexual libido can. Eros brooks no long postponement and asserts its rights even without the participation of consciousness. The ego imposes the pleasurable stimulation of the erogenous zones even in the most adverse conditions. Aggression, by contrast, must for long stretches be content with phantasy. Perhaps this is the heritage of thousands of years of communal life, which permits no daily murderous *actions*, and an expression of the body's threshold of pain, which puts a limit on sadistic satisfaction on one's own body. We might want to add that this could have been one of the reasons for the interlocking of the drives: the aggression that could no longer impose itself directly sought to link up with sexual satisfaction in order to be able to convert some of its energy into pleasure after all, even if it was tamed by the libido. In any case, sadism itself, because of its *capacity for postponement*, seems to lend itself to social exploitation. Hostility, after all, is immediately and usually without restriction ready for action when it is given the chance to act (in deadly peril, in defense, on the hunt, in war, and so on).

We thus might say that the listlessness springs from *frustration*. When aggression is promoted only to be postponed, no wonder it cannot contribute to the psychical gain in pleasure! The only possible objection is the one I have already mentioned: the gain in pleasure is not a function of physical satisfaction but largely a psychical variable. Although it does multiply when a suitable physical stimulus supports the activity of phantasy—and the *pulsional aim* is always a physical one—pleasure arises already in the *excitation of the wishes*. The procedure of deriving profit from the activity of phantasy should thus not be an unsolvable task and no reason to reduce pleasure for sadism, which must put up with this restriction elsewhere as well. Usually, of course, the wishes must clear the hurdle of inner censorship; ultimately, drive, ego, and superego share in the factual satisfaction, in the act as in phantasy. Every wish fulfillment is a compromise in which various forces—differing as to their origin, quality, and aim—*convert their energies into affects*. The psychical apparatus, if you like, can be conceived of as a device that converts somatic stimuli and tensions into affects. This function of the psychical alone is what stands in the way of the social utilization of the pulsional energy.

We now unwittingly find ourselves contradicting our own assertions. Earlier we said that dominion channels the pulsional energy off before it can bind itself to these wishes, and now we name the subjective affects as the source of the surplus of energy from which power draws but equally note that these very affects are socially undesired. A way out is afforded by the idea that *pulsional satisfactions are possible without the participation of conscience* after all *but that instead of being particularly pleasurable—since they are relieved of the sense of guilt—they become rather unexciting*.

Insofar as the pulsional wish aims at something that, although it runs counter to the infantile commandments of the superego, conforms to precepts of cultural morality that say the opposite, a conflict arises within conscience. Quite a few neurotic developments stem from an irresolvable split between conscience and external seduction. Usually, the dilemma is sorted out by the ego either submitting to the inner voice or by silencing it and adapting to the external morality. Both [solutions] leave traces in the psychical organization. But it is also possible that the superego adapts to the demands of reality, such that the contents of its demands are indistinguishable from those of the external world; in satisfactions that take place in keeping with cultural morality (however pulsional they may be), no inner conflict arises. We have our eyes on a third [possibility], however: in the psychical, there is a path past the superego, provided that an action's pulsional character can be eliminated and its conclusion entails no pleasure. If we suppose that the satisfaction in question is pulsional but takes place without participation of the ego and instead through a direct alliance between id and reality, then the superego is temporarily paralyzed. It has nothing with which to oppose this union since its defense strategies are designed to restrict and protect *the ego*. At the same time, the conversion process of the displacement from pulsional energy to the objectivized forms of satisfaction dispenses with the subjective pleasure quality. The superego does not defend against the pleasure but rather diminishes it precisely through its own paralysis. Only *post festum*, once the secret conversion process has taken place—which manifests *subjectively* in increased cathexes in all *internal* representatives of power, not least in the superego itself—will it attack the ego. The ego thus earns guilty reproaches for a satisfaction that procured it little pleasure and whose actual beneficiaries exist outside it. Insofar as individual socially conditioned excitations can be made conscious, what appears in analyses is thus not anxiety or self-accusation but *intense shame* because of the pleasureless pulsional inundation.[10]

It will rightly be objected that the affects pleasure and unpleasure depend not only on economic factors but also, among other things, on a particular quality of the *stimulus tension*. Freud distinguished between pleasurable tensions and unpleasurable relaxations.[11] Starting from the observation that pulsional satisfaction can be bound both to increases as well as decreases of stimulus quantities, he postulated the "Nirvana principle." This tendency to eliminate the tensions in psychical life represents the intention of the death drive.[12]

The rule of the absolute reduction of tensions is superordinated to the pleasure principle, which seeks to maintain a vital level of tension. And both the Nirvana principle in the service of the death drive and the pleasure principle representing the demands of the libido must assert themselves against the necessity of external reality, represented by the psychical reality principle. While the pleasure principle lays out the conditions under which a tension qualitatively becomes a pleasure, the Nirvana principle strives toward a linear abolishment of the tension. I, however, recognize in this tendency to diminish psychical tensions an intention that instead testifies that *the operation of concrete, nameable practices of a social power* are the action of the death drive. When in a system of dominion, the majority of individuals' psychical pulsional energies is diverted, when psychical and social, subjective and objective mechanisms are skillfully used by a dominion to time and again extract people's pulsional force (which thanks to the connection with the body is given *ab ovo* and thus inexhaustible as long as life lasts) and accumulate it in objective power, then this *might appear as a tendency toward reducing tension, but in truth it is a loss that is brought about with premeditation*.

Now, though, we have explicitly acknowledged the principle of the death drive and therefore cannot refuse the task of assigning symptoms to it. The death drive is not to remain a mere theoretical speculation. And since I have detached masochism from its connection [with the death drive] and call the "Nirvana" theorem a power-apologetic mystification, I feel duty-bound to rehabilitate the death drive by way of a few observations.

Notes

1. Other views see no connection between masochism and the oedipal conflict. The latter appears as a "form of search for love" (Berliner 1958, 45). Scheunert says: "Unconsciously, the child has grasped that the adult has used and still uses it as an object to release his aggressive strivings. It therefore makes itself such as [the adult] unconsciously wants it to be: unendearing, obnoxious, 'naughty,' whiny, or 'stupid.' The attempt is made, paradoxically, to attain the longed-for love and care by suffering and lament on the one hand, by refusal and objectively malicious actions on the other, in short, by making oneself as unendearing as possible" (1976, 164). For Edith Jacobson, too, the "development of masochists" consists in that "a helpless child with a hostile, rejecting, or smothering mother will do his best to accept and submit to his powerful, aggressive love object, and even give up his own self rather than give up the love object entirely" (1964, 112–13).
2. Freud 1905a, 168. In the same paragraph, however, Freud also says: "What distinguishes the instincts from one another and endows them with specific qualities is their relation to their somatic sources and to their aims. The source of an instinct is a process of excitation occurring in an organ and the immediate aim of the instinct lies in the removal of this organic stimulus. There is a further provisional assumption that we cannot escape in the theory of the instincts. It is to the effect that excitations of two kinds arise from the somatic organs, based upon differences of a chemical nature" (168). He immediately recognizes one of these kinds of excitations to be sexual; the organ in question is designated as the "erotogenic zone" of the partial drive that starts from it. Although Freud notes a few pages earlier "that there is an intimate connection between cruelty and the sexual instinct" (149), he does not want to acknowledge the second kind of somatic excitations to be the aggressive one. The psychical phenomena of sadism and aggression are appreciated at length but are not attributed a kind of stimulation of their own.
3. Freud 1923b, 30n1.
4. Because of the qualitative difference between the two kinds of drive, a direct conversion is out of the question. In the case of reactive ambivalence, too, we stipulate a cathexis-displacement, "energy being withdrawn from the erotic impulse and added to the hostile one." There, however, "a displaceable energy, neutral in itself," is called on for help, which joins the "qualitatively differentiated erotic or destructive impulse." This [energy] is the sublimated, desexualized libido at the disposal of the ego in its integrative functions (Freud 1923b, 44–45). If, however, we hold on to our view that the libido comes with a coefficient of saturation for aggression, which means that there is free, unbound pulsional energy present in the psychical apparatus whenever the libido can no longer take in any more aggression, this would mean that in all cases—and not just in masochism—the "sublimated" energy of the ego was originally the aggression.
5. Freud 1923b, 42. See above, II.11.
6. The intensity of the cathexis of a pulsional wish can be assessed by how much anxiety is co-stimulated in its satisfaction (see Le Soldat 1978, 102–3). Since the pleasure affect is often subject to repression, while the superego, for obvious reasons, will not spare the ego the anxiety, the drive's intensity betrays itself through this unpleasure affect. The connection between pleasure and anxiety, however, is more involved. The superego does not really have power over the anxiety, it rather has guilt affects and shame at its disposal. Anxiety instead *directly* associates with the pulsional energy and is used by the ego also as a sign of alarm ("anxiety as signal").
7. The physical satisfaction of a pulsional wish can for a short while contain the somatic source of the pulsional tension, but it does not in all cases lead to pleasure. If we exclude for the moment that the pleasure is defended against, that is,

that it exists only for the unconscious, the following causes remain: the quality of the pleasure is insufficient or the cathexis intensity is too low, the stimulation of the erogenous zone does not match the aim of the partial drive. The superego, of course, does not determine its reaction according to the effective pleasure but according to the pulsional quality of the wish excited.
8 See, for example, the studies conducted by Parin, Morgenthaler, and Parin-Matthèy ([1963] 1972) among the Dogon in western Africa (Mali).
9 See above, II.8.
10 The obfuscation tactics of the dominant are also manifest in language. We usually call ambivalence both the interlocking of the drives and the unconnected juxtaposition of libido impulses and aggression. A passively submissive position toward a hated opponent counts as ambivalent as much as the tendency to idealize and simultaneously damn oneself does. When a phenomenon that causes tension and unpleasure in the subjective domain is characterized with the same term as its absence, then we may suppose that the subject suspects something correct, namely, the double nature of its drives, but seeks to deceive itself about the effect of its repression. The *absence of ambivalence that continues to be called ambivalence* without having left behind symptoms of lack, that is, the loss of pleasurable equivocalness in favor of two divergent strivings, points to a socially produced disavowal, a "forgetting." If the individual were yet to become suspicious that not its own pulsional ambivalence but, precisely, its *destruction* is responsible for its dependence on the authority, then it would not find any support for its emancipation in language and consequently not in its thinking either.
11 Freud 1924a, 161.
12 Freud 1920, 55–56.

2 Pleasure and duration

If it is thus not the death drive that effects a constant reduction of tension for people but a social dominion that exploits their pulsional energy, we will nonetheless have to acknowledge a different kind of psychical unpleasure that has to do with stimulus diminishment and nevertheless is dictated by the *principle* of the death drive. It does not, however, appear continuously; it does not work in secret; and it does not resist its becoming conscious. Rather, it is so self-evident that we hardly ever have reason to suspect a mystery behind it. I am talking about the impossibility of *maintaining a pleasure unchanged over a longer period of time*.

We conceived of the death drive as a psychical impulse that, coming from the id, compels the faltering and abatement of the pulsional force. We will hardly be able to suppose that this effect occurs only once in life, at the time of death. For the diminishing of pulsional energy presented itself to us not as the final product of a destruction but as the common and immediate consequence of a psychical force, I have called, as antagonist of id gravitation, the centrifugal force in the id.[1] If the death drive describes the principle by which pulsional pressure is diminished in *every* pulsional process, then the centrifugal impulse in the id indicates the *force* the death drive makes use of. Psychoanalysis causes much confusion by naming its variables with intuitive concepts that describe their contents. Thus, the superego, of example, seems to be superordinate to the ego. Yet we were able to show that occasionally, the superego is subjected by the external world and its ally, the ego, or subjected without contradiction to the pulsional demands. The "death drive" seems to designate a pulsional urge whose aim is the extinction of pulsional tension and self-destruction. The force Freud characterized with this self-explanatory concept seems to admit no other interpretation than precisely this, that it is a drive toward death. My claim, however, is that although the death drive is a force that unmistakably articulates itself in psychical life, it does not condition death—not, that is, the *temporal limitation of life*—but sets a meter or rhythm of the flow of pulsional energy. This [force] has the effect of a *temporary restriction of pleasure*. In that sense, the "death drive" is not a dynamic drive but rather an axiom or basic law of the psychical. The reasons for nonetheless sticking with the name are purely historical.

Pleasure and duration 227

We are easily tempted to mistake the apparent diminishing of the drive immediately following a satisfaction for the effect of the death drive. It seems entirely "natural" to us that a displeasurable tension is alleviated once the stimulus is removed and that a pleasurable tension is extinguished in the moment of its satisfaction. The limitation of the duration of the pleasure by its fulfillment, however, must be attributed to the pleasure principle; and this does not lead to a collapse of the pulsional intensity either, because what is happening is not a "pulsional satisfaction" but the production of a perceptual identity in phantasy as the physical tension resolves. Even a "satisfied" wish is still an acute wish cathected with pulsional energy. The pleasure principle *aims* at the physical satisfaction and *effects* a conversion of pulsional energy into affects, but it leaves the pulsional pressure untouched. The apparent psychical tension reduction after a wish fulfillment has other causes. It probably is not even correlated with the pulsional process but is attributed to it because it *temporally* coincides with it. It appears merely as an *easing of the pulsional tension*, but in truth it is a *loss of the drive as such*. After we learned from psychoanalysis that we are controlled and dominated by unconscious drives, we will now have to get used to the idea that these drives determine us by their presence as much as by their absence.

A pleasurable tension, an enjoyment or a pleasant excitation, but also—something we notice less—the same internal unpleasure cannot be put off at will without the drive faltering. It is certainly no coincidence that Goethe's Faust offers Mephisto his life and servitude in the beyond in exchange for a *pleasure whose eternal duration he yearns for*. "Pleasure wants eternity,"[2] and yet it must falter, in every pulsional process, during or after a successful satisfaction, even if external and internal conditions were to remain favorable for a long time yet. The pleasure dies off although the body could take in the stimuli and no prohibition inhibits, no defense pretends listlessness. The drive abates for moments, for minutes, and no physical manipulation, no psychical busyness can bring it back to life. The effect of *Faust* consists in having *stretched* this intimate, as it were microscopic process temporally and to have associated it with guilt conflicts. In this way, the pleasurable is reaffirmed formally and the ego's integrating tendency to interpret its own foundations psychically is placated: what brings us down time and again are not the *unforeseeable, sudden invasions of the pulsional force*, we do not fail in every single wish fulfillment because we no longer feel the pleasure; we rather entangle ourselves in an interconnected, dramatically escalating guilt conflict. The poet here operates an illusionary reversal of painful reality that resembles the one we discussed via Freud's interpretation of the "three caskets." What time and again puts an end to Faust's pleasure is not a neutral and therefore unrelenting principle in psychical life, it is *Faust himself* who no longer enjoys sensual pleasure and internal stimulation! The sovereignty regained consoles him, and the replacement of the uncanny pulsional force by the familiar sensations of pleasure, desirability, and desire is just as reassuring. The *summum bonum*, however, which to Faust seems [to lie] in the *perdurability*, and not in some particular quality of the pleasure, also makes him certain that Mephisto cannot fulfill his task in this life. The death drive enters no bargains and commands the silent faltering of pleasure in time.

Our suspicions, of course, are allayed by the fact that Faust is *old*, and that death is already reaching for him.[3] We should think that his desire is of a sexual kind or at least of a subjective nature. The unconscious understanding has long come up with a different thought. Although Faust dies a multiply guilty man, although at the end he prefers succumbing to an illusion to accepting the annihilation of his work through the forces of nature, in allowing Mephisto to triumph—"the poor wretch" who wanted to hold on to "this final, mediocre, empty moment… lies here on the sand an old, old man"[4]—he ultimately has nonetheless subjected himself to *one* power, that of the death drive. It really seems as if we would rather endure anxiety and guilt than confront the *uncanniness of the fluctuations in the life of the drives* that have no relation whatsoever with unconscious processes and certainly not with consciousness.

Just as the effect of the death drive sets in in the psychical, just as the drive runs dry, without people being able to add anything or do anything to oppose it, so they must tolerate, powerlessly as it were, the inevitable *subsequent increase of pulsional quantities*. Recall that we conceived of the death drive as a principle that must measure its force against that of the pleasure principle. Within an excitation, pleasure principle and death drive fight over the intensity of the cathexis, more precisely: the impulse of the death drive adds itself to the striving of the pleasure principle, which gives rise to a *rhythmic, staccato-like course of the cathexis* in all pulsional processes. The oscillations or the "cathexis flicker" will be all the greater the more the death drives gains power over the pleasure principle. Especially in the case of a libidinous satisfaction in which pleasure could establish itself, there will be a noticeable diminishing of the pulsional energy at the next impulse of the death drive, [a diminishing] we would like to attribute to the "satisfaction," as its effect, although the easing of the tension it prompts is the success of the pulsional pressure with the opposite polarity.

All this yields four factors for the restriction of pleasure: the social reduction of tension with the aim of displacing energy; the function of the psychical defense mechanisms, which for contentual reasons curtail, delay, or dynamically conclude (via countercathexis) the pleasure; then we must also consider, beside the current relationship between pleasure principle and death drive, the effective intensity of the centrifugal impulses of the id. Yet if we allow [this intensity] to coincide with the pulsional energy, with the effect of the gravitation of the id, then we are no longer able to explain why, in libidinous or in aggressive satisfactions, a longed-for fulfillment gives way to a vexing emptiness after just a short while. That the absence is *secondarily* endowed with affects and integrated to form a conflict changes nothing about the fact that what, for a moment, became visible, unveiled here was the work of the death drive. The disavowal of the insight into the coercive force and necessity of the death drive ("Ananke") leads Faust to his unfulfillable wish for persistent pleasure.

Notes

1 See above, Chapter II.12, pp. 156–64.
2 "Yet all joy [*Lust*] wants eternity" (Nietzsche [1883–1885] 2006, IV.12: 264).
3 Eissler on the contrary holds that the desire for the enjoyment to last forever is "a concealed call for death" [Eissler 1984, 34]. On his reading, Goethe, through the saving effect of Gretchen's appearance in the Walpurgis Night, says "that the process of socialization develops in the detour via aggressive-destructive actions and that an internalization of the destructive deed leads to ethical elevation." For Eissler, this is a "surprising anticipation" of guiding ideas in Freud's *Totem and Taboo* (Eissler 1984, 49).
4 [Goethe, *Faust II*, in Goethe (1808/1832) 1994, ll. 11589–92.]

3 The object of identification

The Faustian wish—"I will tell the moment: Tarry, remain!"[1]—presented itself to us as the result of a two-fold defense. To evade the insight that the perpetuation of the pleasure is opposed by a *psychical law*, the principle of the death drive, Faust denies that unconscious powers let a drive abate at will. *He* himself wants to be the one whom nothing excites anymore. His failure appears as the consequence of his entanglement in guilt, as a drama of old age, greed, and the unfulfillability of wishes. Yet the unification of pleasure and duration is objectively and absolutely impossible. Faust rebels against a basic condition of the psychical. The poet creates a liberating compromise by preferring, as a displacement-substitute for the *chaotic flow of pulsional energy*, one of its effects, the *constant striving for pleasure*. Moreover, he places Mephisto at Faust's side, and thereby the illusion that, if the quest for pleasure bears no fruit, at least malice and sadism might defy the internal compulsion to diminish [pleasure]. The pleasurable reversal concerns the deal in which [Goethe] abandons [the possibility] for Faust of sexual and intellectual enjoyment as untenable but insists that aggression is hard on his heels and will not let go of [Faust]. This is meant to save at least some solid emotional ground. Yet destructiveness is neither a secret ally of the death drive nor one of its derivatives.

In keeping with Freud's theory, I see in the death drive the antagonist of the sexual drives; yet I do not oppose libido and destructiveness to each other but conceive of aggressive and libidinous strivings as usually inseparable components of the sexual drive, which in turn is subject to the pleasure principle and the death drive principle simultaneously. I think that the impossibility of keeping a pulsional impulse constant for more than a few moments although the cathexis quantity remains undiminished must be attributed as an effect not to the pleasure principle but to its opponent, the death drive. In this way, *the death "drive" is really a pulsional antagonist*. As a common pulsional component, aggression is subordinate to the struggle between these two principles. In the case of masochism, I see no reason to postulate a particular influence of the death drive.

This brings us back to the masochistic development that in Part II we left at the onset of the oedipal conflict. Psychoanalysis speaks of an Oedipus conflict when in the course of psychosexual maturation, around the fourth year of life, the persons of the external world become essential objects of the pulsional wishes but the infantile impulses come up against social taboos. The incestuous wishes are directed at the mother, murderous impulses strike the father. As in the preoedipal period, the actual aim of the drive is a satisfaction in one's own body; the real objects, however, no longer count merely as instruments or inhibitions for the physical relaxation but are included in the wishful phantasies as a new category of aims. Because of the pulsional ambivalence, vis-à-vis the love object, the hostile strivings must be repressed, vis-à-vis the rival the tender-passive strivings. This usually makes the resolution of the conflict easier since the return of the aggression favors relinquishing the love object, [while the return] of the erotic binding to the father favors submission. Yet we found the situation to be different in masochism. An early [quantitative] shift of the cathexes from libido to aggression has become irreversible and leads to the emergence, beside the usual ambivalence, of great quantities of unbound destructive energies. We note an ambivalence that largely tends toward sadism and does not allow an ambivalence-tension to arise. What for the others is the aim of the defense efforts, namely, the containment of the *consequences of the ambivalence*, for the masochist becomes, in the *absence of the ambivalence tension*, a cause of unpleasure and defense.

An ambivalent position toward the rival, the so-called feminine, homoerotic tendency of the boy, is one of the sources of *castration anxiety* that ultimately causes the internal failure of the oedipal demand. The absence of ambivalence, then, should create better preconditions for the masochist. That is not the case. First, we learned that the intensity of the anxiety is largely caused by one's own sadism, which is being projected and then internalized again. Second, in the psychical, the commandment of the pleasure principle always takes precedence over the binding to the object. Since the maturation demands an orientation toward the persons of the external world, whereas the pleasure principle insists first of all on the interlocking of the drives, *object cathexis and the rehabilitation of pleasure are fighting each other*. For, the non-alloyed pulsional components together contribute much less to the gain in pleasure than ambivalent cathexes. Repressing a part of the ambivalence does cause an unpleasure-tension, and the labor of defense, too, is subtracted from the gain in pleasure, but what suffers an unbearable loss due to the lack of ambivalence is the *quality of the pleasure*. Only the alloying of the pulsional components creates that tension in the wish cathexes whose excitation can be qualitatively converted into pleasure affects. When we now turn to contentual analysis again, we will thus remember that one factor has changed in comparison to the normal parameters of the oedipal conflict. The pulsional ambivalence is not first a disturbance in unfolding the wishes and then an aid in relinquishing [the wishes] but on the contrary an element missing in the cathectic energy and therefore in competition with the objectal interests. When masochistic patients seem fixated on the oedipal situation, we will interpret their conflict-inclination as a holding on to the infantile demands, but in so doing, we should not forget that they are concerned, much more than with embarrassing pulsional strivings, anxiety, and guilt affects, with the consequences of the low [degree of] ambivalence tension. Unbound aggression, to be sure, manifests in the wish cathexes and in ego activity as well and thus is also directed at the objects. The *course* of the conflict, by contrast, proves that *in masochism, the pleasure principle does not chiefly work to fulfill the incest wishes but primarily to restore the pleasure quality*.

In the analytic cure, we usually have no reason to be concerned with anything but contentual conflicts. The experience of the unconscious takes place in the medium of object cathexis. Formerly intense wishes are repressed thanks to unpleasurable phantasies and embarrassing experiences, their striving to become conscious establishes symptoms, and in the transference relationship, wish, defense, and the persons involved in the conflict come back to life in a multiply condensed and disguised form. Freud reports the dream of a patient who "was pulling a woman out from behind a bed"; this man was giving a woman, presumably the mother he loved incestuously, *preference* over the father, whom he hopes to have found again in the person of Freud.[2] Another patient of Freud's who "dreamt that he was an officer sitting at a table opposite the Emperor"[3] confesses his wish that the physician treat him "man to man," give him orders, as is custom between emperor and subject. Fritz Morgenthaler recounts the case of a server who told him that on her day off, she dreamt she was serving him coffee as she was already doing every day in reality. The woman thereby reveals her wish exhibitionistically to uncover herself before the admired man.[4] In these phantasies, we see an objectal wishful impulse caused by the oedipal conflict.

The "acrobat," too, had an entire series of dreams with what seemed oedipal content:

> It's in a room. A woman and a man. They want to sleep together. They are very horny for each other. It's very exciting. Then a second woman comes in, she has pitch black hair, with a white streak in it, as if sprayed on, a straight line, it looks incredibly beautiful. Like a bird of paradise. She asks if she can join in. Then they're having a threesome, and it's very exciting.

The seductive tendency we already observed in the patient in another instance here extends to a situation with three people: a man and two women. If we hadn't been warned, we might be inclined to impute to the dream an oedipal wish fulfillment only slightly disfigured by the defense. The parents are doing it, she comes in, and instead of being chased away, she is allowed to join in. This is what a successful compromise might look like. She relinquishes the incestuous wish and the murderous intention and in return is welcomed into the bed. The "acrobat" even provides us with an association to confirm the point. Her older sister, of whom she was extremely jealous, always wore black clothing, though she dyed her hair red. If the sister functions as a displacement substitute for the mother, then hypocritically calling her "beautiful bird of paradise" instead of "black witch" would not be a bad disguise for the rivalry aggression. The man and the woman at the beginning of the dream, however, are the patient herself and I; we are the oedipal pair that brooks no interruption. The external circumstances—an incident with another analysand that had impinged on one of her sessions and some youth really spraying pornographic graffiti outside our window—were the day's residues for the formation of the dream. I notice two small details, though. Both the rape dream reported at the outset (Chapter II.1) and this one begin with three elements. Here we find (1) a room, (2) a woman, and (3) a man, there we had (1) a cathedral, (2) the black robe, and (3) the red tambourine. There's nothing yet I can do with this observation, but I tell the patient about it—along with the second peculiarity. If three elements determine the first sequence already *in* both dreams, then we can probably also expect *three*, not two, dreams that *belong together*.[5] I then learn that the "hypocritical" dream preceded the one about drumming in time but that the patient did indeed have a third dream *between* the two others, one she dislikes telling. She calls it "unimportant and banal":

> I see you [the analyst] in the city. You have a new car. I'm really looking for a parking spot for my car, but I see that yours is much more beautiful. It is red and black, black on top and at the bottom it has very wild, red stripes. We decide that from now on, we'll continue the analysis there. My car, meanwhile, has broken down, is banged up somehow and already taken away.

The remark about the formal oddity has had the effect of an interpretation. What *in the dream* is once the woman (2) and once the black robe (2) was defended against in the transference process: the second of the three dreams, "the one in the middle," was missing. Since we know that the patient is ashamed of "the middle of her body," that is, her penislessness, we know that in her sleep, she slowly approached the "terrible thing." The hypocritical enthusiasm about the "incredibly beautiful" line in the hair reveals itself to be disgust at the genital cleft amid the *black* pubic hair. The *red* color of course recalls menstrual blood and establishes the connection with the idea of castration. The term "bird of paradise" mirrors mockery and ridicule both of her own anatomy and of the embarrassing memory that, "like a bird of paradise," namely, all dressed up, she tried to seduce both the analyst and the father. Now, however, [the analyst] is berated as a "bird,"[6] and [the patient] denies the horror caused by the genital excitations during the sessions on the couch. The dream-work pleasurably inverts a fear: I can satisfy myself! The wishful tendency of the last dram, masturbation, fully imposes [the tendency] of the second dream: the patient demands that the analysis now concern itself with *auto*eroticism.[7] What stands out, though, is that the "acrobat" neither knows how to drive nor has ever owned a car [*Auto*]; accordingly, the censorship assesses the latent wish to be entirely impossible [to fulfill]. While I hear the indication that in her autoeroticism, she is "banged up and broken," I cannot see much more in it than her idea that she is castrated and wants to be made new and whole. To unfold the conflict, let's turn once more to the third dream, which, however, was told first. Its theme at the time seemed to be the rape, but now the very first scene already opens up a repressed autoerotic dynamic. The huge empty dome of the cathedral is her vagina, and there, sexuality is "drumming." The pulsional demand is about genital satisfaction by means of the hand, and in the hectic busyness that immediately sets in, the manifest dream is meant to deny her obvious helplessness before the genital excitation. In the context we are dealing with, however, this can only mean that a latent conflict has led to the patient being unable to masturbate pleasurably.

All three dreams share the wish to be masturbated by the analyst, but from this dream presented as a symptom, I expect elucidation of *why* the patient so urgently needs my "help." We now understand better that the subsequent exciting ideas that all concerned masturbation primarily served to defend against the embarrassing admission. It is evident that the lack of a capacity to resolve the sexual excitation for herself is as worthy of censorship as the fact of masturbation. The shame of depending on external cooperation in any case had up to now prohibited the patient from talking about the topic. In analysis, we in this situation expect the return of memory; once the resistance has been worked out, indications should arise as to what events and conflicts blocked the natural talent.

In the course of childhood, Stephanie discovered that her father was not a faithful man. She often observed him with woman strangers, and when at a party, his father was flirting with a lady, [Stephanie], full of jealousy and of intense pity for the mother, came at her father with a knife. She had "blown a fuse." She was punished by being locked up in a dark room. At the time, the light had often gone out in the house, she believed ghosts to have done it, but she had been told the "old fuses" were responsible. She had played with the fuses. Back then, those were small white conical ceramic objects, with a metal thread running through them that held a little red head at the top. "Blown" meant that there was too much current on the line and the head was cast off. We may suppose that the child was afraid in the dark and tried to calm herself by means of a genital stimulation; we may further suppose that she employed the used fuses as masturbation aids. Yet since, via the ceramic fuse, the idea that if one is "charged" too much, something is cast off "in front"—the idea, that is, of an endogenous castration by the aggression—was associated with an anger affect concerning the father, everything seems to come together in a common oedipal castration threat. *Because* you were jealous, you were punished radically. We remember, however, that the "acrobat" presents the three dreams and the corresponding ideas to the analyst while she feels betrayed and abandoned by her, in a way similar to the father back then. Her impulse can only be to kill the therapist or to leave her. That, however, she cannot do because in her mind, [the analyst] has long become a displacement substitute

The object of identification 235

for the missing member. Murdering the analyst would mean castrating herself once again. The oedipal anger for the father did not stem from frustrated love but from the claim to possession; the father was interesting only insofar as he was an unavoidable appendix of the desired object. In the course of the analytic work, the *infantile wish for a penis* is transferred to the analyst, and it is the intensity of this wish that is responsible for the disruption of the ability to masturbate.[8]

While in hysteria, for example, the two pulsional components would have developed two forms of transference one after the other, an embarrassing, forbidden love with the wish to receive *from* the analyst a replacement for what was missed as well as, later, a guilt conflict, what arose here was a claim *to* the analyst *as replacement*. It is onto her that the patient has projected the idealizing cathexis, in the inner psychical world, she exists exclusively as *incorporation of the lost penis*, as "bird of paradise." The idea is rather supported by the objectal form of the transference, where the analyst as the beloved mother is out of the question in any other form than *with* a penis. The *third element* in the dreams, I now think, is thus not the oedipal rival but the missing member. The triad of the dreams, too, points in this direction.[9] If this is the case, however, then we must understand the fuse phantasy as a defense against guilt. If the little girl thought to have injured herself through aggressive masturbation (the "beating" of the drum), then she must have found solace in the idea of the fuses: I didn't do anything, it happened by itself; it wasn't anything big, just a little thread; and after all, it can always be replaced.

The multiplication of the men in the dream pleasurably inverts the uniqueness of the one woman, who now *is* her own member. In its therapeutic intention, the transference relationship has restored the relationship she had developed with the internal image of the missing member during the oedipal conflict. The patient is caught in the dilemma of aggressive sexual excitation. If she leaves or kills—for the unconscious, these are identical—the analyst, she will have castrated herself once more; yet fully taking possession of her is of course as impossible as changing the genital anatomy. In the drug addiction, she tries to transfer the dependence from the projected body part onto the pills, which can be purchased and are available at any time. Similar to the rapists in the dream and the small dildos in childhood, the pills, via the oral path this time, were meant to make her whole again. Later, when she became suicidal, she turned the aggression against herself. Yet only in the dream of the drum does she find a solution that also corresponds to the rest of her character. She *defiantly* turns against her wishes: I don't need you; you depend on my help. I'm not touching myself at all, and anyway, my member isn't gone, it's just "floppy."[10] The turn to defiance allows for an economic relaxation, since aggressive quantities are employed, beside the defense, in maintaining the ego functions as well.

Although it has now become more understandable why the young woman cannot satisfy herself, the interpretation of the dream is not yet entirely complete. *Masturbation would appear to her as an admission of penislessness and as final relinquishing*.[11] That, however, neither explains how she nonetheless achieves relaxation nor does it spell out the unconscious wish fulfillment of the dream. In the manifest dream content, we find the phrase: *You are cynical and unbroken, I am powerless and passive*. We cannot expect that the dreamer thereby intends to give a description of the real relationship between her and the analyst. The dream has worked out a compromise that is surprising and witty. While she is not allowed to look down at herself, her *phallic wishes* are unbroken. She has displaced the body representative of the penis onto an external object but in no way has she given up the corresponding pulsional demands. She must thus make a separation where usually there is an unquestioned unity, namely, *in* the ego. A part of the ego takes upon itself the mutilation that it ascribed to itself as a result of the aggression, while another share in the ego remains sadistic and phallically aggressive. It would be incorrect to consider this second area in the ego to be a function of the superego; yet neither is the ego share identical with the repressed aggression impulses. The split in the ego, rather, is the effect of a *cathexis displacement*. We now reencounter the phenomenon that within the pulsional wishes we conceived of as disentanglement of pulsional wishes, in the differing cathexes of two large areas in the ego. Where otherwise, ambivalent energies cathect the self-representative,[12] here an aggressive and a primarily libidinous part oppose each other. The latter has taken on the alleged consequences of aggression *instead* of the genital, supports passive, libidinous pulsional aims, and leaves the pursuit of sadism and hostility to the other part. The censorship agency, however, faces the paradoxical task of associating the two ego shares via feelings of guilt although it ought to promote the repression of the ambivalence. When in the dream, the superego pushes "you," the aggression, and "I," the passive sexual excitation, toward the same vicissitude, then the perpetuation of the difference is initially pleasurable. As the dream events develop, of course, the penis wish imposes itself, and under the conditions of the dream-state—something that does not succeed in waking life—the coincidence of the two pulsional components becomes a source of pleasure. The "rapists" then are nothing but genital orgasms. A continuous, long series of men rape her and yet can't "finish" her off. Since we know that for the unconscious, negation does not exist, while a series of equals only represents something singular, very special, the translation of the latent dream wish fulfilled in the last turn of phrase can only be this: I finally managed to finish [*schaffen*] a real orgasm!

We may be surprised to discover the motor of the complex dream work to be a more or less banal and, in itself, harmless wish. Yet since the wish is not about a particular quality of the pleasure but has genital satisfaction in general in mind, there can be no doubt that this [satisfaction] is not impeded by repressions alone. One part of the ego has identified with the penis given up for loss. The ego has submitted to the coercive force of reality and accepts the penislessness; at the same time, it has introjected the object given up on and raised it up again in the inner world. In the process of identification, the ego spares itself the unpleasure of the work of mourning by identifying itself with the lost love object and allowing it to go on living unchanged in the inner world.[13] This leads me to assume that the identification can go to a love object as much as to the phantasized penis. What is mourned is not a body part that really has come off—like baby teeth, for example, that often symbolize [the penis]—but a phantom member or a fetish: the *phallus of the woman*. As content of the ego identification, it acts as if it had physically existed.

I notice that the defense in the dream has reached a regression to anal modalities. A defiant attitude predominates, and the final scene recalls the anal intercourse with her boyfriend. The patient thereby refers to the exciting and pleasurable manipulations on her anus operated by the mother trying to remove a tapeworm. She thus equates the penis with the stick of stool and garners a triumph that in the dream she hypocritically refers to as "the worst": she herself is the "producer" of what she misses, she can bring it forth from herself, and the mother, whose love she believes she must relinquish because of, precisely, her penislessness, is assisting her.[14] Although in some cases, the regression of the drive contributes to restricting the gain in pleasure, the "acrobat's" anal fixation nonetheless does not suffice to explain the inadequacy of the genital masturbation.

In Friedrich Hebbel's *Maria Magdalena*, we find an example of a masochistic fixation on oral partial drives. Clara's monologue appears as an angry self-laceration:

> I want to wait on you, I want to work for you, you need give me nothing to eat, I want to support myself, I want to do sewing and spinning for other people at night, I want go hungry when I have nothing to do, I would rather bite a piece out of my own arm than go to my father and let him suspect anything! When you beat me, because your dog is not at hand, or because you have kicked him out, I would rather swallow my own tongue than emit a cry which will betray to the neighbors what is going on. I cannot promise that my skin will not show the welts caused by your whip, for that is not in my power. But I want to lie about it, I want to say that I fell head foremost against the cupboard, or that I slipped on the floor because it was too smooth—that I want to do before anybody has time to ask me where the black and blue marks came from!—Marry me! I shall not live long! And if it lasts too long for you, if you do not care to meet the expenses of the divorce proceedings necessary to get rid of me, then buy some poison of the apothecary and put it somewhere as if it were for your rats. I want to take it without your even nodding to me, and tell the neighbors with my dying breath that I took it for pulverized sugar![15]

What might seem to be a masochistic seduction tactic, perhaps also a submission before a sadistic superego, is—viewed psychopathologically—the *dialog between two irreconcilable parts of the same person during the unsuccessful masturbation*. Without exception, the self-accusations that sound as if a cruel object or the own angry superego must be appeased serve *phallic impulses*: I want to, I will, I go, I buy, I will show, I will say, I want to do... We witness the internal process *after* the cathexis displacement in the ego. One share is identified with the castrated genital, powerless and helpless, another share of the ego continues to be phallically active and orchestrates the events. The superego has succeeded in the idealizing cathexis of the projected genital assuming sadistic traits and in the pulsional aims having to regress to orality. Through the "marriage," the pulsional components could be connected again, the identification of the ego be abandoned, and the projection be nullified. Yet what actually happens is an increased excitation (cathexis increase) of aggressive phantasies. While for the "acrobat," the defense guides the aggression toward anal modalities, aggression in Hebbel's Clara appears displaced by a hysterical mechanism, from the bottom to the top, as *oral sadism*. The overpowering speech itself and the elements it makes use of (eating, hungering, biting into, swallowing one's tongue, emitting cries, taking poison, and so on) prove the aggression cathexis of the oral zone.

I now add to *pulsional defusion, which I acknowledged as the first masochistic symptom*, the *identification of the ego with the threatened genital*, which I affirm to be the *second neurotic symptom of masochism*. While we are unable to give a purely psychical reason for the excessive aggression, the ego identification with the abandoned phallus of the woman is the correlate of and addition to the oedipal identification with the aggressor. It serves to defend against the unpleasure that insight into women's natural penislessness would generate. Although it now seems as if this were a phenomenon of female development alone, *for boys, too, the internalization of the female phallus counts as insurance against the consequences of castration*.[16] Boys thereby deny not the illusion of a hope but the evident confirmation of their fear. The projection of the idealized penis onto an external object as well as the cathexis displacement between a sadistic and a powerless and threatened district in the ego, that is to say, the repression of a pulsional share, is the clinically visible consequence of primary identification.

Whereas usually, we expect an identification with the aggressor, coerced by castration anxiety, to conclude the oedipal conflict, under the conditions of masochism, we find in addition to the internalization of the aggression the introjection of the "victim," of the castrated penis. It is questionable whether the strength of the drive—and, accordingly, of the anxiety—alone deserves the double repression. Presumably, the identification also lends itself to the demanded relinquishing of the soothing and in many regards *pleasurable idea of the "phallic woman"* and is convenient in *sparing oneself the work of mourning*.[17] In that case, though, the introjection of the idealized penis would not only apply to both sexes in masochism, it would not depend on the neurotic conditions at all. It would always have to be possible to detect it, but only in the particular quantitative amplification in masochism would it be recognizable as a symptom of suffering.

Notes

1 [Goethe, *Faust II*, in Goethe (1808/1832) 1994, ll. 1699–1700 (modified).]
2 Freud 1900, SE 5, 409.
3 Freud 1900, SE 5, 409. However, Freud is not discussing transference here but the representation through words in the labor of dreaming.
4 See Morgenthaler 1986, 72–76.
5 It was Morgenthaler ([1978] 2020 and 1986) who pointed out how important formal criteria are in the interpretation of dreams.
6 The expression "bird," *Vogel*, condenses the sexual association *vögeln*, "to fuck," with the insult common among us, "You *are* a bird," roughly in the sense of "useless idiot." The patient thereby repeats her aggressive seduction strategy, as when she said I was a "monkey." The insult is instead to be seen as a *conjuring*; I am to treat her that way even if it is disgraceful.
7 The "sister" with the red hair and the black dress is a cover memory or displacement substitute for the bleeding vagina.
8 In what follows, we will realize that this cause must be joined by the special—masochistic—resolution of the oedipal conflict.
9 Numerous examples from the interpretation of dreams show the number three to symbolize the male sex; see Freud 1900, SE 5, 358; Freud 1916–1917, 10th lecture: "Symbolism in Dreams," SE 15, 149–69. [See also above, #]
10 She thereby refers to the "floppy hat" in the dream [above, #]. The hat, once more a male sexual symbol, is well suited to housing a recompensation phantasy. The idea of the "acrobat" that her genital is not destroyed at all, that it just turned out to be a little small or [that it is] floppy and will soon straighten up forcefully again, is a familiar form of female disavowal.
11 In keeping with the animist organization, for which the love object has acquired the character of a fetish, to relinquish once would be to relinquish always. Giving up hope once would mean giving up forever.
12 The ego structure names the psychical agency, while the term "self-representative" designates the reflective psychical element within the ego structure. If the ego is for the largest part unconscious, then the self-representative, too, has repressed shares.
13 See Freud 1916.
14 This image will not come as a surprise if we know that in the anal phase of development, stool is held in the highest esteem.
15 Hebbel (1844) 1914, 3.2:65–66 [modified]. Karl Abraham cites this passage as well, albeit as the masochistic phantasy of a *hysterical* patient (Abraham [1910] 1982, 217).
16 There are good reasons to suppose that the castration idea is not directly associated with the observation of female penislessness, but that the latter has a motivating effect once sadistic wishful impulses of one's own occur. The child wants to punish, actively and itself, the frustrating and unfaithful beloved by means of a genital mutilation.
17 "But why it is that this detachment of libido from its objects should be such a painful process is a mystery to us and we have not hitherto been able to frame any hypothesis to account for it. We only see that libido clings to its objects and will not renounce those that are lost even when a substitute lies ready to hand. Such then is mourning" (Freud 1915c, 306–7; see also Freud 1916, 244–45).

4 A forgotten cultural achievement

It will have been noticed that I have not yet completed the task of naming a reason for the masochistic restriction of masturbation. Yet one thing gives us occasion for another culture-critical excursus. It is hardly a coincidence that time and again, I am citing *female* examples of masochism. Is there some truth to the *on dit* that suspects there to be an intimate relationship between women and masochism and asserts passive submission to be the source of women's sexual pleasure?[1]

So far, I have not discussed male and female developments in masochism separately, and I see no reason to do so as we continue. The psychical effect of aggression and castration anxiety remains the same whether the phantasized consequence of masturbation is projected into the future (for boys) or whether it appears (to girls) as a fact of the past. There is also no difference in the coercion of reality that does not spare children insight, be it on their own bodies, be it in consciousness, into women's penislessness. I have already pointed to the advantage of binding aggressive energy to the subjective perception of the male genital. It cannot be denied, of course, that the oedipal crisis usually comes with a transformation whose results differ between the sexes. Incestuous wish and rivalry make the mother become the *love object* for the boy, the father the love object for the girl. For male children, this development is less problematic to the extent that they can *hold on* to the original object of the early years and *expand* their interest to a second object. Girls, by contrast, are supposed to *relinquish* the first love object, *transform* love and dependence into hatred, and orient their libido *anew* toward the father. Psychoanalysis has given this process of female genesis the title "recathexis." We observe that four- to five-year-old girls prefer the father and rival with the mother. It is also assumed that the change of love object comes with a change of erogenous zones (from the clitoris to the vagina). This is joined by the turn from "activity" to sexual "passivity," that is to say, a change in the pulsional quality and in the pulsional aim. No one is really able to name causes for these innovations, except maybe the maturation of biological functions. Although oedipal recathexis blatantly contradicts the otherwise continuous persistence of the libido—only just now, we saw how much suffering the ego takes on itself to spare itself relinquishment and work of mourning—girls'

A forgotten cultural achievement 241

turn toward their fathers, at least, seems to take place without coercion and internal turbulence. Nor can a look at female homosexuality change anything about the thesis of the originarily opposite-sex orientation of sexual interest, since there, penis envy and castration anxiety are denied but nonetheless fully intact.[2]

Various reflections that I would like to lay out in what follows have led me to a different assessment of the female change of object. I think the fact of the recathexis cannot be doubted, yet [I also think that] the *female heterosexual object choice* has the *quality of a neurotic symptom*. The motive of wish formation, which I acknowledged to be the production of a perceptual identity with earlier satisfactions, is likely to be generally applicable, and thus should neither be varied according to sex nor be admitted for childhood but denied later. If for men, the first love object, the mother, remains associated with the easing of the pulsional tension of the first period of life, then we won't be able to postulate other developments for women. The *originary* object of the pulsional wishes, of the libidinous as well as of the hostile ones, is in every case the mother, whom other objects must first *repress*.[3] Psychologically, the female heterosexual object choice thus has the same status as the male homosexual [object choice]. Both are *compromise formations* between an originary pulsional demand and a series of conflicting forces.[4] Yet while male homosexuality is exclusively defined by internal conflicts, represents an appropriate solution of the oedipal problem, and indeed makes do without symptoms of suffering, the female change of love object appears as a *cultural artifact* and as coerced by conditions other than psychical ones. The sex-specific recathexis in early childhood—girls *ought to* perform the displacement, boys not—may count as the result of a social force. The change of object is operated by children in the service and under the impression of an intention that is foreign to them and of which they have no consciousness of any kind, and it is coordinated with their own conflicts and aims only secondarily. The perpetuation of the cathexis displacement succeeds only as long as the external force remains effective and via a work of defense that [children] must perform to repress the unpleasure associated with the relinquishing. The oedipal recathexis cannot be undone, whereas it is sometimes possible to spare oneself the effort of repression insofar as the larger share of the motivation to change objects is made conscious.

Such claims, of course, call for clarification. Let's once more turn to the masochistic development in hopes for information. Twice already, we have been able to use our theory to shed light on general problems, on the death drive, and on the question of the aggressive cathexis of the genital. Yet although I otherwise declare the change of object to be, at bottom, optional for girls as well, in *masochism*, we must postulate an *obligatory and unavoidable oedipal recathexis for both sexes*.

In the oedipal crisis, the masochistic phantasy about masturbation is particularly significant. The little masochists imagine the difference between the sexes to have emerged from the effect of aggressive masturbation, more precisely, the aggression cathexis of the genital and the excitation of sadistic wishes during the physical manipulation. Girls reproach themselves with self-mutilation, boys fear that in watching an erection wearing off, they are witnessing the damage *in statu nascendi*. In this situation, of course, the *father* is the only possible love object because he is not tarnished by penislessness. He is respected as bearer and possessor of the idealized member and admired for his taming his drives; yet, properly speaking, he is not a *love object* because the appreciation that really concerns his intact male member is merely transferred onto him. He is loved *because* he is in possession of the phallus. We saw (in the case of the "acrobat") that it is possible for the idealization to be refocused on the genital and the father to be tolerated as a necessary evil and appendage of his member. Despite the intense anxieties, the sex of the mother, too, attracts attention. In the runup to the oedipal conflict, in the phallic phase of development, the pressure exerted by the maturation of the incestuous wish prompts sexual curiosity to turn toward the mother. The early childhood idea that the mother has a penis as well can of course no longer stand up to the strengthened reality testing. The solution we supposed for this moment is an *identification with the member that in reality has been given up on*. But matters cannot end here: once it has arisen, the incest wish demands being fulfilled. Under different preconditions, the wish takes the form of wanting to sexually possess the mother and beget children with her, an intention that can be actualized only "over the dead body" of the father. The father's alleged revenge is being re-introjected and—with the threat of castration—silences the pulsional wish even if it does not calm it. In masochism, however, castration anxiety is not one of the reasons for the solution of the conflict but the precondition [of the conflict]. The content of the incest phantasy is always to return her penis to the mother and to equip her as "phallic woman." *The oedipal aggression in turn is given the goal of castrating the father and putting his penis at the mother's disposal.* The incestuous wish is now active, projecting one's own masturbatory ideas onto the mother, now passive, expecting genital satisfaction from, precisely, the mother's phallus.

Yet reality testing, combined with the effect of fear of the father's revenge, leads to a *double aggressive projection*. The mother is reproached for having mutilated *herself* through masturbation.[5] The suspicion quickly becomes the content of the castration anxiety: if the mother is as excitable and sadistic as I am, she will not hesitate to use her anger against me. The alleged victim of the castration becomes its executrix, the *mater castrata et castrans*. Simultaneously, the desired member of the father appears aggressively charged and threatens to take revenge on the little rebel. The child cannot endure this double external danger for long, and a new phase of aggressive re-introjection sets in. At a certain moment that can be defined quantitatively, there is a qualitative switch in the cathectic flow. While the projection onto the mother diminishes only in intensity and one's own aversion toward her in turn increases, the pleasure principle is afforded an occasion for placing passive

A forgotten cultural achievement 243

libidinous energies in the cathexis of the father. It is supported in this by consciousness of its anatomy, that is to say, by the reality principle. This results in a constant inclination toward cathexis displacement and, ultimately, a surplus of the libidinous binding to the father. The crisis comes to a preliminary halt but is by no means resolved. The new devotion is not ill-suited to defending against the anxiety about the revenge—the child, after all, sought to rob the father's most valuable possession—and we must not think that the originary impulses are abandoned. We may note, though, as a result, that beside the ego identification with the female phallus, a recathexis has taken place, that is, a displacement of the libido from the first love object onto the father. This definitively attributes the castration impulse to the mother, and she becomes the oedipal rival for both sexes. The common masochistic position toward the love object, if you like, corresponds to the heterosexual position of women and the male homosexual position. This statement, however, can in no way be reversed.

In their internal dynamic, neither the female genesis nor male homosexuality share anything with masochism. Yet if it *seems* nonetheless as if more women than men, and among them those more so who have found a particular solution to the Oedipus conflict, become masochistic, this judgment is not a consequence of psychopathological ignorance but of a well-grounded *social intention*. The false consciousness here serves the interests of a, for us, everyday dominion, that of men. In the association of masochism and sex, of devaluating a psychical clinical picture and scorning socially discriminated groups, men's claim to dominion imposes itself. In examining "voluntary" servitude, I have tried to explain in what ways those who suffer under a cultural ideology (I spoke of political, economic, and religious power) keep this ideology alive.

We are not concerned here with the fact that the *patriarchy*, too, seeks to justify its claim to power with the "submissiveness" of women and homosexuals. Our attention, rather, is on two new factors we have not heeded much so far. In the context of the form of dominion of the patriarchy, we notice that its being replaced by the subjective power of its representatives (the "men") must have still other and deeper reasons than we suspected. This question, however, I will delay a little longer.[6] The problem, in turn, which role conscience plays in the change of object, has not been fully resolved. When I assert that girls continue to be attached to their mothers and turn to the male object only under coercion, then the instrument of the recathexis would have to be the superego. I have denied that there is any biological necessity, and the psychosexual development at the very least makes the change of object appear optional. The regularity, one might argue, is the consequence of a superego identification. While little girls see the father as rival in their love for the mother, they later acknowledge his strength, not least because of the difference between the sexes, and submit to him. They desire the former opponent with the same ardor, albeit with a changed pulsional aim, as the first object. This process corresponds to the *"negative" outcome of the oedipal conflict*, and I think it characterizes the *common female solution* that seems normal to us.[7]

Yet if the recathexis is the result of the identification with the aggressor, then it cannot simultaneously be the precondition of the oedipal submission. We thus find ourselves compelled to assume a preoedipal change of object that is emphatically confirmed and thus doubled by the regular internalization, at the end of the crisis, of the aggression directed at the father. Yet why be so cautious? One answer results from taking the female feelings of guilt into account that are repressed along with the incestuous wish. One stratum of the sense of guilt concerns the embarrassing heterosexual phantasies of being genitally satisfied by the father, conceiving his child, being able to play with his penis, and so on, while the mother is eliminated. A deeper stratum of repressed oedipal wishes, however, is attached to the incestuous wishes directed at the mother, and the reproach is *to have betrayed and abandoned the mother*. Yet if the *first oedipal repression* concerns the homoerotic relationship with the mother, followed by the recathexis and finally the exclusion of the disapproved demands on the father by the second thrust of repression, then the female superego is of particular significance.[8] The unconscious guilt refers to the infantile *murder plans*, yet it does not concern the rivalry between the women but on the contrary the *betrayal* of the first love.[9]

A second answer to why the caution of a double confirmation of the change of object seems well-advised might be that men, without conscious intention but with latent seduction tactics, intervene in the female development because they fear for [their own] sexual rights. One might also think that the patriarchal ideology has prevented consciousness of the truth about the change of object. The not at all inconceivable alternative of perpetuating the libidinous bond to the mother and transferring it to female replacement objects without relinquishing pleasurable sexual intercourse with men would hurt men's vanity.[10] The availability of female sexual objects would be restricted; moreover, men would have to give up a good number of occasions for the pleasurable deployment of sadism and cruelty. No ideology, however, could settle its proponents with such burdens.

While dominion cannot be indifferent to the subjective loss, such a loss cannot be the cause of the amnesia. This notion, though, brings us back to the idea that forces other than psychical ones participate in the female recathexis in early childhood as well. Insofar as we focus on *economic* aspects and neglect pulsional quality as well as the sex of the object, this is what we find: the double turn of women's oedipal development, that is to say, the countercathexis of the first incestuous wish, [in addition] to the defense against oedipal strivings that must be performed in any case and is demanded of men as well, creates a *quantitative surplus*. The *pulsional dynamic* surplus has three sources: the additional work of defense, the pulsional quantity of the repressed complex, and the insufficient pleasure quality that issues from it. Obviously, men, too, are engaged in unconscious guilt conflicts, yet what is essential is that in the female development, there is a—let's not be shy about saying it—very slight but regular *additional burden of defense*. The performance of the *female psychical surplus labor*, however, goes to the dominion of men in the form of power. We are looking at an example of "voluntary servitude." That individual men profit from the frustration and guilt of women is of little importance when we consider that the increased work performance effects a pulsional economic displacement between the sexes from which not men but *the law of the patriarchy* benefits. This is not to say that women are "weakened" or disadvantaged because of the psychical burden. The subjective defense work is immediately converted into an addition to the objective power of the ideology it serves. The pulsional energy that can no longer be bound to the repressed complex is invested in the new object relationships and affirms the dependence. After all, the energies that are quite capable of imposing a pulsional aim and reach physical excitation but in so doing succeed only insufficiently in transforming into pleasure-affects because of their qualitative lack (the missing perceptual identity with the original wish) constitute the energetic reservoir that the dominion of men siphons off.[11] The unbound pulsional quantity cathects ego activities (actions, thoughts, positions) that the patriarchal ideology, via socialization, has already channeled and that only confirm the superiority of the men. Emancipation, equal rights, and the reversal of the relationship in individual cases change nothing about the fact that between women and a society organized by the law of men, there is a relationship like the one between subject and tyrant in La Boétie's essay. Preoedipal repression, recathexis, and heterosexual object choice are the commandment of the patriarchy and are fulfilled by the women to their complete disadvantage. The constant cathexis displacement between the sexes then appears as women's "masochism," and the conversion of the female psychical performance into the *objective law* of the existing form of society [appears as] "natural," at most as rendered necessary by the internal conditions of psychogenesis.

When we take the standpoint that the psychical causes do not suffice to explain the consequential "slump" in the line of female development, that neither coitus nor pleasurable heterosexual practices would need to be relinquished if the emotional binding were handed down to female replacement objects and not to men, we realize that the individual has no freedom of choice. The double repression is dictated to oedipal girls not just by internal conflicts; the main burden of causation is borne by objective coercive forces. It seems as if psychical processes that are barely noticeable and subjectively usually unfold unconsciously, necessarily increase the value of an established cultural ideology. If we assume a *hypothetical schism*, then the male demand for love will create social institutions as instruments to impose itself, whereas the female repression performance gives rise to objectivized forms of itself that turn back on the subjects and continue to condition the "voluntary" submission. The subjective pulsional demands nolens volens must adapt to such conditions; the pulsional vicissitude then testifies to the degree of restriction or promotion an unconscious impulse experiences from subtle objective coercive forces. Meanwhile, the symptomlessness with which the channeling of the drives takes place—and this was our starting point—may not be surprising where the men are concerned: they enjoy the advantage of an unbroken development and are privileged as shareholders of the objective power. Yet where women are concerned, it can be explained only if we accept a *historical thesis*. There must once have been a historical struggle between patriarchy and matriarchy that the matriarchy lost. The new rulers insisted on the tribute paid to the victors, and the defeated henceforth were obliged either to die for their habitual pulsional aims and objects or to assimilate.[12] The violence has long been replaced by nonsuspicious social institutions and a general cultural ideology no longer recognizable as a prescription of dominion, yet the *obligation* has been perpetuated for each individual woman in the long succession of generations of women since the downfall of the matriarchy, [the obligation] to *repeat*, in the object choice, *the submission* and to *confirm the law of the victors*.

The unconscious impulse at the beginning of the oedipal crisis to change *objects* does not stem from an internal necessity; little girls, rather, thereby react to a correctly assessed objective supremacy in the external world. In a way that resembles the command of the reality principle to relinquish the penis wish, to repress it, and to cathect other passive sexual aims, reality testing suggests to them giving up their original love object and to turn toward the father. The recathexis becomes a compromise between pleasure principle and insight into real necessity when the submission is followed by wishes as embarrassing as those aimed at the mother. Yet the regularly "negative" outcome of the oedipal conflict, that is to say, women's heterosexual inversion, perfects the defeat by internalizing the law of the father, tabooing the aggression against him. It also shows, though, that reality did not succeed in imposing the relinquishing and that the disapproved love object is now newly established internally, together with the repression of the incestuous wish. Girls then relinquish the originary object like they do their penis wish, namely, not at all. In consciousness and in reality, they bow to the law of men, but in the unconscious, they hold on to their claim to the mother as well as to the demand for an intact genital for both [themselves and the mother].

The *objectivized male-oedipal pulsional demand* thus has created for itself the *form of dominion of the patriarchy* that now *demands of women a cultural tribute*. As the defeated in a long-forgotten societal struggle, which was unable to change the genuine pulsional structure, women must, on the one hand, acknowledge the reality and orient their object choice accordingly (they thereby repeat the historical subjection in the pulsional vicissitude), on the other hand, they cannot escape the internal compulsion of the pleasure principle and will uphold penis wish and mother-object in the unconscious. The repression performance, however, which is to prevent the return of what cannot be reconciled with reality, creates the conditions for perpetuating the defeat. In the unconscious psychical work, the objective power of men's dominion finds one of its energetic resources, and the individual relationships profit from projections that were supposed to take some weight off the repression. When children transfer their penis wish onto the new object—which, psychically, makes a lot of sense—the triumph of the historical victors and the seemingly "voluntary" submission are perfected. Girls desire men the way they wanted the missed member to please the mother; they become dependent on and addicted to them. The oedipal development, however, began with a *relinquishing* that must be considered a *cultural achievement*.

To sum up: Women's male love choice is an assimilation to historical-social conditions; it contradicts the originarily phallic pulsional aims of the oedipal demand and the fixation to the first love object. Under the dictate of the reality principle, girls relinquish the object the way they are later prompted by castration anxiety to give up the incestuous wishes. They must perform a double oedipal repression that endows their development with a characteristic "slump." The result of the first repression is the recathexis, and the second defense concerns the internalization of the aggression. The regular female inversion solution of the Oedipus conflict obfuscates the two-time defense effort. Externally, women have found the male object, but this object is simultaneously idealized as the core of the superego. On the one hand, the object is protected by the erotic binding; on the other hand, it has become inviolable through the internal inhibition. This is opposed by the repression of the penis wish and of the original love object. The pulsional quality is still phallic, the pulsional aim is still autoerotic or homoerotic, but the wishes bow to reality and let the ego guide them secondarily onto genital-passive tracks. The cathexis displacement within the pulsional aims, like the recathexis, is undoubtedly a *cultural achievement*, but it is much more likely than [the displacement] is to become the object of neurotic conflicts on which more than merely subjective displacement depends.

Notes

1 As Helene Deutsch [e.g. Deutsch (1931) 1944], Sacha Nacht, or Karen Horney explicitly do. Passivity, submission, enduring pain, for example in childbirth, are listed as female pulsional aims. [It is difficult to ascertain which publications by Nacht and Horney Le Soldat has in mind: In the work by Nacht Le Soldat lists in the bibliography, Nacht presents such positions in detail but emphatically criticizes and explicitly rejects them (Nacht 1938, 243–44). As for Horney, the bibliographic information in the first edition is incorrect: the text cited there, "The Problem of Feminine Masochism," appeared in 1934 but contains only the abstract of a lecture given in 1933, which was then first published as an original article in English in 1935. The references instead cite Horney's 1926 article, "The Flight from Womanhood." What has been said for Nacht, though, also holds for Horney: in both of the texts referenced—as generally in her work—Horney is skeptical about, or even opposes the supposition of a primary female masochism.]

2 The supposition is that the female homosexual choice of object proceeds according to the narcissistic type. A choice according to the model of the first, maternal love object would be more obvious. Yet even there, one will have to acknowledge that the love object is much more connected with the introject, the secretly harbored phallus of the woman, than with the figures of childhood.

3 "Mother" is of course not to be understood biologically. Remarkable are those cases where the emotional function of the first object is performed by a man. I only once had occasion to see a patient whose mother died shortly after his birth and who was taken care of during the first years by his father alone. I could see no deviation from the development posited here since the consciousness of female penislessness arises in any case. For this patient, the father had become the bodily confirmation of his idea of the "phallic woman." In the oedipal conflict, the boy struggled against his uncle, the father's older brother, for the love of the "mother." As an adult, he was a philanderer and had innumerable, exclusively heterosexual relationships. For him, only a woman could be his analyst. What he was seeking thereby, though, was not the return of his deceased mother, with whom he had few ties. While the unavoidable oedipal disappointment of love in the father and the defense against the homosexual inclination that had arisen as the result of the inversion solution did favor the defiant and counterphobic turn toward women, they could not explain it completely. The addictive character of his relationships rather suggested that castration anxiety motivated his search for a partner. He was compelled by the superego (the interiorized aggression toward the uncle) to time and again picture what would happen to him if he did not give up his claim *to the father*. In conquering women, he identified with the inner aggressor, treated him the way he had expected from the uncle, and each time confirmed to himself that "nothing happened" to him after all. The corresponding analytic transference appeared "masochistic"; he treated me as sadistic uncle or devalued me as castrated woman. When the patient later began wooing me, it became clear that his "masochism" did not display an important symptom, the recathexis. He had now developed a classic *male hysteria*. He tried all the tricks in the book to actively seduce me. It was beyond doubt, however, that he identified me with the father, unquestionably considered me a man, and that his incestuous wish was no longer opposed by the anxiety about genital self-destruction or about contamination by the female "castrate" but by the re-introjected aggression. We may thus conclude that the actual sex of the infantile love objects plays a subordinate role. When the father figures as the first love object, he is not seen as a "father" but as a particularly desirable, because not castrated, mother. Phantasy will always find ways and means to conceive, beside him/her, of a "castrated" woman or a further "father" as oedipal rival and representative of the castration threat.

4 We could also call the object choice according to the anaclitic neurotic since it corresponds to a *fixation* of the libido onto its first object. The expression, in this context, is not used psychopathologically but points to the increased inclination toward conflict and the resilience of a compromise symptom over against the greater flexibility of other solutions.

5 In *hysteria*, the reason for the penislessness of the woman is that the father has injured or castrated the mother during coitus, that is, it coincides with the sadistic coitus theory of the early, preoedipal period. This idea supports the *projection of the aggression*: if the *father* treats the mother this way, then she—like me—deserves it as punishment for a misdeed, and the father is in a position to exercise his justice on me as well. (The example cited, too, conforms to the "classic" hysterical phantasy of conquering the mother and killing the father. The masochistic variant of castrating the father and of satisfying active as well as passive wishes with the conquered trophy, that is, to have intercourse with the mother or presenting her with the penis in order to be copulated by her, shows, first, the *central conflict about the difference between the sexes* and, [second,] the preferred use of introjection and identification instead of repression.)

6 [See below, III.6, esp. #239–45.]

A forgotten cultural achievement

7 See on the contrary, Freud 1931, esp. 239–40. On the concept of the negative oedipal outcome, see Freud 1921, 105–6. [This passage, however, does not feature the term "negative." While the reference might be erroneous, it can already be found in the draft JLS-Maso-7, note 36 on page A 78].
8 Freud, too, held that the female superego differed from the male one, but for him, that was because "[i]n girls, the motive for the demolition of the Oedipus complex is lacking" (Freud 1925b, 257). We have reached the opposite conclusion that the difference is conditioned by a *double repression*.
9 Matters are confusing because the content of the girl's positive oedipal position consists of homoerotic pulsional aims. The inner conflicts of female homosexuality, meanwhile, are wholly different from regression to love for the mother.
10 As far as I know, such solutions are acceptable in matrilinearly structured societies.
11 See my elaborations above, II.8 and 9.
12 Although among the "vanquished," there must of course have been men as well (we are not thinking of a community of Amazons, after all), the women were the defeated because *they* had held power before.

5 Splendor and misery of the superego

We noted for the female development that the *recathexis* obeys neither a pulsional nor a biological necessity but rather emerges only in the detour via a memory preserved in social conditions. We heard that women's passive, seemingly masochistic tendencies are not the cause but the consequence of the infantile change of object. A social process, by contrast, makes use of a factual historical event, in which there were victors and defeated, and exploits the unconscious psychical processes of the subjected in the service of the winners, to consolidate—across generations—the right to dominion of those who once were stronger. The recathexis is *first* of all a cultural achievement in so far as it allows for enduring a subjective unpleasure for the sake of the community. *Secondarily*, the drives seize the object and the aims reality prescribes to them; the traces of the compulsion, of course, can never be erased. There is nothing on the male side to correspond to the psychical effort of a life-long perpetuation of a repression that targets the originary pulsional facilitation. Men *can* keep their first love object; women *must* give it up. I am aware that the additional effort, compared to the other repressions cultural life demands of both sexes, is minimal, and also that the striving for pleasure will not hesitate to take advantage of the new situation as well. And yet the *regularity* of the unconscious change suffices to achieve the *quantitative* displacement of forces that appears as feminine "masochism."[1]

There is no reason to postulate a sex-specific pulsional constitution. Women are no less sadistic than men, and neither the inclination toward passive sexual wishes nor the impulse to phallic activity takes anatomy into consideration. When after the recathexis, different pulsional vicissitudes emerge for the boy and the girl, insight into physical givens has the slightest share in the process. For, what becomes psychically effective is not the *difference between the sexes* in itself but *consciousness of its existence*. While the phantasies that are being associated with it, that is to say, castration anxiety, produce the internal condition of the structural change (of the superego) for both sexes to an equal extent, the *law of the reality principle* is responsible for the bifurcation of the pulsional vicissitudes. Under the impression [of this law,] the little girl turns to the new object, and she does so initially with an undiminished phallic attitude. She tries to seduce the father no less actively than the boy tries to seduce the mother. After the recathexis, too, all children disavow female penislessness. The *phantasy* about how this [penislessness] has come about, how this might happen to him as well, leads the boy to internalize the aggression, whereas in the female development, the same phantasy—since the girl, too, feels herself in possession of a very small or hidden penis—leads to the same goal only via a characteristic detour—we must qualify the point and note that it psychically structurally leads to the same aim, since the detour will not be without consequences for the function. Although the drives enter into a compromise and accept a substitute rather than relinquish satisfaction entirely, at the height of the conflict, the original constellation imposes itself once more against the defense. The mother is the only desired object, and phallic-homoerotic aims once again appear in undiminished intensity.[2] The hatred is turned against the father, who disturbs, who prevents this love, and whose penis one intends to rob. The anxiety about his revenge, however, compels resignation. The incestuous wish is repressed a second time. Up to this point, the motive, the castration anxiety, is identical for the outcome with the male variant. With the introjection of the hostility against the father, the superego emerges. What up to now had been the *achievement of the recathexis is now taken over by the submission of the ego to the internal authority: the taboo on attacking the victor, on desiring his sexual objects, and on refusing to give in to him.* The inversion solution for the boy, under the impression of the pulsional ambivalence and taking quantitative factors (e.g., the intensity of the anxiety) into consideration, is preferable, for the girl is categorical: *the rival becomes the love object*. While the inversion is convenient for the passive strivings of both sexes, the reality principle makes it inescapable for the woman. The insight into penislessness links up with the perception of men's social supremacy. The girl thinks she has been punished, that is, castrated, *by* the father *because of* the forbidden relationship with the mother. It is essential that—unlike the castration *threat* during the crisis—this phantasy can arise only after the relinquishing, for what manifests here is not only the first effect of the superego, guilt, but also the return of the penis wish in a form agreeable to the patriarchy. If the father has castrated me, then he will also be able to redress the injustice in me! While heterosexual binding of the man must impose itself *against* the now internal danger, that of the woman is perpetuated *by* the castration threat. The *penis wish*[3] works in the interest of the dominant cultural ideology, and the fact that the pleasure is restored in the new object cannot hide that the alignment of the drive[s] with the interests of Power is being paid for with the subjective unpleasure of an additional defense effort.

Denigrating the secret effort of women as "masochism" is a criticism only in appearance. The thesis is more about exculpating its beneficiaries than it is about devaluation. It may be that a suspicion arose in men, who profit from their dual status as love object and authority when they siphon off the cultural work that has become unconscious, that they personally have not merited so much privilege. They are not wrong about that, and the reflection, too, that declares the symptoms of this socially disavowed defense to be female masochism is not entirely absurd. While no one will want to attribute one and the same neurosis to all women, it is clear nonetheless that the psychogenesis of woman and masochism each have a characteristic breaking point, the recathexis, which is reason enough to suspect a kinship. The intersection of two lines of development at a prominent point—in the zenith of the oedipal crisis—and accordingly the similarity of some manifest symptoms, however, should not impress one's judgment. The fact is that the female recathexis is coerced by the dominant cultural ideology, that is to say, comes about because of the *reality principle*, while the masochistic change of object is the immediate consequence of the *pulsional economy*, that is to say, of the unfavorable relationship between aggression and libido.

While for woman, the cathexis displacement is a psychical necessity, which the drives initially resist and which emerges only because of a compromise, through the mobilization of psychical work, for the masochist, the recathexis is a dynamic relief and an economic gain. In the conflict of the little girl, the pulsional wishes *follow* the cathexis, that is, given the new conditions, other perceptual identities must be formed as well. In the case of masochism, in turn, the change of object is not a question of the orientation of the libido but of diminishing the aggressive projection onto one parent and increasing it onto the other. We may thus indeed assert that it is a *defense* for the masochist as well, albeit not in the service of reality.

In masochism, the projection onto the mother is amplified; she appears as bearer of the castration intention. The father is seen as the knight in shining armor who is to yield the secret of how to obtain a penis or keep it intact. The peace, of course, is deceptive. Just as definitely as the recathexis was necessary, it deteriorates again after a short time. Deception of love and the unavoidable re-aggressivization of this component, too, entail hatred, mortification, and feelings of shame, and the *originary double aggressive cathexis of both objects* reemerges. The ego sees itself beleaguered from all sides, by the sadism of the drives, by the reproach that it is destroying itself through masturbation, by cruelty and revenge, which it projects onto the objects. The levels of anxiety and aggression rise in the ego such that the situation converges in a repetition of the earlier trauma. To protect against a pulsional inundation, the ego deploys an *emergency function*. Suddenly and radically, *all pulsional energies are withdrawn from the object cathexes and the projections are given up*. The ego thus attains a strengthened position vis-à-vis the id, yet it relinquishes its claim to the objects of reality. The withdrawal, of course, cannot be compared to a psychotic consequence because reality testing and perception remain untouched. The relinquishing corresponds to an appropriate, active defense that must be considered an autonomous achievement.

In detail, though, the recathexis deteriorates *first*, *then* castration anxiety acquires an unbearable intensity, and finally, the objects are dismissed as far as the inner reality is concerned. This sequence is essential insofar as it becomes, first, the condition of a further characteristic masochistic symptom, the objectal regression, and, second, the economic basis on which the masochistic superego establishes itself. There is no need to dwell on [what] the deterioration of the recathexis [means] for the object relations. Because they regress to the binding to the mother, masochistic women appear homosexual; they seek to conquer women although their *pulsional wishes*, because of the genuine orientation toward the phallus and the short phase of love for the father, rather have to count as heterosexual.[4] Genital passivity and penis wish unite in the phantasy of being satisfied by the "phallic" mother. Men, in contrast, after a period of homoerotic love for the father, return to the originary incestuous wish. We must not, however, suppose that the pulsional quality has remained unchanged. Thanks to the recathexis, the masochist, too, now wishes *to obtain a pleasurable satisfaction in a homosexual practice from the mother who is also equipped with a phallus*. These objectal ideas are henceforth the model of all masturbation phantasies.

We are now able to better localize their genetic origin, even if the contents of the wishes have nothing new to tell us; the *genesis of the superego* is extremely remarkable. I will repeat here only the bare minimum to capture the difference from the masochistic path more clearly. The child associates erotic wishes with the mother and aggressive [wishes] with the father. Although both objects are ambivalently cathected, the contrary pulsional component is repressed so far, or shifted crosswise, that in the first phase of the conflict, love and hatred appear clearly distinct. Under the effect of the castration anxiety, however, the frontlines are blurred once more. The mother is reproached for her penislessness, and contact with the "castrated" one is feared; the hatred toward the father turns back on the attacker as revengeful threat of punishment. Love deception and anxiety create so much unpleasure that the ego represses the pulsional demand and internalizes the incriminating aggression.[5] Both processes unfold simultaneously, and we have to picture the ego as using the very aggressive energy it withdraws from the father to establish the repression. The ensemble of the internalized aggression becomes the core of the superego, whose content is associated with the object of the father and with the wishes referring to him, but whose energy comes from one's own aggression drive.[6]

We will have to view what is happening in masochism differently. If both parents have to bear an aggressive projection, the mother the threat of castration and the father the revengeful anal or oral overpowering, yet [if] the child withdraws the cathexis from both objects at the apex of the conflict, then there exists nothing but this withdrawal to count as superego introjection. The totality of previously projected (that is to say, bound to the object representatives) aggressions is freed in the ego and unites to form the new structure. The content of the masochistic superego is inconspicuous, since, as usual, it derives from the aggressive oedipal strivings. And although there is nothing enigmatic about its connection with the pulsional source and castration anxiety as the occasion of its emergence, the agency displays two particularities. It cannot aim its censorship directly at the incestuous wish, since this wish was already withdrawn from the ego in the *first* thrust of repression, in the course of the recathexis. The superego confirms the defense and strengthens the countercathexis. Most urgently, however, it turns against the striving that has *replaced* the forbidden love wish, against masturbation. While previously, the aggressivization of all functions impeded masturbation, too, in the short time between cathexis withdrawal and the formation of the new structure (by means of libido that was freed and "narcissistically" attached to the ego) the opportunity arose for pleasurable masturbation. The establishment of the superego, however, reestablishes, via a detour, the preoedipal condition. *Sadism-turned-morality ruins masturbation.*

The infantile masturbation of the latency period usually enjoys a certain mildness of censorship because the superego sees in it a sign of relinquishing the incestuous demand. The superego contents itself with rejecting all too forthright phantasies and with tempering the pleasure. The masochistic superego, however, rightly considers masturbation not a defense but a *substitute of the incestuous wish*, and the taboo strikes all of autoeroticism.

The structural progress, though, entails a further disadvantage, and this names the second peculiarity. It will come as no surprise to anyone that the masochistic superego is a strict and sadistic one. After everything we have said about the aggression surplus, the lack of pulsional alloying, as well as the constant presence of unbound aggression energy in the ego, it cannot be otherwise. The masochistic super-ego is vicious and cruel, yet at the same time, it is *weak, deficient, and barely able to fulfill its function*.

We probably already suspect why that is, but let us once more seek advice from clinical practice. Recall the dream of the "kitchen fairy." At the beginning of her analysis she reported having dreamed that I (the analyst) was "pissed off"—*stocksauer*—at her for being late for her session.[7] We said that the latent content expressed her wish that it may not be too late for her to marry and that she yet wanted to have children. The meaning of the word *stocksauer* remained unclear and no opportunity to analyze arose subsequently.[8] I now want to make that up. The patient was known among her friends to be friendly and sociable. In analysis, she showed another side of herself. She was defiant, cold, and for a long time, the analyst had to endure scornful ridicule that was hard to top. She devalued all interpretations. She disliked my appearance and my office, and she met psychoanalysis with contempt. She reported on incidents with business partners whom she trusts but quickly ends up quarreling with. She then always has to give in, [she said,] she cannot bear conflict. As soon as she wants to make peace, however, she is miserably rejected by the other. The analyst, too, is greedy for money, quarrelsome, and is only out to humiliate her, but won't succeed. She herself is stronger and smarter, the other person a coward, and so on. Of course, we think that the patient in her everyday position has developed a reaction formation against defiance and negativism. In the transference relationship, this defense is replaced by the identification with the failing internal agency. She fears being ridiculed and then berates me the way the superego usually terrorizes her.

The "kitchen fairy" had grown up in a stable, middle-class family. As an adult, she avoided all contact with her parents. She talks about the mother from a cool distance. The defense, however, changes in the course of the analysis, and the aversion turns into hatred. She reproaches the mother with malevolence and neglect. At the same time, she talks about current events. She complains that her boyfriend does not want to sleep with her, that he probably doesn't love her at all, and so on. Once it had become clear to me, though, that she had chosen her boyfriend according to criteria that unconsciously reminded her of her *mother*,[9] her resistance could be explained only as a reaction against an embarrassing, homoerotic-incestuous longing. This, of course, meant that one secret of her virginity had disappeared. If the man at her side was a replacement substitute for the mother, then in living together with him, she pleasurably perpetuated the oedipal situation: she has won the mother for herself and eliminated the father. This "mother," however, has miraculously obtained a phallus after all. Yet what brought the patient into analysis? She casually remarks that late in life, the father had to undergo an appendectomy. Although the surgery was harmless and went smoothly, she has since then lived with an inexplicable fear that the father might die. It was impossible for her to visit him at the bedside. Her father is a candid, kind man. He suffered a lot during the world war and came into the country as a refugee. He never succeeded in fully feeling at home. He took a job that did not correspond to his artistic capacities. He was an extremely tender and attentive father to his daughter. He played a lot with her and would never have prohibited anything or refused to grant a request. In the unconscious, though, the "kitchen fairy's" most hostile feelings were directed at this father. She could not understand why the mother gave her love to this "picture of misery" instead of her, the able and brilliant one.

The repressed aggression against the rival showed itself [directed at] a substitute object, the grandfather. She was often sent to him on nights when the parents wanted to go out. A musician by profession, the conductor of a men's choir, he too seems to have loved and fostered the girl but only earned her contempt. She considered him old, ugly, and stupid, and she particularly resented that he did not conduct his choir bare-handed but needed a baton to do so. She thought it a sign of weakness. The baton reminded her of crutches—something unworthy of a "real man." She also thought the grandfather was too fat, ate too much, above all that he had no manners, smacking his lips and slurping. When she was bored at his place, she went into the garden, wandered about, and when she felt no one was watching, she indulged a secret passion. She dug into the earth looking for grubs, which she collected, examined, and buried again, albeit not individually but gathered into big piles. One day, the grandfather caught her, and although he did not understand what she was doing, he recognized her bad conscience and talked to her parents about it. The parents confronted her, and shortly afterward, the adults forgot the insignificant affair. The girl, however, felt exposed and denounced by the grandfather. She plotted revenge and thought to herself, "I hope you burst, you old pig [*Sau*]!"

For a while, she hassled the grandfather until he did in fact get angry. When he then berated her, she triumphed internally, and again she thought: "I hope you burst with anger!" Yet when he was taken to the hospital because of an upset stomach, she suddenly felt guilty and feared that her wish had come true, that the grandfather really had "burst" and she would be recognized as his murderer.

The nightgown in the dream[10] is an allusion to the white, long gown of the grandfather in the hospital, but also to his burial gown had the attack on him succeeded. The compound word *stocksauer* is a condensation of *Stock* ["stick"] and *Sau* ["(female) pig"]; you will recall the grandfather's conductor's baton, which now threatens her. The "pig" seems to be the grandfather who is to be blamed for his own illness because he eats so much; at bottom, however, she herself is the "sow" digging through the earth for grubs. This action is to be regarded a masturbation replacement. She has maintained the structure of the excited digging and drilling in the vagina as well as the quality of the pulsional, which is immediately evident to the adults without their grasping the meaning of the action: the girl was looking for the lost penis. Her looking *in the earth* is a compromise. The aggression forbids her pleasurable masturbation, she fears destroying herself even more. For the purpose of nocturnal relaxation, she has developed a practice we already know. She refrains from touching herself with her hands, which she considers aggressive and destructive. By digging into the earth and not into herself, she bows to the superego prohibition. Yet if the earth is a replacement for the body of the mother (the "Mother Earth"), then in her phantasy she is playing the mother's genital the way she was hoping for from her for herself. The action becomes particularly exciting through the fact that she defiantly presents the forbidden to the grandfather/father: Look! This is how little I care about the taboo!

Yet there is something else to the *Saustock*, the "pig stick." It of course symbolizes the penis. Her longing for the idealized member has turned into angry contempt. Once reality had taught her that her hope was pointless, a radical turn took place in her. She now wanted to have nothing, nothing whatsoever, to do with the penis, with men, and with the difference between the sexes. In her phantasy, she devalued everything connected with what is male. In the unconscious, she denied that there was anything like it at all. During adolescence, she intensely fell in love with another girl at school; superego formation and social considerations, however, barred the path to homosexuality. There was thus nothing left for her but to choose a man who was sufficiently passive and reticent to spare her the "pig stick." That worked for a while, but the former wish inevitably transferred to the boyfriend/mother as well. She wanted to conquer and love the man the way she wished for with the mother, namely, phallically, with a penis of her own.

We understand that she could not confess *this* wish with the same ease as her worry it might be too late for her to marry. We also recognize that the patient is operating a father transference onto the analyst. In the sessions, she treats the analyst the way she considered herself scorned by the father, the way she herself finally provoked the grandfather. We may expect that because of the therapeutic regression, the devaluation will make way in the analysis for a broad idealization and penis transference. (I presented this process in detail for the "acrobat.") The result would then be that in the patient, increased aggressiveness, or rather the displaced relationship between aggression and libido has led to an emphasis being placed on defiance and negativism, that she is homoerotically fixated on the mother, and that she is caught up in a sadistic conflict with the father and all that is male. The superego profits from the aggression, unmitigated by any admixture of libido. Undeniably, the "kitchen fairy" suffers quite a bit from the scorn and ridicule of the internal censorship agency. She is tormented by reproaches, and some of her phantasies can only be seen as self-punishments, the way she acts can often be seen as repentance. The superego can be characterized as sadistic and malicious. And yet I'm not entirely happy with this diagnosis. Several things do not fit this picture. Although we now understand better what she means by *stocksauer/Saustock*, by "pissed off"/"pigstick," it remains unclear what significance is to be attributed to the idea that she is "too late" and *therefore* I am angry. The father's illness becomes the occasion for undergoing therapy. She feared—and hoped—her murderous wish had finally come true, that the father had "burst."[11] The similarity of the symptoms, the grandfather's enteritis and the father's appendicitis, to be sure, lends some credence to the reactivation of the infantile neurosis, but it seems a little thin to me. We learn that the patient associates various pleasurable phantasies with the idea that the belly becomes bigger and bigger until it finally bursts. The superficial sadistic birth phantasy is: if the mother betrays me with the father, then she is a pig, and it only serves her right if her big belly bursts.[12] More important is the soothing idea that something big is hidden in the belly and is becoming bigger, the penis growing back, that will one day "jump out." In connection with men, it is a satisfaction for her to think that underneath the night gown, they too, are just "big," inflated girls, as it were. And the passive sexual excitation has operated a small displacement from the penis's capacity for erection to the swelling of the belly, where the "bursting" is to stand in for the orgasm. While she denies the existence of the male member, she transfers its impressive ability to erect to the neighboring region of the belly.[13] The conflict between phallic striving and penislessness, between passive wishes and the deadly contempt for the penis, however, does not suffice to explain her symptoms of suffering.

We know that the censorship draws its energy from the id, that is, it uses pulsional quantities to convert [them] into feelings of guilt. We may say that the sadism directed at the inside is a pulsional satisfaction as well. While the ego does not participate in the pleasure, the generation of affect, nonetheless, *economically* is a gain for the entire psychical apparatus. I add one further observation, though. At the beginning, I thought that the ego of the "kitchen fairy" submits unconditionally to the internal tyrant. I saw her, identified with the superego, mocking the analyst.[14] I hear from her that she feels exposed to a psychical compulsion constantly to punish herself. In the course of the superego/father transference, however, the patient not only becomes fearful and, in reaction, malicious, which would indicate the identification, but also combative in a particular way. She berated me and could not endure my remaining silent; she provoked me and was content when I seemed upset. Her angry wrath, meanwhile, was almost unstoppable, the triumph obvious, when the analyst had to admit she was right in a certain respect. The *pulsional* quality[15] of her pleasure was unmistakable, and it is hard to believe that the gain was due solely to a defense.

In this phase of the analytic relationship, the "kitchen fairy" has established *between us* the *internal* relationship between ego and superego. She projects the sadism of the superego onto me and through identification subjects to its power. Simultaneously, *she of course has not stopped being sadistic herself* and torments the analyst/superego pulsionally and pleasurably. Masochists are commonly recognized by the unrelenting pressure of conscience, by constant feelings of guilt, by a "masochistic" ego that submits to a cruelly strict superego. Yet we should not let ourselves be deceived by the manifest clinical picture. The unconscious can never be visible *directly and unadulterated* in the symptoms. The clinical leitmotif of masochism, the suffering and submissiveness of the ego, cannot simultaneously be the cause of the neurosis. If the ego finally acknowledges, before the superego, the defeat before the reality, the oedipal rival, then over time the capitulation acquires a *demonstrative* character. The influx of additional aggressive quantities into the ego does challenge the verdict of the superego, but it strengthens the economic situation of the ego to such an extent that a "balance of terror" emerges. In consciousness, the ego bows to the seeming supremacy; silently, it has allied with the drives and deploys aggression against the tormenting internal agency the same way it did in the oedipal war against the father. Insofar as the superego is hostile and, thanks to the castration threat, powerful, it can block *actions*, repress *phantasies*, and curtail pleasure. In becoming active, it produces, through the guilt affects, *unpleasure*. Yet in no case can it prevent that the ego is cathected by aggressive pulsional energy and that these then turn against it. The excitation of the ego functions, above all the guilt-defense, is an aggressive satisfaction, associates regressively with the repressed phantasies of the oedipal plans for murder, and undoubtedly generates *pleasure*. The ego will seek and take up the same fight with the superego as the oedipal child did with the father. The sadistic pulsional strivings, whose path to the body and the external world is blocked precisely *by* the censorship, have the alternative of binding itself to the superego raging against the ego—or of allying with the ego against the prohibiting agency. In both cases, pleasure is generated that is kept secret, with different justifications, from consciousness. It is, at bottom, astonishing that the pleasure of conscience in tormenting the ego is so rapidly apparent while it took us a lot of time and effort to acknowledge the mere possibility of besieging the superego with pulsional energy, and subsequently the advantage of the ego in doing so. The motif of disavowal, in turn, can be produced only by the superego, and we are unlikely to be wrong in suspecting here the intention of keeping its own vulnerability secret. Yet the *pleasure affect in the ego* is nothing but the consequence of a *genuine aggressive pulsional satisfaction*. Like most postoedipal wish fulfillments, this satisfaction does without a physical activity and the real presence of an object, and [it] draws the gain in pleasure from exciting, in phantasy, pulsional cathexes that are as broad as possible.[16]

In its triumph, the masochistic ego benefits from an unexpected consequence of the inclination toward aggressiveness in the id. The internalization of the moral agency took place in the abandonment of the double hostile projection onto father and mother. We recall that the child could not endure the internal threat of the drives, projected castration anxiety onto the mother and pulsional anxiety (in the form of anal and oral phantasies of overpowering) onto the father, but was finally compelled to give up all object cathexes. This gave rise to a superego with an undiminished aggressive charge, whereas remainders of the libido cathexes could be bound narcissistically in the ego. In this way, however, the superego loses one of its essential functions, that of the *ego ideal*. Where usually, the ambivalence toward the rival leads to the superego assuming a Janus face—conscience represents the prohibition to do as the father does as much as the commandment to become like him[17]—in masochism, the libidinous cathexis of the censorship agency is almost entirely absent; that is why [censorship] lacks the ability to draw boundaries for the ego and to serve it as a model. The masochistic superego is sadistic but finds itself incapable of obtaining the ego's admiration and voluntary conformity. *The superego becomes inadequate to the same extent that it is strict*. The defect is in no way one of morality, that is, it is not to be interpreted contentually; it is an economic defect. *The hostility of the ego is directed against the lack of the superego's ideal function*. The ego will miss no opportunity to upbraid its internal opponent for this weakness. Economically, however, the ego profits from the missing libido binding. The more the superego's energy cathexis is displaced toward aggression, the more quickly the saturation degree of the ambivalence is attained and the more "free" aggression energy remains for the ego. We must suppose that in the choice between investing itself in the superego and taking the path through the ego to the objects, the aggression drive will usually choose the internal agency.[18] The ego seems to be abandoned without resistance to the power of conscience. But now we learn that a minimal change in the pulsional economy has unimagined consequences: *maximum strictness of morality* and *sadistic pleasure in the ego to torment the judging agency*. I go a step further and assert that the intention of the ego, and the aim of the aggression drive after the oedipal internalization, consists in eliminating the superego structure from the psychical apparatus once more. This intent is usually thwarted by the agency's ambivalent cathexis, which is able to bind sufficient aggressive forces. The rest is repressed, channeled, and socially consumed. Only in the case of masochism does the pulsional aim become visible at all, though of course, it must not become conscious. The superego certainly cannot admit the possibility of its own abolition. Although there is no chance at any point in the psychosexual development to bypass the formation of conscience or to avoid its consequences, the ego's demand *to liquidate the superego* (and not just the more harmless variant of *disregarding its commandments*) in the interest of the drives is an outrage. That the masochist attempts nothing short of just that is evinced by bitter struggle, waged with equal weapons, between ego and superego.

One would be hard pressed to imagine a less appropriate interpretation of masochistic symptoms than the thesis that masochists submit to the superego and enjoy the suffering. The opposite is the case. The demonstrative repentance of the "kitchen fairy," the loudly proclaimed *mea culpa* of the "physicist," and the apparent capitulation of the "acrobat" in her addiction are *compromise formations* between sadistic morality and the ego's uninhibited pleasure in attacking the moral agency. Only in the analytic transference, however, does the true suffering unfold, and it does not concern the guilt conflicts, neither the compulsion to submit nor the sadistic triumph, but the withered libido. In presenting the internalization of the superego, I concluded that it turned primarily against masturbation. The resulting restriction of pleasure is evident. Beside this, I claimed that the incestuous wish is "repressed" prior to this, in the recathexis phase. I must now correct this statement, since repression is not yet an option of defense at this point. The capacity for countercathexis arises only with the superego: the repression is established and maintained *in the service* and largely *by means* of the superego's aggression energy. Yet the result of the introjection cannot already define the defense at the beginning of the conflict. If projection and identification are ruled out, and if disavowal and denial appear too weak to keep an intensive pulsional wish away from consciousness, we find ourselves in an embarrassing situation. The course masochists' analyses take shows that the originary incestuous demand toward the mother is "repressed" *prior to* the recathexis—long *before* the hostility toward the father is internalized. I saw the defending force to be the castration threat. There can be no doubt that from that point on, the disapproved wish is *dynamically unconscious*, it imposes itself effectively for a moment only one more time, at the apex of the conflict, and must otherwise be considered "repressed." It also makes sense that the oedipal repression of masturbation *once more* strikes the claim on the mother connected with it. However, a pregenital defense must have been in operation that is apt at securely keeping the mother incest from realization, in the female development, and, in the case of masochism, [preventing] the active castration impulse.

In Freud's posthumous writings, there is a note on the "Splitting of the Ego in the Process of Defence" that might be helpful in addressing our problem:

> Let us suppose, then, that a child's ego is under the sway of a powerful instinctual demand which it is accustomed to satisfy and that it is suddenly frightened by an experience which teaches it that the continuance

of this satisfaction will result in an almost intolerable real danger. It must now decide either to recognize the real danger, give way to it and renounce the instinctual satisfaction, or to disavow reality and make itself believe that there is no reason for fear, so that it may be able to retain the satisfaction. Thus there is a conflict between the demand by the instinct and the prohibition by reality. But in fact the child takes neither course, or rather he takes both simultaneously, which comes to the same thing, He replies to the conflict with two contrary reactions, both of which are valid and effective. On the one hand, with the help of certain mechanisms he rejects reality and refuses to accept any prohibition; on the other hand, in the same breath he recognizes the danger of reality, takes over the fear of that danger as a pathological symptom and tries subsequently to divest himself of the fear. It must be confessed that this is a very ingenious solution of the difficulty. Both of the parties to the dispute obtain their share: the instinct is allowed to retain its satisfaction and proper respect is shown to reality. But everything has to be paid for in one way or another, and this success is achieved at the price of a rift in the ego which never heals but which increases as time goes on. The two contrary reactions to the conflict persist as the centre-point of a splitting of the ego. The whole process seems so strange to us because we take for granted the synthetic nature of the processes of the ego. But we are clearly at fault in this, The synthetic function of the ego, though it is of such extraordinary importance, is subject to particular conditions and is liable to a whole number of disturbances.[19]

What Freud calls "this way of dealing with reality, which almost deserves to be described as artful [*knifflig*],"[20] fits pregenitality very well, and we already questioned the synthetic function of the ego in the case of masochism anyway.[21] What consequences for the sexual function, then, can we expect from this defense? When the most embarrassing infantile demands experience no countercathexis, they are not eliminated for consciousness but present in a particular form. They are *preconscious but emotionally isolated*. The incest phantasies do not fall prey to the usual infantile amnesia, they form a secret, pleasurable core in the ego.

It thus seems as if matters turned out well for masochism in the oedipal conflict after all. Reality is not fully acknowledged; in turn, sadistic satisfactions are guaranteed and the incestuous wish is rescued. In the psychical, however, an old Talmudic saying applies: whatever he does, worries follow the poor man like faithful dog. With the internalization of aggression, the castration anxiety is usually repressed, and in its place the tension of the sense of guilt appears in the psychical. Masochists, however, are saddled with the sense of guilt without being able to escape castration anxiety. Their guilt affect draws its force from the pulsional anxiety. The castration phantasy that is attached to the mother and has, along with the sexual wish, evaded repression must be projected once more. This adds an object dependence to guilt and anxiety.

Only the real presence of an "evil" object can allay the internal anxiety. This henceforth indispensable bearer of the projected castration threat is opposed internally by the most intense genital wishful phantasies that, although untouched by repression, have become emotionally unattainable. Masochists have not exchanged the anxiety for the "permanent internal unhappiness" of the sense of guilt[22] but obtained *anxiety* and *guilt* and the feeling of *longing* that, though [its fulfillment seems] within reach, can never be stilled.

To sum up: in the future, the masochistic characteristics will include the ego generalizing this special treatment of reality. The split in the ego remains irreversible. The ego, in any event, has received a further unmistakable masochistic trait. Every time a conflict pulsional wish versus reality or pulsional wish versus superego arises, the ego reacts *by both submitting to the threats and holding on to the pulsional satisfaction*. The longed-for ambivalence has been lost definitively, this time structurally. The libidinous phantasies circling around the idealized phallus are isolated, accessible to the striving for pleasure but not to the emotions, split off from the aggressive impulses. What used to be a necessary consequence of the imbalance in the pulsional quantities now is the sealed outcome of the oedipal structure formation. In not operating the repression of the incestuous wish, masochists, to defend against castration anxiety, remain dependent on the real presence of a threatening object. In what follows, I will refer to them as *perverse objects*.

The "kitchen fairy" had become dependent on the help of an angry ("pissed off") object. The intensification of her genital demands on her boyfriend had prompted her anxiety to increase. The father's illness amplified the anxiety through an increased emotional pressure of guilt but was not decisive for the wish to enter analysis. Instead, she was in urgent need of someone to guarantee the aggressive satisfaction that had to be kept away from her genital at all costs. Her attempts at getting close to men failed under the scorn of the superego that ridiculed her penislessness, and the masturbation ended in panicked phantasies of being mutilated and destroyed. The turn to passivity was blocked by the penis wish and the reproach of betraying the mother. The sexual tension could not be relieved and established the *unconscious wish to enter analysis*. The therapist was to abolish the castration threat projected onto her and finally provide her relaxation with the "pig stick."

Notes

1. I once heard a rich man say: "I speculate on the stock market. In 49.9% of cases, I lose money, in 50.1%, I win. And life hasn't been bad with these 0.2%."
2. Questions of homosexuality that pose themselves in this context are extremely difficult, since male and female homosexuality each take different paths and do not form a unity in themselves. The genesis of homosexuality is no less complex than that of masochism; the homosexual *object* in any case can be no criterion of the internal development.
3. Tellingly, the *female wish for a penis* appears in the literature as *"penis envy."* This, however, not only assumes a male standpoint, which sees the pulsional wish to be aimed at itself. More importantly, a consistent motif of female development is

fixed in a form that it assumes *for a short time*, at the height of the oedipal crisis, in the collapse of the recathexis. When the girl wants to rob the penis of the father to conquer the mother with it, the impulse indeed deserves the name of envy. Prior to that, however, the origin of the penis phantasy is not objectal, and the regular unconscious fulfillment of the wish consists in the idea of the female phallus, which, although it is not visible, exists. After the conflict has been settled, the penis wish once more appears as dependence on a man. Reality and drive have united in one effect, such that fulfilling the unconscious demand is expected no longer from the ego but from the idealized object. Since the alignment [*Gleichschaltung*] is not dictated by internal forces but takes place compelled by and in the service of social dominion, it is the latter's interest that must impose itself in the nomenclature. With [this] *pars pro toto, it prevents consciousness of a further pulsional energetic source of objective power.*

4 This structure was clearly visible in the case of the "acrobat."
5 Establishing the superego comes with the incestuous wish seemingly being given up. The child loses interest in the mother and for short time even in masturbation. In reality, a pulsional wish configured in the unconscious can never be dissolved again. The drive reserves the facilitation it has created for itself, namely, to the extent that pleasurable excitations and anxiety are associated with it. There is thus a defense function to correspond to the retreat from the (effectively *preconscious*) claim; this function is the "countercathexis" performed by the ego in the service of the superego that keeps the disapproved wish *dynamically unconscious*.
6 Freud articulated the connection of morality and drive as follows: "it may be said of the id that it is totally non-moral, of the ego that it strives to be moral, and of the super-ego that it can be supermoral and then become as cruel as only the id can be" (Freud 1923b, 54).
7 See above, II.4 [#].
8 [The etymology of *stock-* in this instance is unclear; as in a number of other compounds it is used here to signify "very." As evoked below, #, it is homonymous with *Stock* or "stick." Meaning "angry" in this case, *sauer*—related to the English "sour"—contains *Sau*, the female pig or "sow."—Trans.]
9 Thus she noticed in the course of the analysis that both names begin with the same sequence of letters and that in calling the boyfriend she always had to suppress the name of the mother. Thanks to a contre-jour photograph, a striking similarity of their figures emerged, as well as the memory of the mother's body odor, which may be more effective.
10 [See above, II.4, #]
11 Swiss German would use the common phrase *es verjagt ihn* [literally, "it chases him away"] here. It designates an outburst of anger ("jetzt hat's ihn verjagt") and, casually, dying as well ("es hat ihn verjagt"). The sexual association we discuss in what follows takes up the male orgasm with ejaculation ("den hat's verjagt"). The German word *zerplatzen*—literally, "to burst"—conveys the nuances insufficiently, triggers much too aggressive ideas. "Es verjagt ihn" plays much more with the ambivalence and the voyeuristic pleasure.
12 This is one of the common *revenge phantasies* of children when they feel betrayed by the mother.
13 In interpreting dreams, we see time and again that the path associations take heeds a thing's external structure less than it does its movement, development, and function. If the salient movement of erection is emotionally essential, it is without hesitation transferred onto belly, eyes, legs, and so on. The causality evident to us, that the male erection is connected with the female belly growing big, is in this case certainly conducive but recedes in the face of the necessity of defending against the voyeuristic unpleasure. The "kitchen fairy" cannot endure the sight of the active penis, must disavow it, must transfer the movement she longs for onto the belly.

14 Already at this point in time, the identification with the "aggressor" is ambiguous. The patient projects her own hostility onto the analyst and struggles against her *in order to* impose her disapproved sexual demands. See also above, I.2.
15 The "made in id" we always grasp. [See above, #153 and #284n56].
16 Let me point out once more—because it is difficult for insight to access—that *pulsional satisfaction* is an exclusively *psychical* matter and conceived by us as the excitation, as consistent and intense as possible, of broad swaths of phantasy. Repression acts as an "interruptor" on the pathway or course of excitation; unpleasure arises from the restriction of conversion of pulsional energy into affects or from the special production of unpleasure affects by the superego. There we observe the curious fact that *too* broad excitation processes, too, generate unpleasure, namely, anxiety. Although the pulsional satisfaction is psychical, the pulsional *wish* is nonetheless categorically directed at a physical fulfillment to be perceived on *one's own body*.
17 The superego's "relation to the ego is not exhausted by the precept: 'You *ought to be* like this (like your father).' It also comprises the prohibition: 'You *may not be* like this (like your father)—that is, you may not do all that he does; some things are his prerogative'" (Freud 1923b, 34, Freud's emphases).
18 In this tendency, the originary oedipal facilitation of aggression becomes visible. While the pulsional wish is turned away from the external object and detached from the internal representative of the father, the pulsional tectonics have not changed completely. In this regard, conscience formation does not enter into a dynamic opposition to the pulsional force but uses its orientation to gather and reverse it.
19 Freud 1938a, 275–76.
20 [Freud 1938a, 277. *Knifflig* may also be rendered as "tricky" in the double sense of employing tricks and of being difficult (to figure out or to deal with).—Trans.]
21 It is supported by the primacy of wishful thinking over reality testing and the emphasis on disavowal over repression.
22 As Freud puts it in *Civilization and Its Discontents* (Freud 1930, 128).

6 Who's afraid of castration?

In our investigation, we now find ourselves in a situation that everyone who analyzes knows only too well. We have put masochism on the couch. We have heard a number of things and understood a few. But we are not content. We cannot rid ourselves of the impression that there is something essential we do not yet know. A central area of the conflict remains closed to us. As in analysis, where in this same situation we make use of the means of information [*Auskunftsmittel*] that is countertransference, let's take a moment and look at the course our explanation has taken. One thing that stands out is that it has taken me an unusually *long time* to grasp the repressed sexual wish. Assuming that it is not due to obtuseness on my part, two resistances can explain this hesitation. Either I have not yet become conscious of a further defense that is active in me and shies away from acknowledging the most profound sexual wish, or the arduousness of the progress *is* the masochistic pleasure. In the latter case, I would in the course of the reflection have identified with the masochist, a procedure that indeed corresponds to analytic practice and precedes conscious insight. However, we then don't know what to do with this new piece of information. Why should postponement and delay be pleasurable? Although psychoanalysis is aware of the significance of "fore-pleasure,"[1] the quality of active tarrying that is becoming clear to me now is entirely different from that. We'll have to postpone the problem and first look at the other thesis.

Once the *double triumph of sadism*—as overly strict morality and as pleasurably waged fight of the ego against the weakened superego—is discovered, we have also recognized *the distress of sexuality*. Masochists do not suffer from despondency and docility, their *aggressive pulsional satisfaction* is more than guaranteed and ready to transfer onto the objects; the *sexual partial drive*, by contrast, is blocked by the neurotic development. The reasons for the frustration have in the meantime become familiar to us. They are of a pulsional economical nature and concern the deficient alloying; they refer to the repression of the masturbation phantasies, which renders physical manipulations pleasureless, as well as to the disavowal, coerced by the castration anxiety, of the difference between the sexes. We found nothing peculiar about the quality of the sexual wish; it is genital, and the physical excitation seeks to be relaxed by masturbation or by the oedipal love object. Conflict arises between ego and superego when masochists try to connect the genital satisfaction with incestuous demands, and between striving for pleasure and reality insofar as for both sexes, the love object can only be a woman equipped with a penis. The inevitable turn to passivity mortifies self-confidence, but it is no longer able to allay the sexual inhibition, since the motive of everything that is happening, the castration phantasy, has long settled [in the inhibition] as well. The passivity, however, is a fixation point of the neuroses, since the excitation of passive wishes satisfies a genuine partial drive and simultaneously fulfills the superego's commandment to make oneself sexually available to the rival. If even this compromise between superego and striving for pleasure, which amounts to an *alliance between unconscious morality and drive*, cannot be maintained, then castration anxiety is, once more, the reason.

Where does the castration phantasy get its power? This seems to be a meaningless question, since the terror of a genital mutilation is intuitively clear to everyone. But I think that the horrendous *content* of an idea does not suffice to find its most general effect. Even if anxiety is constantly kept awake as a way to maintain a threat, even if it has entered into insoluble connections with the most intimate and urgent sexual wishes, that only sheds light on its universality but not on its power.[2] And this power cannot be meager because it is up to anxiety to simply blow up once more an alliance of superego and pulsional demand, as we just saw in masochistic passivity. Castration anxiety, obviously, is a psychical formation—a phantasy—and cannot be kindled by real practices or threats. My claim, though, is that its continued effect as much builds on *internal* motivations as it feeds on *objective interests* in the external world.

Psychoanalytic experience teaches us to take infantile pulsional demands seriously. The child does not pursue the fulfillment of its wishes playfully, say, or merely in the imagination but concretely, materially, and physically. The mother is desired sexually and physically, and the father is threatened with a genuine murderous intention. For the child, the oedipal conflict is not a psychical conflict of the inner world but factual reality. Once we grasp that, we are no longer surprised by the drama of infantile passions; instead, it seems astonishing that there are no known attempts by children to murder the oedipal rival. While the sexual drive has more leeway and children are allowed a number of tender excitations they will later be denied, the intention to kill, though indeed realistic—five-year-olds already are physically and intellectually capable of murder—is referred to phantasy. I do not doubt the ambivalent (for it is also erotic) binding to the father and the anxiety about his revenge, but I think it does not suffice to keep the sexual demand in check, and the murderous intention under control.

During the oedipal crisis, children are assailed by passions—not so the adult. Although unconscious communication inevitably conveys to them, too, the meaning of the infantile excitation, they by no means feel bewildered. We can often observe that the sexual temptation is effective and the parents themselves are caught up in internal turbulence, but they will hardly ever fear for their lives. They can confidently await the outcome of the conflict, since everything works out as if by itself. The Oedipus conflict, I say, fails because of *internal* obstacles. The greatest among these, however, the castration complex, I now claim, also serves to defend *vital interests of the elder*. Of course, I am not thinking here of a direct causality between infantile demand and parental behavior. In the course of this study, I insisted several times that we cannot assume object relations to exercise profound influence on the pulsional vicissitudes, that the causality, rather, works the other way around. It would be ridiculous now to try and trace the existence of conscience back to pedagogical efforts or to parents' sexual privileges.

Thanks to ethnopsychoanalytic research, we know that the oedipal conflict is a ubiquitous phenomenon whose preconditions and outcomes have culture-specific variations. Neither the murderous rivalry with the father nor the internalization of the aggression is imperative. What in my view happens in every case, however, is an engagement with the difference between the sexes. My next thesis is that the collision between precocious infantile demands with adults' seeming disinterest or incomprehension (which seems inevitable as soon as people of successive generations live together) is invariant as well. If the children were a little older, their strivings would be taken more seriously—but this way, the greatest crisis of childhood takes place without public significance. I do not think this has always been the case. If human beings' *physiological* maturation reaches a stage at around twelve years of age at which children become sexual partners and dangerous opponents, then responsibility for the *anachronism of pulsional development*, on the one hand, lies with the fact that pulsional wish, body, and reality enter only into a loose association—the pulsional formation pays no heed to the possibility of wish fulfillment. On the other hand, the privileged position, which has no psychical justification, of castration *anxiety* entitles us to suspect that the temporal displacement of the conflict—which in reality becomes significant for the external world in late childhood—to early childhood is in the interest of social dominion. *The precociousness of psychosexual development must be considered a success of a social intention that exists to protect the fathers. The castration threat is the instrument of a particular type of society to defend the life, property, and sexual objects of dominion*. If [this type of society] manages to suppress the demands *in statu nascendi* and if in so doing it is able to ally with an internal force, it *spares* itself the otherwise indispensable *physical confrontation*.

We can no longer refuse the insight that the psychical power of castration anxiety stems from a regular turn of the aggressive sexual drive, which in the phallic phase assumes the form of a genuine *active castration pleasure*. What we later expect from others, above all from the oedipal rival, is what first we wanted to do him. The violence of the originary sadism—which, in keeping with the phase-specific sexual interest, in the oedipal conflict is directed at the genital and thus also returns as a threat as well as fear of the revenge—explains the *innerpsychical* privilege of castration anxiety. The maturation of the psychosexual function long before the biological might be attributed to the general irrationality and contradictoriness of the life of the drives, but I prefer pondering the participation of social interests in this respect as well. When we look at the result of the temporal divergence between the psychical, oedipal crisis at about four years of age and purely biological maturation or social relevance at about twelve to fourteen years, the psychical latency period of the ones turns out to be a social *closed season* for the others, whom just now they still sought to castrate and to murder. To the superego's anchoring of castration anxiety in the psychical on one side corresponds the institutionalization of the memory of the outrage (e.g., through religious symbols) on the other, which merely stabilizes the objective power of the elder. But we do not know how that is supposed to happen. Displacing a psychical conflict forward and accelerating it, after all, is something that cannot be compelled by force of will or violence.

I can imagine that a process, which, like "voluntary servitude," is engaged for centuries in the constant displacement of unconscious forces and which, like in female development, was prompted by a factual historical event, could have such an effect. Franz Borkenau in 1957 wrote a well-informed study on Greek mythology from which I take some hints. The Minoan culture of Crete was ruled by a matriarchate. Under the law of the Magna Mater and of special mountain goddesses, women were socially privileged and sacred. They held the economic, religious, and political power. They were free to choose a lover, a *paredros*, who had to bend to their will.[3] In the second millennium BCE, Minoan matriarchy was shaken by two waves of migration from northwestern Greece and replaced by a patriarchal system. Scholars assume that the first wave of patriarchal conquerors from the north in the seventeenth century acknowledged the privilege of women. For a while, the new dominant group appropriated the customs of the subjected. Only the second wave in the twelfth century violently repressed the matriarchy. Significant for us, of course, is the transition period. What consequences regarding the oedipal conflict can we expect from a drastic change in social organization? Does the sex of the rival, too, change with their social status? If it is true that the formation of the superego strengthens the objective power of the established social dominion, then a change that is not ideologically conditioned but tied to sex must psychically have a *structural effect*. The change in the contents of the commandment might release old taboos, demand new ones, something that leads to stable ego assimilations within a few generations; the observation of the difference between the sexes, by contrast, is so fundamental a psychical element that we may assume the perception whether social power is held by "phallic men" or "castrated women" to have far-reaching consequences. The very idea that women are castrated may well already be associated with their social defeat—they could have been punished this way as the ones who lost. Accordingly, in matriarchy, women would be anatomically perfect whereas men would suffer from a genital prolapse. The thesis, of course, does not stand scrutiny. The castration phantasy existed long before the oedipal internalization. Woman, because of the pulsional development, is considered castrated by both sexes. Unavoidable sadistic sexual wishes and the cathexis of genital excitation by the aggression drive lead to the anxiety about damaging oneself. This anxiety is projected onto the women, in whom one thinks to find the obvious confirmation of the phantasy. Female anatomy initially participates in conscience formation as *associative confirmation*, then the guilt reproach concerns the *active causation* of the genital mutilation. Later, the superego creates the *causal connection* between social defeat, punishment, and castration.

We should not assume that the human beings of an archaic culture four thousand years ago found the conditions of their pulsional setup to be different from what we find them to be today. Pulsional quality and the laws of the psychical hardly undergo significant changes. The replacement of one culture by another, however, will slowly and barely noticeably leave traces in the pulsional vicissitudes and in the pulsional tectonics. If the change takes place *violently* and if both the overpowered dominion and the new law are *tied to sex*, then, over the course of generations, upheaval arises in the unconscious phantasies. The formerly subjected *paredroi* take revenge on their former "lords," the mothers, and yet cannot make their own decisions because as members of the old culture, they are subjects of the new lords, the barbarians from Magnesia. That the mothers now become social outlaws does not mean that they lose their power as oedipal rivals. Although there is, to my knowledge, no direct evidence of the psychology of the Helladic-Minoan age, I will venture some speculations.

Under matriarchy, a *woman* occupies the place of the failing object; this woman, in any case, cannot be identical with the psychological mother,[4] she is conceivably a grandmother, aunt, and so on, a person whose subjective interests accord with social dominion and who has an established right to sexual intercourse with the mother. Castration may well have seemed to the little Minoan Oedipus to be the price of incest. We should not be surprised that a woman can be a good representative of the castration threat. Rather than revenge, strivings to take advantage are projected onto her. Something similar can be said for little girls; only relinquishing the penis wish and accepting the idea of having been castrated by the Magna Mater as a punishment allows for defending against the sense of guilt. *Psychically*, the sexual wish is inevitably tied to the condition of castration. Will we find no differences between cultures, then?

In a patrilinear order, where social authority and the freedom to choose one's sexual objects are handed down from the father to the son, the infantile incestuous wish reaches for the father's privileges, and the aggression aims at his murder. When the father takes the child's urging seriously, he finds himself compelled to defend his property, his potency, and his life; he has good reason to think that only his *castration* can be the aim of the adolescent strivings. His sexual organ is what the aggression is focused on, it is the obstacle to the fulfillment of the sexual wish. When the father defends himself, he defends vital interests, and his violence becomes institutionalized in the *incest taboo* and in *parricide guilt*.

In matriarchy, by contrast, incest will hardly be blocked by lethal sanctions. The union of mother and son must instead appear as a commandment and—in the service of securing offspring—take place under the eyes of the Magna Mater. The taboo is more likely to concern the willful overpowering and *rape of the mother*. At the same time, the murderous intention cannot take recourse to the castration of the female rival but will demand her sadistic *impalement*. This is associated with a number of psychological consequences. The reciprocal conditioning of preoedipal anxiety and conscience formation is rendered more difficult. Castration and impalement both imply death by means of a genital devastation, but they exclude each other. While the projection of the castration phantasy succeeds onto the female rival, too, the re-internalized aggression has a different aim. It is unclear how the superego is to condense both ideas into *one* threat, and it is very much questionable whether this gives rise to a *guilt* affect. And the incest taboo does not strike particular objects but the *quality* of the genital drive.[5] If, however, the alloying of the pulsional components becomes fatal, this once more affects the relationship between ego and superego. The superego is economically weakened, its position vis-à-vis the drives becomes indecisive, and thus it also becomes more difficult to establish social power that relies on the taming of individual pulsionality. Maybe it was this psychical refinement, not just the social defeat, that contributed to the worldwide demise of matrilinear systems.[6]

The unsolvable internal contradiction in patriarchy exists between incestuous wish and sense of guilt, and the preferred neurotic structure it thereby generates is that of hysteria. We can only speculate about the conscience conflict in matriarchy; in any case it is more likely to have been maintained by pulsional anxiety, the repression-worthy wish more [likely to have been] of an aggressive than of a libidinous nature. It thereby moves closer to masochism, insofar as the superego formation is concerned, but it is of a completely different kind when it comes to the blocked pulsional component. I can imagine that in the period of the transition from the Minoan matriarchy to the new culture, former psychical taboos became social practices, especially in the destruction of the Great Mothers. In adults' historical memory as in infantile phantasies, the anxiety about [the Mothers'] revenge conquered the castration phantasy and was defended against with a *secondary* eroticization of the relationship.[7] Caucasian myths about *rock births*, for example, the legend of Ullikummi, give rise to the suspicion that killing with hot stones was being considered. But we may suppose that the phantasy of inserting something into the vagina with a sadistic intention forms as many different variants as the phantasy about the way in which penis and scrotum were separated from the body. In consciousness, the anxiety about impalement is represented by a reversal, such as a phantasy of birth. Anxiety-affect and the idea of pain are thereby maintained, the sadistic intention, however, is pleasurably inverted into the opposite. Later *Baubo rites* can be understood as condensations of the old anxiety and the younger penis wish. In the patriarchy, the impalement idea yields its violence to castration anxiety and its content comes in to defend against sexual pleasure. This, via a detour, breaks the second taboo, the alloying of the drives, and replaces it with the new patriarchal prohibition, which burdens *objects*, not pulsional aims. For the psychical economy, this is undoubtedly a gain.

Even after profound social subversion, a newly established power has no reason to address infantile pulsional demands. *Children's* latent sexual wishes and oedipal plans for murder never represent an *objective* threat.[8] Culture and power only find an opponent in the *unconscious* inclinations of adults, which of course derive from those wishes and plans. Insofar as patriarchal law defines the cultural ideology, the antinomy of sexual drive and castration anxiety converges in incest taboo and parricide guilt. In matriarchy, by contrast, we must suppose that the same intention, namely, to defend the elders' pulsional satisfaction privilege, would prompt the internalization of the little female rival's impalement aggression. Conscience then does not become the threatening and punishing agency we are familiar with but an intrusive agency of control—a turn we have observed in our social organization. There, of course, the intrusive rather than punishing tendency is not an indication of a change of dominion but the result of an energetic displacement among the drives on the one hand and, on the other hand, between the power of subjective pulsional demands and the objectified forms of their satisfaction. We will have to verify, however, whether this is true to the same degree for the transition from matriarchy to patriarchy. We heard that "voluntary" servitude is handed down in a subtle chain reaction of unconscious phantasies and social laws. When two dominion ideologies are at war, little changes for those who are dependent insofar as the mechanisms largely endure—once the old potentates have been overcome, the defeated culture transfers its mode of action onto the contents of the new power without great difficulty. In a sex-related change of power, however, the fact that the unconscious phantasies primarily revolve around the *difference between the sexes* does have some significance. After the first phase, in which the old and the new dominion let others fight for them, something outrageous will happen instead of the usual resignation before the new lords: the adolescent *paredroi* contest the dominion of the men, and do so in a way as if they had no conscience, no inner censorship that paralyzes them before the authority. How is that possible? Like all dependents, they counted on the downfall of the mothers, and the foreign attack succeeded in what the cohesion of objective power with their unconscious anxiety definitively denied them. The *missing association between castration or impalement and the male object opened the way for the real and uninhibited struggle against the male rivals*. For the innerpsychical establishment of castration anxiety, we must thus assume, beyond the psychical causes concerning the pulsional defense, a historical situation in which the real interest of dominion and the imposition of the infantile wishes intersect not just in phantasy but indeed in the social reality. It takes a third step, the violent suppression of the unique "unconscionable" rebellion, to associate the new lords with the idea of genital annihilation as well. Decisive for this process are not the real sadistic practices but the internal process that adds the harmony of content, of preoedipal anxiety and oedipal aggression, to the economic advantage of conscience formation.[9]

We still haven't reached the end, though. The drive is not soothed but rather stimulated by a satisfaction; power is not content with a victory. The usurpers rightly feel threatened by those they violently subjugated and will undertake everything to assert their idea of law and sexuality against the adolescents' phantasies. In this situation, the *temporal advancement of the struggle between the generations* makes concrete sense. If power does not wait for the children's physical maturation but intervenes already at the first clear stirring of aggression and rivalry pleasure with an unequivocal demonstration of violence, it will not have to fear a conflict later. If the *paredroi*'s intention was to castrate the men, then children will be threatened with just that. Internally, the initially concrete, later latent threat enters into connection with the genuine castration anxiety of very early childhood that cannot be dissolved again. The little Minoan defeated are thus integrated in a new cycle of "voluntary" servitude. The pulsional development's oedipal precociousness takes place without external influence; the *consolidation of the castration anxiety* in the resolution of the crisis by contrast can only be explained by the subtle unfolding of the interest of dominion in the psychical. Dominion has conquered its position by means of physical violence, imposed sexual practices by means of coercion, enacted the incest-taboo to privatize privileged sexual objects, and put a stop to the rival's threats by advancing the confrontation from puberty to early childhood. It is understandable that power shows no great interest in keeping this career in consciousness. Disavowal and amnesia are made easier by the fact that, subjectively, entirely different causes lead to the same repressive intention. Although the infantile impulses still remind dominion of its violent origin and although it no longer seems to undertake anything to defend itself, it enjoys the fruits of the painstaking work of displacement that has been going on for centuries.[10] In addition, it relies on the effect of secondary affects—shame, sense of guilt, and mortification—that take the relay of the primary anxiety and expunge the infantile defeat from consciousness.

In her collection of dreams from the Nazi era, Charlotte Beradt tells the dream of a sixty-year-old Berlin lawyer, a Jewish man whom the political developments had deprived of job and security and who suddenly found himself declared an "under-man":

Two benches were standing side by side in Tiergarten Park, one painted the usual green and the other yellow. There was a trash can [*Papierkorb*, lit. "paper basket"] between them. I sat down on the trash can and hung a sign around my neck like the ones blind beggars sometimes wear—also like those the government makes "race violators" wear. It read, "I Make Room for Trash If Need Be."[11]

We cannot look to the dreamer's associations for help, we do not know when and in what circumstances the dream emerged, nor why it was recounted and recorded. I will nonetheless venture an interpretation. The castration anxiety, we just heard, draws its power from a two-fold source: the unconscious phantasies about the difference between the sexes and the historical interest of dominion that, too, has long become unconscious. The *sexual drive* thus confronts a coercive *internal* limitation—which appears as completely absurd—and a subtle *social* restriction whose commandment is all the more evident. Might it be possible to claim just this kind of social genesis for the additional obstacle to the sexual in masochism? We saw that to sufficiently explain the symptom of suffering, the psychical inhibitions do not suffice, neither quantitatively (concerning the pulsional intensity) nor in the content of the neurotic conflict. That is why we address the *question concerning the social conditioning of masochism* to an example whose accidental causation is abundantly clear.[12] The dream can be directly characterized as masochistic. The dreamer yields to the external power, anticipates its intention, and humiliates himself the way that he is afraid of being abused by it. That, in any case, is the manifest content, the success of defense, and secondary elaboration. What could the repressed be? What unacceptable wish has disturbed the dreamer's sleep? There are *two* painted benches in Tiergarten Park. I think that the separation between Jews and Aryans enacted in reality is to represent in the unconscious the polarization between women and men. On a deeper level, it becomes an allusion to the irreconcilable pulsional components.[13] *Tiergarten*, literally "animal garden," is a multifaceted allusion to sexuality: as a pleasure district in Berlin, as the place where the "animals" (the drives) are locked up, as erogenous zone of the body, the genitals. "In Tiergarten Park" means "down there," where the animal-pulsional is. (The dreamer assumes an ironic and distanced position toward the genital, as does, for instance, the "acrobat.") The two benches between which he sits down can be interpreted as heterosexual and homoerotic tendencies. In deciding in favor of neither one nor the other, he seeks to construct a compromise between the phallic strivings, which are dangerous in the external world, and the homosexual strivings, which are disapproved internally. The dreamer instead sits down on the trash can in between: he has identified with the penis, and the dream denotes the regression to masturbatory phantasies. He subsequently devalues the member as blind, as a beggar, thin and worthless like paper, similar to the "physicist" who abuses his member as a "corpse."

The dream's placid, even cynical surface, however, cannot deceive the judgment that this is a description of an *acute anxiety dream*. At the center is the phantasy of the "race violator." The unconscious, which does not care about political ideology, conceives of the social prohibition as an *exogamy taboo*. Unlike the superego, which places lethal sanctions on incest, reality takes the stance that *only* endogamy is permitted. The unusual conflict between external world and conscience on the question of incest leads to the invigoration of the repressed. Might the oedipal wish finally be fulfilled? By "*race* violation," the unconscious, however, understands something different from what reality does. For the id, it means the prohibition to unite with the *other* sex, which is equivalent to a binding rule of homosexuality. This usually cannot please the internal censorship, which appeals to the public conscious and infantile anxieties. *Castration anxiety prohibits what reality secretly demands on pain of death*. There is only one way out: resexualizing the superego, projecting the anxiety, relinquishing the phallic wishes, and eroticizing the dependency on the murderously hated authority.

For masochists, however, there is another path as well. The conflict gets the "artful" treatment we are now well familiar with going: bowing to the danger without relinquishing the wish fulfillment.[14] Where others make a regressive compromise, whose symptom consists in sexualizing aggression, masochists, on the basis of their neurotic structure, are able simultaneously and unscrupulously both to satisfy disapproved wishes and to make a gesture toward the superego. The contradiction between internal commandment and (unconscious) public morality does not particularly confuse them. A psychical scandal for the others, the dichotomy for them is part of the neurosis. Their special resolution of the infantile crisis has destroyed not the incestuous wish but the ability to derive pleasure from genital excitation. Aggressive satisfaction is possible and a daily occurrence, incest phantasies are not repressed and almost freely accessible, yet the connection between drive and body is abolished and prohibited. Let me emphasize that despite all efforts, I have not yet understood this last fact. Usually, guilt affects and anxiety affects defend against the pulsional pleasure, which can, however, be restored by dissolving repressions. In masochism, by contrast, the formation of the superego has not only led to guilt conflicts; the pulsional tectonics has been changed in such a way that, while the psychical pulsional satisfaction is guaranteed, the connection with the physical excitation is lost. In this situation, the idea that there are *Triebtäter* will become intriguing because it designates people whose pulsional condition is so exclusive that they accept no substitutes and risk their lives rather than relinquish a very specific kind of physical, concrete wish fulfillment.[15]

In the phantasy of the "race violator," sexual wish, sadistic components, and the longed-for connection with the body condense: I contravene all laws. I have intercourse with whomever I please, I "violate" whomever I want. (The "violation," like the "rescue"/"murder" discussed earlier, takes up the infantile, sadistic idea of coitus.) My urge is so strong, my excitation so intense that no father, no government will be able to hinder me. The dream thus pleasurably inverts a two-fold helplessness. The external distress needs no explanation. The dreamer defiantly turns against the social denigration, which the unconscious does not conceive of as a life-threatening aggression. For the id, rather, it counts as a desirable repetition of the infantile state. Yet the ego cannot act nearly as vigorously in confronting the other affliction. It feels excited and angry and at the same time helplessly dependent on external participation to relax the sexual tension. The phantasy of being a *Triebtäter* fulfills the wish for the pleasurable excitation of the body and its autonomous satisfaction. The dependence on a "perverse" object[16] (the "sign" he begs for) is mortifying by itself but becomes, the moment all of reality offers itself for projection, completely unbearable.

While the external world secretly allies with the incestuous wish and the inclination toward homoerotic passivity, the id wants to impose autoeroticism ("I do it myself").[17] That is why it is understandable that the internal censorship becomes active at *this* point. In the secondary elaboration, it compels disavowals and a reparation. I've done nothing, I haven't masturbated and "violated" anyone, I'm not potent at all (instead, I'm "blind"),[18] I'm a beggar and still in need of external help. The last phrase, the dreamer making "room for trash" can be considered an affirmation of the masochistic solution we are familiar with: the ego identification with the idealized penis is replaced by the one with the castrated member.[19]

The latent dream thought—"I am a *Triebtäter*"—has presented a wish as fulfilled that both reality and the masochistic conscience disapprove of, albeit with completely different intentions. The terror regime tolerates no freedom of pulsional satisfaction because that would mean the loss of urgently needed energetic resources. The internal prohibition is directed against autoeroticism because within the dynamics of the drive, [autoeroticism] has taken the place of incest.

What masochists seek to prevent with all their defense measures, namely, the sexualization of the aggression, is loudly and publicly advanced by the environment. For others, the subjective cathexis displacement means an economic relief,[20] but for masochists, it becomes synonymous with the pulsional danger. That is how they become *rebels against their will*. Prior to all rational reasons and ideological reflection, their neurotic structure does not allow masochists to conform to a sadist regime. This will surprise us. We like to think of masochists as particularly willing subjects. Yet insofar as the social intention of alignment exploits the tendency of people to assimilate to spare themselves conflict, masochists *cannot* submit to an aggressive reality.

What is fatal for them in the maelstrom of social violence is not, as it is for others, the sexualization of aggression—masochists have developed sufficient protection against this pulsional danger in their neurosis—but the seduction to project the castration anxiety. We heard that for them, a superego has emerged that is sadistic on the one hand but on the other hand is weak and defective. From the former derives the continued existence of the inclination to project the genital anxiety, from the latter [the fact] that idealization needs external objects. The lacking ambivalence tension, however, commands the pleasure principle to cathect one and the same object with the expectation that it relaxes the sexual tension and simultaneously endure the aggression.

Our question concerning the social conditioning of masochism is given a clear answer. External coercion, violence, and accidents can neither generate nor decisively promote masochism. On the contrary, the seeming submission turns out to be a latent sadistic readiness for combat. The object dependency serves the autoerotic intention alone and will not let itself be displaced toward aggressive aims. The conditions masochists find in a terror regime do not differ essentially from those that they, thanks to their pulsional vicissitude, are familiar with from their inner life. The calm masochists sometimes experience in an accident or in suffering from an openly violent reality is in no way to be attributed to their enjoying their suffering. Nor do they clinch a punishment from the superego/vicissitude, as Theo Reik, for example, thinks.[21] Masochists in these cases appear calm because their *habitual neurotic defense* against the new reality is adapted—by coincidence, we must say—to the new reality. The structure of the neurotic defense prevents the social alignment that aims at sexualizing the aggression. Masochists are sufficiently burdened with the disentanglement of the drives and cannot endure any further reduction of the ambivalence. What we found confirmed in the supraindividual, namely, the historical and social roots of castration anxiety that reach all the way into the present and remain psychodynamically active, cannot simply be transferred onto subjective events. Reality contributes less to the etiology of the neurosis than reason and intuition want to acknowledge.[22] Then where does the rumor come from that masochists are willing victims not only of private oppression but of tyranny as well? We don't need to look for an answer for very long.[23] In the service of an apology of power, consciousness once again operates a reversal of causality. Not the masochists are victims, the victims are masochists.

One last effort remains. I began this contribution with the suspicion whether the masochistic sexual wish might not be defined by a particular pleasure *quality*. Now that [we have seen that] neither the psychical conflict nor the external conditions suffice to explain symptoms of suffering, that it is still incomprehensible to us how the censorship agency can succeed in disrupting the connection between drive and body, we will have to solve the masochistic "riddle"—or our work so far will have been in vain.

Notes

1 In 1905, Freud thought that "fore-pleasure" designated pleasure through excitation of erogenous zones, while "end-pleasure" was given by the satisfaction-pleasure of sexual activity; fore-pleasure was what the infantile sexual drive produced and what became end-pleasure only under the conditions of puberty (Freud 1905a, 210–11; see also Freud 1938b, 152–56). In our context, the concept "fore-pleasure" means the pleasurable *buildup of tension* or the pleasurable tension itself. The end-pleasure, which insists on the psychical wish fulfillment and on physical relaxation, it seems to me, cannot be tied to the biological functions and reserved for adulthood. All conditions of genital end-pleasure are already met by infantile masturbation.

2 In the oedipal conflict, any and all anxiety is irreversibly associated with the sexual function.

3 The proud, downright arrogant attitude of the "Prince of the Lilies" from Knossos (see Evans [1921–1935] 2013), according to Borkenau [1957, 3–4] a *paredros* of the Magna Mater, can be seen as the defense and the reversal of the anxiety of a doomed man.
4 The "psychological" mother is the caring person of the first years of life.
5 Here and in what follows, it is unclear how homosexual strivings would be treated. The tabooed pulsional alloying would have to come out.
6 Of the few matrilinear structures still in existence, the majority functions only constitutionally, for example among the Minangkabau people on Sumatra, who practice *matrilineal succession* but socially are under the influence of Islam and thus, in their unconscious phantasies, are castration-oriented.
7 I think that the younger female idols, Šauška, Ishtar, and Atargatis, emerged only at this moment. They were the idealization, displacement substitute, and reparation for the mothers who had been overthrown and murdered. So far, we have unquestioningly supposed that castration dominates the preoedipal processes, too, with the idea that something is genitally torn from us. Perhaps we now ought to broaden our horizon and acknowledge impalement, too, as a form of genuine pulsional anxiety.
8 It would be a fallacy to claim that biological fathers object to the adolescents' impositions. While individual struggles do indeed create subjective repressions, they are not suited to forming the basis of the general structural formation.
9 There is no reason to consider a society's sadistic penal practices to be the direct expression of unconscious anxiety; anxiety *and* pleasure *and* political opportuneness are required for them to emerge. When for Borkenau [1957, 12–13] even the myth of Oedipus has little to do with castration but instead with the then common *slighting*, he confuses cause and symptom. In the myth that Freud found in Sophocles, [Borkenau] thinks he can show displacements and reinterpretations of historical events that know only one motivation: the repression of the historiography of the defeated by the victors. The memory of historical punishments, however, that both victors and vanquished want to eliminate (slighting, execution [by hanging] "from the feet"—Oedipus's club foot, sacrifice by means of poisoned thorns, stoning), is linked to the unconscious anxiety by association, not as a simple depiction. The cathexis-displacement in the unconscious does not arise *in* the changes in public murder practices but from the subtle connection between sexual wish/sexual taboo, aggression intention, and their internalization.
10 I speak of displacement *work* because perpetuating the status quo requires an energetic effort from both sides. See above, II.7–9.
11 Beradt (1966) 1968, 135. The ellipsis replaces the Beradt's interpolation, "in those days, Jews were permitted to sit only on specially painted yellow benches."
12 In 1905, Freud established a "complemental series" on neurosis formation that connects the constitution and accidental childhood experiences, disposition and traumatic events (see 1905a, 239–40.)
13 We do not know why the dreamer speaks of benches (bench = bank?), of the Nazis as "green," or of paper (paper money? emigration documents?).
14 [See above, #234.]
15 [*Triebtäter* literally means "pulsional perpetrator," which is the sense Le Soldat is working with here. It is most commonly used, though, as a colloquial expression that roughly corresponds to "sex offender."—Trans.]
16 The expression is not a moral one but a terminus technicus. We heard that the *perverse object* is being idealized as displacement substitute for the defective superego, that it is to represent the externalized castration threat and, simultaneously, that it is to effect the relaxation of the sexual tension. Characterizing it as "sadistic"—in the popular opposition sadism versus masochism—seems rather paltry to me.

17 [Le Soldat is referring to the lawyer's hanging the sign around his neck himself.]
18 "Blind" is a condensation of the negation "I do not see any difference between the sexes" and the result of the castration, of which blinding is an unconscious symbol.
19 My interpretation has had to rely on formal factors and missed out on all plays on words and the entire labor of the dream *work*.
20 An explanation of this advantage presupposes a psychoanalytic theory of fascism that we do not have.
21 See Reik (1940) 1941.
22 In a different context, Anna Freud comes to a similar conclusion. In 1945, together with Sophie Dann, she writes about the development of six heavily traumatized children from the Theresienstadt concentration camp, whom she had taken in at Bulldog Banks: "That the children were able to attach their libido to their companions and the group as such, bypassing as it were the parent relationship which is the normal way to social attitudes, deserves interest in relation to certain analytic assumptions. In recent analytic work the experiences of the first year of life, the importance of the relationship to the mother during the oral phase, and the linking of these experiences with the beginnings of ego development have assumed great significance. Explorations in these directions have led to the belief, held by many authors, that every disturbance of the mother relationship during this vital phase is invariably a pathogenic factor of specific value. Grave defects in ego development, lack or loss of speech in the first years, withdrawnness, apathy, self-destructive attitudes, psychotic manifestations, have all been ascribed to the so-called 'rejection' by the mother, a comprehensive term which includes every disturbance within the mother relationship from loss of the mother through death, permanent or temporary separation, cruel or neglectful treatment, down to lack of understanding, ambivalence, preoccupation or lack of warmth on the mother's part" (Freud and Dann [1951] 1973, 227–28).
23 See above, II.6.

7 Unavoidable pain

The connection of the psychical to the body is one of psychology's trickiest problems. If we assume theoretically that a physical process that is being *perceived* is already a psychical content,[1] then we can presuppose a reciprocal conditioning of psyche and body and turn to elucidating the activity of phantasy. I have done nothing different in this study so far. I have assumed that a pulsional process begins in a physical tension and is directed at a bodily satisfaction; the drive, however, is an exclusively psychical factor. I see no reason to modify this conception.

Symptoms of illness accordingly appear in a two-fold dependence. For the theory of neuroses, somatic changes (a symptom act, parapraxes, rituals, tics, and conversion characteristics) are significant insofar as they are consequences of a psychical conflict. Two opposing strivings, usually the pulsional tendency and the superego prohibition, unite to form a compromise. The pulsional wish, for example, demands an exhibitory satisfaction, the superego says no! and threatens castration. As a compromise, a genital eczema emerges. The treatment by a physician this calls for fulfills the embarrassing impulse, the sensation of displeasure allays the need for punishment. In this sense, hysterical and obsessional-neurotic symptoms are *expressions of sexual activity*.

Maybe my presentation of the three masochistic patients has created the impression that they developed no manifest erogenous symptoms. That is not the case. The "acrobat" achieves sexual satisfaction when, with her hands and feet tied to the bedframe, unable to move, she is being masturbated by a man. The "physicist," too, lets himself be tied up, whipped, and anally satisfied with a fist; he lets himself be gagged and manhandled by his lover with hot needles. The "kitchen fairy" can masturbate pleasurably only when, in addition to the genital manipulation, she attaches an apparatus to her leg that exerts painful pressure and scratches the skin open.

Of course, it will be asked why I have not reported these very details. Once some obstacles are removed for them, the patients in any case do not hesitate to describe their ritual at length. It is the first thing they offer for interpretation. If we keep in mind the concept just mentioned, that symptoms of suffering are compromise formations of unconscious strivings, we will hardly

DOI: 10.4324/9781032666273-38

be tempted to try and understand the events intuitively, but we will perceive the subsequent analysis from a specific position. The confusing ritual is a compromise formation, it testifies to the striving for pleasure as much as to the need for punishment, and it will clear up as soon as one succeeds in bringing its pulsional dynamic conditions and its connection with the life-story to consciousness. The search for pain seems particularly suited to suspecting an increased tendency toward self-punishments. Readers will not have missed that the "drumming dream" of the "acrobat" can be effortlessly linked with her bondage practice. The ritual of the "kitchen fairy" can be associated with her phantasy of a punishing "stiff as a stick" penis. And the "fish farm [*Fischzucht*]" of the "physicist" appears as an allusion to his being disciplined [*Züchtigung*] (the *hot* needle being replaced by the *cold* fish).

Had I begun my study with the manifest symptoms, the path toward the unconscious conflict would have been cleared and the comprehension of the individual design of the rituals made easier. I would not have been able, however, to elucidate why the pain becomes indispensable for the sexual pleasure. Now that we are familiar with the psychical genesis of masochism, the sexual symptom or the *perversion* seems only more obscure and the transition from unpleasure to pain entirely incomprehensible.

Let's pause for a moment. We mustn't think that we can deeply engage with psychical events without showing reactions ourselves. In psychoanalytic therapy, the "countertransference," that is to say, analysts' unconscious reaction to their patients' communications and demands, is the most reliable instrument of understanding. In analyzing masochism, my situation was not much different. Through the trick of bringing up the perverse ritual not at the beginning but only at the end, I placed myself in an opposition to the masochist and thereby revealed a defense. To interpret this, there are number of possible suppositions. I gave consideration to seemliness and modesty, I was shocked myself, I didn't want to seem voyeuristic, and so on. Yet when we get to the bottom of the defense, only one *identification* is possible: Look, I don't even need to spill the intimate details, I can pin down masochism "freehand," purely with the help of imagination and theory, I can postpone the tension again and again, and the solution of the riddle, the body-symptom, is nothing but a superfluous appendage of the mental effort! I observed the tendency toward identification earlier already.[2] I thought that if there is nothing unusual to characterize the content of masochistic pleasure, then perhaps [this pleasure] consists in the slowness, the delay, and the arduousness of the process itself. Yet insofar as masochists' prompt readiness to talk about the perversion is itself a defense, the identification of the analyst has revealed the unconscious.

I now benefit from what my preparatory work has achieved. I no longer *need* the symptom to understand the unconscious. For the continuation of our reflections, I relinquish something that masochists have come to depend on in a particular way: *masturbation*.

As a result of my study, I realized that the masochistic neurosis destroys the ability to masturbate. That, of course, is not a harmless conclusion.

Unavoidable pain 281

We acknowledge that psychical conflicts can severely damage and diminish the gain in pleasure of masturbation. We resolutely resist the insight, however, that the capacity for the most intimate of activities could be lost as such. I am convinced that the unwillingness even to consider the possibility of the *annihilation of sovereignty over masturbation* is the more profound reason why psychology has not understood masochism. The disavowal of the dependence on masturbation recalls the resistance against insight into the psychical's being conditioned by the sexual drive. While that resistance negates the source of the excitation, the "masochistic misunderstanding" serves to defend the possibility of being able at any time to allay, manipulate, or satisfy the sexual excitation ourselves. We project onto the masochists who suffer from a shattering of the capacity for masturbation the torments we expect for ourselves if we had to relinquish th[is] secret support. The freedom to masturbation, and be it with little gain in pleasure, is one of the earliest and most reliable achievements of psychosexual development. The theoretical possibility alone that it could be not only restricted but abolished excites obvious internal upheaval. The didactic "trick" of not revealing the secret and of delaying the tension at will is thus to be considered a substitute for and mental conjuring of masturbation. We proved to ourselves that what must not be, cannot be, and we denied the *commanding dependence on masturbation*. Such an illusionary procedure would really be unforgivable if rendering it conscious did not procure us a great advantage. Now that we no longer feel tied to the masochistic symptom, neither for the theoretical understanding nor for our emotional defense, we can fully elucidate it.

The psychical conflict corresponds to a common neurotic formation. An early, possibly constitutional displacement in the pulsional alloying in favor of aggression has created a series of psychical peculiarities.[3] The emphasis on the difference between the sexes and the perils of aggressively cathected masturbation compel a particular solution of the infantile oedipal crisis. The ego does not submit to the internal agency but has already long identified with the idealized penis or the phallus of the woman, and [it] intrastructurally continues the embittered oedipal struggle. Because of an additional repression (the recathexis), the internal taboo is directed not only at the incestuous wish but primarily against masturbation. The content of the masturbation phantasy is concerned with the idea of being masturbated by the "phallic" mother and to exhibit oneself before her. The internal reproach is: I have damaged the mother, I have castrated her, now the father will take revenge on me in the same way. The *taboo of masturbation* is thereby established pulsional-dynamically and is affirmed economically. When the aggression is internalized, a sadistic but defective superego emerges that cannot exercise its ideal function. Secondarily, the castration threat, too, is projected again. The saturation tolerance of the alloying of the drives makes it such that not all energy can be bound and a secondary inclination toward pulsional disentanglement appears. In the wishes, there are no ambivalent cathexes but instead polarized and irreconcilable quantities of libido and aggression. While the superego can dispose of repression for the purposes of defense, it makes use of the economic situation to spare itself an elaborate effort (the countercathexis) and restricts the drives by isolating them.[4]

The *psychical symptoms* testify to a forceful effort of the *sexual and aggressive striving for pleasure* to resist the intervention of the superego and to make up for the economic lack. But we will have to consider them a particular kind of neurotic compromise formation. While usually, the sexual demand and morality agree on a settlement and the symptom condenses both tendencies, masochistic pleasure consists in the unabbreviated *both. . . and*: pulsional impulses assert themselves in the ego together and simultaneously with impulses of the superego. In no way has the neurosis abolished the pleasure principle; instead, it has given expression to the opposing strivings not in a compromise but in a kind of *conjunction of drive and prohibition*.[5]

The masochistic taboo, meanwhile, strikes the instrument of pleasure: the physical excitement. Although "pleasure" is undoubtedly a psychical category and the "gain in pleasure" consists in relaxing affects that emerge in connection with particular processes in phantasy, [pleasure] nonetheless is conditioned by two factors of physical satisfaction. According to the principle of perceptual identity, the wish fulfillment must be connected *associatively* with the pleasurable phantasy. Moreover, the pulsional process should be *synchronized* with the somatic *excitation*. While we will expect the *pulsional pressure* to be constant—with the restriction I ascribe to the effect of the death drive—the *pulsional process*, on the one hand, is characterized by a particular rhythm, and the *somatic excitation*, on the other hand, is characterized by its variations.

We seldom have occasion to engage with questions of temporal coordination since the psychosexual development joins pulsional process and physical tension together and condenses two components, libido and aggression, in the pulsional quality. The study of masochism, however, teaches us that different processes apply to the two kinds of drives. While libidinous pleasure demands from phantasy repetitive cathexis relationships, aggression wants a once and for all fulfillment. With regard to the pulsional aim, the body's erogenous zones, cathexis process, and bodily tension usually fit together. In the sensorial zones (the mucosa and the surface of the skin) the excitation unfolds in the shape of a sinus wave; the building up of tension already is pleasurable in itself, and the satisfaction calls for repetition. The somatic aggression excitation, by contrast, goes for a one-time relaxation, it maintains an even, high level, breaks off steeply when satisfaction occurs, and recovers just as quickly. In adults, the differences are hardly observable, since sensor and motor zones no longer constitute independent pulsional aims.

In masochism, the masturbation wish undoubtedly condenses the partial drives and is genital.[6] It does not make any unusual sexual or aggressive demands. Yet while the neurotic constellation has established a taboo on masturbation, an, I want to say, technical difficulty renders somatic relaxation almost impossible. The defense has compelled sensorial ("passive") wishes and aggressive impulses to be bound to separate phantasies of body areas. If the ego is identified with the idealized phallus, then the genital is cathected exclusively passively and the hand is the organ of aggression. For phantasy, the simultaneous satisfaction of both strivings—that is, the continuation in the somatic [domain] of the conjunction solution practiced by the psychical symptoms—is identical with castration.

By contrast, *bondage* creates a somatic situation in which the motor system is mobilized (in the resistance against the ties) and genital satisfaction can nonetheless take place masturbatorily, in phantasy or with the help of an object. The ritual of the "acrobat," accordingly, is a successful setup to outwit the prohibition on masturbation and its economic consequences.

The *pain* the "kitchen fairy" inflicts on herself has a different function, since she pleasurably manipulates the genital. Quickly the suspicion arises that she simultaneously punishes herself for doing this to preempt, in the sense of the superego, a worse consequence. We obtained a different conception, though. In the ego, the "kitchen fairy" has identified with the castrated genital and accordingly devalued [herself]. The meaning of the masturbation is that of a (male) homosexual act; in her phantasy, there is a penis hidden in her vagina, and her hand is cathected as an idealized phallus. Simultaneously, in another body area, with her foot, she wages a pleasurable aggressive struggle against an opponent. The pain in no way indicates a punishment but marks the physical limit of the aggressive pleasure. In this case, the ritual does not serve to outwit the prohibition—which the "acrobat" pays for with object dependency—but to, illusionarily, overcome it.

We discover the deeper meaning of the masochistic ritual in the "physicist's" habit of having himself whipped. Few will want to compare the pain stimuli of a lashing with those that limit the aggression pleasure, especially since the "physicist" suffers them passively. An interpretation like the one for the "kitchen fairy" is out of the question. And yet there is no denying that the whiplashes are a source of pleasure for him. In his case, the phallic sexual wish is aggressively cathected. An earlier masturbation technique [of his] tried to materially separate penis and hand from each other.[7] *The function of the pain he now actively inserts in the pulsional process is to place retarding moments in the path of satisfaction.* Since the masturbation phantasy is to fulfill exclusively aggressive demands, the corresponding erogenous zones are excited; these also include the penis. Yet as it unfolds, an aggressive relaxation is able neither to build up a sensorial excitation in the genital nor to satisfy [such an excitation]. The issue, we might say, is to prolong the pleasure. Yet it is more likely that the "physicist" tries to hold on to the sadistic phantasy (he wants to genitally injure his sexual object with the penis) and at the same time forms and shapes the physical tension by means of the pain stimuli until a rhythmical process emerges that resembles the [tension] of a libidinous wish. In this way, the ritual completes somatically what the neurosis has torn apart psychically. In the somatic genital excitation, the alloying of sensor and motor tension succeeds even if it remains hopeless for libido and aggression in the psychical. The pain unmistakably asserts its unpleasure character, the course the masturbation tension takes by contrast is fully satisfying somatically. In this context, we also finally understand the latent dream wish of the "kitchen fairy" with which she began her analysis, the wish that it not be "too late" for her. She wants a delay—a lateness—not of the sexual satisfaction but of its aggressive component.

As was already the case in the discussion of the death drive, we once more, though from an entirely different angle, come to consider the temporal dimension in the psychical. It is astonishing, really, that this factor could remain concealed for so long. Even if we rightly suppose that unconscious, pulsional processes themselves know no time, their unfolding is subject to timing. The quality of the two kinds of drive, libido and sadism, can be distinguished as much by their respective aims—the excitation of sensorial or motor satisfaction phantasies—as by the course the tension of the cathexis energy takes. Libido is repetitive, it oscillates around a probably congenital average value; aggression tension by contrast runs ahead of the rhythm of the libido, collapses abruptly when satisfaction occurs but recovers much more rapidly than erotic excitation. When the drive is alloyed, we need not worry about the libido lagging behind. In masochism; however, the delaying—that is to say, the synchronization of the course of the cathexis in phantasy and in the somatic excitation—becomes the meaningful and pleasurably attained intention of the neurotic, perverse ritual.

After the fact, of course, neither superego nor pulsional demands hesitate to make use of the masturbation practice for their own purposes; it is being "overdetermined."[8] The pain appears as punishment for prohibited action, the fetishes used and the object at issue are linked to castration. Passive dependency wishes cling to the superego taboo, and aggression is deployed in self-reproaches, shame, and new murderous intentions. The erogenous masochism, however, is not understood; the attempt to capture it via a contentual interpretation of the symptoms only attains the effects, not the cause.

Masochists themselves learn very quickly to use unpleasure and pain, the way one learns to use fork and knife to eat. At bottom, they know of the indispensability and, when you think about it, psychical neutrality of their aids. What bothers their internal censorship is not their ritual but the sexual intention it is to facilitate: pleasurable masturbation. It is of course in the nature of things, first, that sometimes the delaying and synchronizing function of the sexual practice fails and, second, that the neurotic conflict is denied whereas the technique draws all the attention. Sense of guilt and shame are displaced onto the "perversion," and the infantile conflict forms anew around the somatic syndrome. The symptom of suffering properly speaking emerges when, due to the secondary development, the ritual is cathected with anxiety. Then the pain no longer appears as an aid to pleasure but serves to project the threat of castration. Sexual relaxation is thus no longer possible via this route. Prior to this, the lack of a connection between phantasy and physical manipulation already destroyed the psychical gain in pleasure.

This is the point where the work of psychoanalytic therapy begins, and here my effort comes to an end.

If psychoanalysis is able to produce the consciousness that the sexual practice is an instrument with which the excitation process can be controlled pleasurably, and if this insight then leads further to the conflicts about infantile masturbation and about aggression, all the way to elucidating the particular resolution of the oedipal crisis, then it has done everything it has the right and the power to do. A therapy that boasts to have "cured" masochistic symptoms was not therapy; in [masochism], the perversion is an indispensable part of sexuality. The displacement in the relationship of the kinds of drives, too, cannot be repaired, the ambivalence not be achieved, the superego never again be reliably integrated.

One last remark. In my investigation, I followed Fenichel's example.[9] I asserted that psychical suffering is conditioned socially and, now that we have come to know the intimate, sexual causation of masochism, I still see no reason to revise that judgment. The fact that psychical conflicts alone lead to neurosis and the perversion symptoms seems to give social dominion no power over them. Contrary to the view that masochists are docile subjects, we even understood that the special neurotic defense against the current social tendency to sexualize aggression forms an unmistakable inner barrier. Precisely because of their neurosis, masochists are more immune than others to the seductions of power. The work on masochism thus has brought me a conviction that I do not quite know what to make of yet.

What appears as the symptom of the disentanglement of libido and aggression is not individual, neurotic masochism but a different—a social—phenomenon: the expansion of service economies. The divergence between treatment and advice on the one hand and the claim to aid and support on the other becomes the social norm, where on the individual level the satisfaction of the (tamed) sadism of individuals is rewarded whereas as the satisfaction of the passive libido must be paid for. That is the case when the sexualization of aggression is not only subjectively advantageous but also politically, militarily, and economically profitable. Over against this stands the sexual libido, which generates nothing but a subjective pleasure affect and thus becomes disruptive and superfluous in the social construct. Previously, power suppressed this part of sexuality, which is unproductive for the perpetuation of dominion. Now it seems as if, although passive dependency wishes are economically exploited, the gain in pleasure is left to the subject. The satisfaction of the subjective demands, however, has long been integrated into the subtle process of displacement between psychical wish fulfillment and the objective forms of pulsional satisfaction, whose symptoms we recognized, here "voluntary" servitude, there the idealized power of religion, of a particular notion of the state, and so on. For the subject, the displacement process could lead as much to the aggressivization of the libido, which would become all the more pleasurable, as to the sexualization of aggression, but the interest of dominion prevents the first outcome. In a hierarchically organized service-oriented

286 Voluntary Servitude. Masochism and Morality

society, the secret belief in the omnipotence of those one surrenders and submits to does not merely procure the idealized helpers and rescuers a gain in power. While the latter do profit from the sexualized passivity of the others, the unstoppable translation of both—of both sadistic and passive—subjective wish fulfillments into autonomized forms of pulsional satisfaction is more important. The organs [of these forms of satisfaction], such as large hospitals, trade unions, and welfare institutions, finally enter into the service of political power as instruments of dominion. In service-oriented societies, it is not masochism/sadism that becomes the social norm but the pleasurelessness both of aggressive satisfaction and of passive submission. Yet since they are involuntary and pulsionally conditioned, it will not be possible to perform acts of "voluntary" servitude, which is how the subjective enactment of sadism now appears as well.

The mocking judgment of masochists quite obviously does not rely on their inclination to submit but on their blatant, desperate struggle for the right to masturbation. The prospect of losing the freedom to masturbation must induce anxiety, namely, to the extent that passive wishes make the object dependency appear pleasurable. The defense against both demands generates the soothing illusion that we are all the less a manipulable object the more we know how to master our excitation. The subjective denial of the autoerotic dilemma, however, is congruous with the social power's obfuscation tactics. Insofar as this power is out to exploit the pulsional energy, the reduction of tension—whose symptom is pleasurelessness—acts in the psychical like sexual activity that is prohibited (by the internal censorship) and nonetheless prescribed (by conscience).

At the beginning of this study, we learned to understand a dominant social tendency as the one that promotes the sexualization of aggression and that relaxes the sexual libido (which is no longer of use for its interests) for the purposes of private amusement. The study of masochism has shown its salient characteristic to be the absence of pulsional ambivalences. The hypocrisy toward aggression, which I interpreted as the symptom of a social amnesia, repeats itself in the neurotic development that leads to masochism. Neither public consciousness nor masochists want to be reminded of the secret supremacy of the aggression drive. Yet the analogy between the disentanglement of the drives, which takes place in the interest of social power, and the pulsional vicissitude in masochism is misleading. The intention of dominion and the neurotic process intersect, like at a crossroads, in the same psychical phenomenon. The sexualization of aggression, of course, is the instrument of perpetuating power, while for masochism it is what must be avoided, the repressed. Dominion forces the splitting of the drives to make it easier for itself to exploit the psychical energy. It will do everything to keep the split open and allow no bridging. The psychosexual development in masochism, too, forces a pulsional defusion. Sexualized aggression quantities explode the usual ambivalence, whose satisfaction serves the pleasure principle. Yet this very striving for pleasure does not tolerate the demise of the now passive sexual libido. The masochistic symptoms of suffering turn out to be measures to restore the original alloying of the drives. The demands of power thus come up against an unexpected barrier in the masochistic disposition.

Contrary to the elaborations by Étienne de la Boétie and other authors, who suspect a "subjective factor" to be the cause of voluntary servitude, I found a secret energetic displacement process between subjective pulsional wish fulfillment and objectivized forms of the drive. The insight into the subtle processes taking place between individual and society, between subjective interests in pulsional satisfaction and the defense against unpleasure as well as the interest in obtaining and perpetuating social power, is hindered by internal resistances as much as by social disavowals and prohibitions on thought. I recognized the thesis, in particular, that the *subjective factor*, that is, identifications and passive submission tendencies, is the motive of social processes, to be a symptom of a social amnesia. It serves to obfuscate what is actually taking place between subject and society and effects an assignation of guilt to the individuals, whose unconscious and irrational forces are held responsible for the status quo. In fact, though, a process is in operation from which power does indeed benefit, which it does indeed promote, but which has slipped the grasp both of the individual and of the demands of dominion.

One of the essential traits of masochism I was able to establish is the deficiency of the superego. The restriction of masochistic morality is threefold, pulsional-economical, structural, and contentual. Psychically, morality draws its strength from the incest taboo, and it becomes unreliable when the prohibition—and be it only in phantasy—is constantly breached.[10] The sense of guilt regresses to the somatic threat and becomes castration anxiety once more. With regard to mollifying the internal censorship, the unreliability of sexual morality would be a rather desirable result insofar as it would be accompanied by a strengthening of conscience, which is turned toward the external world. But the weakness of the superego, its deficient separation from the aggressive pulsional forces, and its insufficient ideal function make masochists all the more susceptible to external threats. No matter how we look at it: if conscience is incorruptible and strict, the individual in internalizing violence and morality becomes the accomplice of dominion; if it is negligent, people remain bound to the external authority by physical anxiety.

Notes

1 Perception of course does not limit itself to consciousness. In the emergence of psychical contents, preconscious (i.e., descriptively unconscious) perception, especially, is decisive.
2 See above, III.6 [#236].
3 There are no studies on the *usual* relationship between libido and aggression. Insofar as they acknowledge aggression as a pulsional component, authors presuppose a balance within the ambivalence or mostly grant the libido priority.
4 The countercathexis interrupts the energetic flow among the wishful phantasies. The cathexis displacement effects qualitative changes in the pulsional energy. Disavowals work by manipulating internal perception. And isolation separates the

wish into its component parts, the idea from the affect, the pulsional aim from the energy quality. The result is at least as successful as that of repression. While each for itself, the isolated parts of the disapproved wish are capable of becoming conscious, they are no longer available emotionally and therefore excluded from the gain in pleasure.

5 "The existence of a masochistic trend in the instinctual life of human beings may justly be described as mysterious from the economic point of view. For if mental processes are governed by the pleasure principle in such a way that their first aim is the avoidance of unpleasure and the obtaining of pleasure, masochism is incomprehensible. If pain and unpleasure can be not simply warnings but actually aims, the pleasure principle is paralysed—it is as though the watchman over our mental life were put out of action by a drug" (Freud 1924a, 159).

6 The aggressions I observed, for example the anal fixation of the "acrobat" or the voyeuristic pleasure of the "kitchen fairy," concern cathexis displacements within the pulsional process whose genital aim remains unchanged.

7 See above, II.13 [#173].

8 We speak of overdetermination when different unconscious motives participate in the same symptom (see Freud 1900, SE 4, 283/SE 5, 569, and Freud 1916–1917, SE 15, 228–32).

9 See above, I.7.

10 See above, III.6. See also Freud 1933, 64 ["Close investigation has shown us, too, that the super-ego is stunted in its strength and growth if the surmounting of the Oedipus complex is only incompletely successful." See also JLS-Maso-3, page 143, where on this topic, Le Soldat quotes the passage "if the surmounting of the Oedipus complex is only incompletely successful," but gives no reference].

Appendix

Two unpublished prefaces from the first version of *Voluntary Servitude*[1]

Preface I: A warning

This book is not really about masochism but about society.

Readers expecting to catch on to secret perverse phantasies will be disappointed.

The author urges readers to interrupt the reading often, very often. Perhaps it is a good idea to begin by reading the first, then the last chapter, and then to look around in the middle. Otherwise, the study has a simple structure: it traces the path of masochism from the originary trauma to the formation of manifest symptoms.

Preface II: An explanation

There are three pictures on my desk: on the left, a portrait of Freud, a copy of Ferdinand Schmutzer's well-known drawing from 1926; in the middle, the reproduction of a drawing by Matisse, a woman, lost and sad. On the right, there was, for a long time, a photograph from the volume by Margaret Bourke-White, the picture of a young man, a survivor of the Buchenwald concentration camp.

In the fall of last year, I don't recall whether it was before or after, in any case, it was around the time that Fritz Morgenthaler, whom I revered and admired, died in Addis Ababa—he was involved in the release of young journalist taken hostage—the photograph of a beaming Rudi Dutschke, taken from the cover of his book, *Geschichte ist machbar* (*History Can Be Made*), suddenly got the spot to the right on my desk.

In working on this book, I am keeping a promise I made to myself when I heard the song of the Jewish resistance fighters in the Kraków ghetto for the first time.

> S'brent, brider, s'brent!
> Di hilf is nor in aykh aleyn gevendt!
> Oyb dos shtetl is aykh tayer,
> Nemt di kelim, lesht dos fayer,

290 *Voluntary Servitude. Masochism and Morality*

>Lesht mit ayer eygn blut,
>Bavayzt, az ir dos kent!
>Shteyt nit, brider, ot azoy zikh mit farleygte hent,
>Shteyt nit, brider, lesht dos fayer! Unzer shtetl brent!
>
>Fire! Brothers, fire! Help depends only on you: if the town is dear to you, take the buckets, put out the fire. Put it out with your own blood—show that you can do it! Don't stand there, brothers, with folded arms! Don't stand there, brothers, put out the fire—our town is burning![2]

My heartfelt thanks to Madeleine Senn for typing up the manuscript and to my friend A. F. G. for his patience and support.

Judith Le Soldat-Szatmári, Zurich, January 1985

Notes

1 These prefaces, contained in the typescript of the masochism book's first version, are preserved in the archives of the Judith Le Soldat foundation (shelf mark JLS-MASO-2).
2 [The quote is the fourth stanza of the poem and song "Es brent" by Mordechai Gebirtig. The translation is a slightly revised version of Murray Citron's rendering (Gebirtig 1936). Special thanks to Ken Moss and Anne Eakin Moss for revising the transcription and advice on the translation.—Trans.]

Bibliography

Abraham, Karl. (1910) 1982. "Über hysterische Traumzustände." In Abraham 1982, vol. 1, 203–31.
Abraham, Karl. (1913) 1982. "Psychische Nachwirkungen der Beobachtung des elterlichen Geschlechtsverkehrs bei einem neunjährigen Kinde." In Abraham 1982, vol. 1, 180–83.
Abraham, Karl. (1922) 2018. "The Rescue and Murder of the Father in Neurotic Phantasy-Formations." In *Clinical Papers and Essays on Psycho-analysis*. Edited by Hilda C. Abraham. Translated by Hilda C. Abraham and D. R. Ellison et al., 68–75. Abingdon: Routledge.
Abraham, Karl. 1982. *Gesammelte Schriften in zwei Bänden*. Edited by Johannes Cremerius. Frankfurt: Fischer.
Adorno, Theodor W. (1946) 2018. "Social Science and Sociological Tendencies in Psychoanalysis." In *Dialektische Psychologie: Adornos Rezeption der Psychoanalyse*. Edited by Wolfgang Bock, 623–42. Wiesbaden: Springer VS.
Adorno, Theodor W. 1952. "Zum Verhältnis von Psychoanalyse und Gesellschaftstheorie." Translated by Rainer Koehne. *Psyche* 6, no. 1 (April 1952): 1–18.
Adorno, Theodor W. (1955) 1967/1968. "Sociology and Psychology." Translated by Irving N. Wohlfrath. *New Left Review* 46 and 47 (November–December 1967/January–February 1968): 67–80 and 70–97.
Adorno, Theodor W. (1966) 1970. "Postscriptum." In *Gesammelte Schriften*. Vol. 8: Aufsätze zur Gesellschaftstheorie und Methodologie. Edited by Rolf Tiedemann, 55–62. Frankfurt: Suhrkamp.
Adorno, Theodor W. (1969) 2005a. "On Subject and Object." In *Critical Models: Interventions and Catchwords*, Translated by Henry W. Pickford, Adorno 2005, 245–58. New York: Columbia University Press.
Adorno, Theodor W. (1969) 2005b. "Marginalia to Theory and Praxis." In *Critical Models: Interventions and Catchwords*, Translated by Henry W. Pickford, Adorno 2005, 259–78. New York: Columbia University Press, 2005.
Adorno, Theodor W. (1969) 2005. *Critical Models: Interventions and Catchwords*. Translated by Henry W. Pickford. New York: Columbia University Press.
Adorno, Theodor W., Else Frenkel-Brunswik, Daniel Levinson, and Nevitt Sanford. (1950) 2019. *The Authoritarian Personality*. London: Verso.
Aisenstein, Marilia. 2014. "Destruction of the Thought Processes and the Negative of Sublimation." *Revue française de psychosomatique* 46, no. 2: 9–20.
Aisenstein, Marilia. 2018. "An Introduction to Michel Fain's Thought." *The International Journal of Psychoanalysis* 99, no. 2: 495–509.

Aisenstein, Marilia. 2022. "Primal Erotogenic Masochism." Presentation. New York. July 2, 2022.
Alexander, Franz. 1929. "The Need for Punishment and the Death-Instinct." *International Journal of Psycho-analysis* 10: 256–69.
Aloupis, Panos. 2017. "Bodies of Women, Feminine Bodies." *Revue française de psychosomatique*, 1, no. 51: 21–34.
Amigorena, Horatio, and Vignar, Marcel. 1977. "*Entre le dehors et le dedans: l'instance tyrannique.*" *Critique* 363–64 (August–September): 790–98.
Anders, Günther. (1959) 1962. "Theses for the Atomic Age." *The Massachusetts Review* 3, no. 3 (Spring): 493–505.
Arendt, Hannah. 1963. *Eichmann in Jerusalem: A Report on the Banality of Evil*. New York: Viking Press. (1964)
Arendt, Hannah. 1976. *Die verborgene Tradition*. Frankfurt: Suhrkamp.
Arendt, Hannah, and Karl Jaspers. (1985) 1992. *Correspondence 1926–1969*. Edited by Lotte Köhler and Hans Saner. Translated by Robert and Rita Kimber. San Diego, CA: Harcourt Brace.
Aristotle. 1984. "Politics." In *The Complete Works of Aristotle: The Revised Oxford Translation*. Translated by Benjamin Jowett. Edited by Jonathan Barnes. 4th ed. Vol. 2, 1986–2129. Princeton, NJ: Princeton University Press.
Arkin, Frances S. 1960. "Discussion [of Leon Salzmann, "The Negative Therapeutic Reaction]." In Masserman, ed., 1960, 314–17.
Bachofen, Johann Jakob. (1861) 2006. Johann Jakob Bachofen and, *An English Translation of Bachofen's* Mutterrecht (Mother Right) *(1861): A Study of the Religious and Juridical Aspects of Gynecocracy in the Ancient World*. Abridged and translated by David Partenheimer. Lewiston, NY: Edwin Mellen Press.
Bacon, Francis. (1597) 1861. "Of Great Place." No. XI of *Essays or Counsels Civil and Moral*. In *The Works of Francis Bacon*. Vol. 6: Literary and Professional Works 1. Edited by James Spedding, Robert Leslie Ellis, and Douglas Denon Heath, 398–401. London: Longman.
Barrère, Joseph. 1920/1921. "La Boétie et Marat." *Actes de l'Académie nationale des sciences, belles-lettres et arts de Bordeaux*, ser. 4, 4: 151–58.
Bataille, Georges. (1963) 2012. *Eroticism*. Translated by Mary Dalwood. London: Penguin Classics.
Benjamin, Jessica. 1985. "The Bonds of Love: Rational Violence and Erotic Domination." *Feminist Studies* 6, no. 1 (Spring): 144–74.
Beradt, Charlotte. (1966) 1968. *The Third Reich of Dreams*. Translated by Adriane Gottwald. Chicago, IL: Quadrangle Books.
Berliner, Bernhard. 1958. "The Role of Object Relations in Moral Masochism." *The Psychoanalytic Quarterly* 27, no. 1: 38–56.
Bernfeld, Siegfried. (1929) 1996. "Der soziale Ort und seine Bedeutung für Neurose, Verwahrlosung und Pädagogik." In Ders.: Antiautoritäre Erziehung und Psychoanalyse. Ausgewählte Schriften, Bd. 1, hg von Lutz von Werder und Reinhart Wolff, Darmstadt, S., 198–211.
Bernfeld, Siegfried. (1932) 1938. "The Communistic Discussion of Psychoanalysis and Reich's Refutation of the Hypothesis of the Death Instinct." *The Psychoanalytic Review* 25, no. 3: 220.
Bernfeld, Siegfried. 1996. *Ausgewählte Schriften*. Vol. 2: *Antiautoritäre Erziehung und Psychoanalyse*. Edited by Lutz von Werder and Reinhart Wolff. Weinheim: Beltz.

Binswanger, Ralf. 1985. "Die Währung in der Psychoanalyse und die Währung in der Politik." *Journal des Psychoanalytischen Seminars Zürich*, special issue, 12–13.

Binswanger, Ralf. 2016. "(K)ein Grund zur Homosexualität: Ein Plädoyer zum Verzicht auf psychogenetische Erklärungsversuche von homosexuellen, heterosexuellen und anderen Orientierungen." *Journal für Psychoanalyse*, 57: 6–26.

Binswanger, Ralf. 2021. "Mehr Klarheit beim Reden über Sexualität! Ein dynamisches Modell zur Strukturierung sexualwissenschaftlicher Diskurse." *Zeitschrift für Sexualforschung* 34, no. 1: 15–27.

Bischof, Karoline. 2008. "Orgasmusstörungen der Frau." In *Leitfaden Sexualberatung für die ärztliche Praxis*. Edited by Peter Gehrig and Karoline Bischof. Zurich: Zürcher Institut für klinische Sexologie & Sexualtherapie. https://www.ziss.ch/site/assets/files/1045/orgasmusstoerungen_der_frau.pdf

Blarer, Arno von, and Irene Brogle. 1983. "Der Weg ist das Ziel: Zur Theorie und Metatheorie der psychoanalytischen Technik." In *Deutung und Beziehung: Kritische Beiträge zur Behandlungskonzeption und Technik in der Psychoanalyse*. Edited by Sven O. Hoffmann, 71–85. Frankfurt: Fischer.

Bonaparte, Marie. 1952. "Some Biopsychical Aspects of Sado-Masochism." Translated by John Rodker. *International Journal of Psycho-Analysis* 33, no. 4: 373–84.

Borkenau, Franz. 1957. "Zwei Abhandlungen zur griechischen Mythologie." *Psyche* 11, no. 1 (April): 1–27.

Borkenau, Franz. 1981. *End and Beginning: On the Generations of Cultures and the Origins of the West*. Edited by Richard Löwenthal. New York: Columbia University Press.

Borneman, Ernest. 1974. *Sex im Volksmund: Der obszöne Wortschatz der Deutschen*. 2 vols. Reinbek bei Hamburg: Rowohlt.

Bourke-White, Margaret. (1946) 1979. *Deutschland, April 1945*. Munich: Schirmer-Mosel. Translation of *Dear Fatherland, Rest Quietly: A Report on the Collapse of Hitler's "Thousand Years."* New York: Simon & Schuster.

Brainin, Elisabeth, and Isidor J. Kaminer. 1982. "Psychoanalyse und Nationalsozialismus." *Psyche* 36, no. 11 (November): 989–1012.

Braunschweig, Denise, and Fain, Michel. 1971. Éros et Antéros. Paris: Payot.

Brenner, Charles. 1959. "The Masochistic Character: Genesis and Treatment." *Journal of the American Psychoanalytic Association* 7, no. 2 (April): 197–226.

Breuer, Josef, and Sigmund Freud. 1895. Studies on Hysteria, SE, 2. In *The Standard Edition of the Complete Psychological Works of Sigmund Freud*. Edited by J. Strachey. Translated by James & Alix Strachey, 24 Vols., 1953–1974. Hogarth Press.

Brückner, Peter. 1975. *Sigmund Freuds Privatlektüre*. Cologne: Horst.

Brun, Rudolf. 1953. "Über Freuds Hypothese vom Todestrieb: Eine kritische Untersuchung." *Psyche* 7, no. 2 (May): 81–111.

Chasseguet-Smirgel, Janine. (1964) 1985. "Feminine Guilt and the Oedipus Complex." In *Female Sexuality: New Psychoanalytic Views*. Edited by Chasseguet-Smirgel, 1985, 95–134.

Chasseguet-Smirgel, Janine, ed. 1985. *Female Sexuality: New Psychoanalytic Views*. London: Karnac.

Dahmer, Helmut. 1982. *Libido und Gesellschaft: Studien über Freud und die Freudsche Linke*. 2nd expanded edition. Frankfurt: Suhrkamp.

Dahmer, Helmut. 1984. "'Psychoanalyse unter Hitler'—Rückblick auf eine Kontroverse." *Psyche* 38, no. 10 (1984): 927–42.

Demandt, Alexander. 1978. *Metaphern für Geschichte: Sprachbilder und Gleichnisse im historisch-politischen Denken*. Munich: Beck.

Deutsch, Helene. (1931) 1944. "Feminine Masochism." In *The Psychology of Women: A Psychological Interpretation*. Forworded by Cobb Stanley. Vol. 1: Girlhood, 239–78. New York: Grune & Stratton.

Dutschke, Rudi. 1981. *Geschichte ist machbar: Texte über das herrschende Falsche und die Radikalität des Friedens*. Berlin: Wagenbach.

Dutschke, Rudi, and Ulf Wolter. 1981. *Aufrecht gehen: Eine fragmentarische Autobiographie*. Berlin: Olle & Wolter.

Eidelberg, Ludwig. (1948) 1952. "A Contribution to the Study of Masochism." In *Studies in Psychoanalysis*, 31–40. New York: International University Press.

Eidelberg, Ludwig, ed. 1968. *Encyclopedia of Psychoanalysis*. New York: Free Press.

Eissler, Kurt R. 1938. "Zur genaueren Kenntnis des Geschehens an der Mundzone Neugeborener." *Zeitschrift für Kinderpsychiatrie* 5: 81–85.

Eissler, Kurt R. 1962. "On the Metapsychology of the Preconscious," *The Psychoanalytic Study of the Child* 17, no. 1: 9–41.

Eissler, Kurt R. 1963. "Die Ermordung von wie vielen seiner Kinder muß ein Mensch symptomfrei ertragen können, um eine normale Konstitution zu haben?" *Psyche* 17, no. 5: 241–91.

Eissler, Kurt R. 1967. "Perverted Psychiatry?" *American Journal of Psychiatry* 123, no. 11 (May): 1352–58.

Eissler, Kurt R. 1971. "Death Drive, Ambivalence, and Narcissism." *The Psychoanalytic Study of the Child* 26, no. 1: 25–78.

Eissler, Kurt. 1974 [1962]. "Zur Metapsychologie des Vorbewussten." *Psyche* 28: S. 951–983.

Eissler, Kurt R. 1975. "The Fall of Man." *The Psychoanalytic Study of the Child* 30, no. 1: 589–646.

Eissler, Kurt R. (1975) 1976. "Der Sündenfall des Menschen." *Jahrbuch der Psychoanalyse* 9: 23–78.

Eissler, Kurt R. 1984. "Wette, Vertrag und Prophetie in Goethes Faust." *Jahrbuch der Psychoanalyse* 16: 29–72.

Engels, Friedrich. (1884) 2010. *The Origin of the Family, Private Property and the State*. Translated by Alick West. London: Penguin.

Erdheim, Mario. 1982. *Die gesellschaftliche Produktion von Unbewußtheit: Eine Einführung in den ethnopsychoanalytischen Prozeß*. Frankfurt: Suhrkamp.

Evans, Arthur. (1921–1935) 2013. *The Palace of Minos: A Comparative Account of the Successive Stages of the Early Cretan Civilization as Illustrated by the Discoveries at Knossos*. 4 vols. Cambridge: Cambridge University Press.

Fäh, Markus, and Monika Gsell. 2021. "Einführung in das Denken und die erweiterte Theorie des Ödipuskomplexes von Judith Le Soldat." In *Trieb und Ödipus: Einführung in das Denken und Werk von Judith Le Soldat*, 53–104. Stuttgart: Frommann-Holzboog.

Fairbairn, William Ronald D. 1946. Object-Relationships and Dynamic Structure." *International Journal of Psychoanalysis* 27: 30–37.

Federn, Paul. 1913. "Beiträge zur Analyse des Sadismus und Masochismus. Teil I: Die Quellen des männlichen Sadismus." *Internationale Zeitschrift für Psychoanalyse* 1: 29–49.

Federn, Paul. 1914. "*Beiträge zur Analyse des Sadismus und Masochismus*. Teil II: Die libidinösen Quellen des Masochismus." *Internationale Zeitschrift für Psychoanalyse* 2, no. 2: 105–30.
Fenichel, Otto. (1934) 1953/1954. "The Drive to Amass Wealth." In *Collected Papers*, Edited by Hanna Fenichel and David Rapaport, 2 vols., 89–108. New York: Norton.
Fenichel, Otto. (1934) 1967. "Psychoanalysis as the Nucleus of a Future Dialectical-Materialistic Psychology." Translated by Olga Barsis. Edited by Suzette Annin and Hanna Fenichel. *American Imago* 24, no. 4: 290–311.
Fenichel, Otto. (1935) 1953/1954. "A Critique of the Death Instinct." In *Collected Papers*. Edited by L. V. Ahlfors, vol. 1, 363–72. London: Routledge.
Fenichel, Otto. (1938) 1981. "Psychoanalyse und Gesellschaftswissenschaften." *Psyche* 35, no. 11 (November): 1055–71.
Fenichel, Otto. (1945) 1996. *The Psychoanalytic Theory of Neurosis*. London: Routledge.
Fenichel, Otto. 1953/1954. *The Collected Papers of Otto Fenichel*. Edited by Hanna Fenichel and David Rapaport. 2 vols. New York: Norton.
Fenichel, Otto. 1998. *119 Rundbriefe (1934–1945)*. Edited by Elke Mühlleitner and Johannes Reichmayr. Frankfurt: Stroemfeld.
Ferenczi, Sándor. (1912) 1950/1952. "On Onanism. A Contribution to Fourteen Contributions to a Discussion of the Vienna Psychoanalytic Society." In (1916, 1922, 1950,) Contributions to Psychoanalysis. R. G. Badger, Boston, (1952, 1994), under the title: *First Contributions to Psychoanalysis*. Edited by and Translated by Ernest Jones, vol. 1, 185–92. London: Hogarth Press.
Ferenczi, Sándor. (1912) 1955. "On the Definition of Introjection." In 1916, 1922, 1950) Contributions to Psychoanalysis. R. G. Badger, Boston, under the title: (1952, 1994) *First Contributions to Psychoanalysis*. Edited by Ernest Jones, 316–18. London: Hogarth Press.
Ferenczi, Sándor. (1916) 1950/1952. "Interchange of Affect in Dreams." In (1916, 1922, 1950) Contributions to Psychoanalysis. R. G. Badger, Boston, (1952, 1994), under the title: *First Contributions to Psychoanalysis*. Edited by Ernest Jones, vol. 2, 345. London: Hogarth Press.
Ferenczi, Sándor. (1933) 1955. "Confusion of tongues between adults and the child." In: The International Journal of Psychoanalysis, (30) 1949, pp. 225–230. (In: (1955, 1994) *Final Contributions to Psychoanalysis*. Edited by Michael Balint, Foreword by Clara Thompson, The Hogarth Press; Karnac, London, pp. 156–167; (1999) Selected Writings. Edited with an introduction by Julia Borossa, 293–303. London: Penguin Books.
Ferenczi, Sándor. 1950/1952. *The Selected Papers of Sandor Ferenczi*. Edited by John Rickman et al. 2 vols. New York: Basic Books.
Ferenczi, Sándor. 1955. *Final Contributions to the Problems and Methods of Psycho-Analysis*. Edited by Michael Balint. New York: Basic Books.
Freud, Anna. (1936) 1973. *The Ego and the Mechanisms of Defense*. Translated by Cecil Baines. Vol. 2 of Anna Freud 1973. New York: International Universities Press.
Freud, Anna. (1949) 1973. "Notes on a Connection Between the States of Negativism and of Emotional Surrender (*Hörigkeit*)." In Anna Freud 1973.
Freud, Anna. 1973. *The Writings of Anna Freud*. New York: International University Press, 1973.
Freud, Anna, and Sophie Dann. [1951] 1973. "An Experiment in Group Upbringing." In Anna Freud 1973, vol. 4, 163–229.

Freud, Sigmund. 1895. "A Reply to Criticisms of My Paper on Anxiety Neurosis." In SE 3, 119–39.

Freud, Sigmund. 1898. *Sexuality in the Aetiology of the Neuroses*. In SE 3: 259–85.

Freud, Sigmund. 1900. *The Interpretation of Dreams*. Translated by James Strachey. In SE 4–5.

Freud, Sigmund. 1905a. *Three Essays on the Theory of Sexuality*. Translated by James Strachey. In SE 7, 123–247.

Freud, Sigmund. 1905b. "Fragment of an Analysis of a Case of Hysteria." Translated by Alix & James Strachey. In SE 7, 1–122.

Freud, Sigmund. 1907. "Delusions and Dreams in Jensen's *Gradiva*." Translated by James Strachey. In SE 9, 1–95.

Freud, Sigmund. 1908a. "'Civilized' Sexual Morality and Modern Nervous Illness." Translated by James Strachey. In SE 9, 177–204.

Freud, Sigmund. 1908b. "On the Sexual Theories of Children." Translated by D. Bryan. In SE 9, 205–26.

Freud, Sigmund. 1909. "Analysis of a Phobia in a Five-Year-Old Boy." Translated by Alix and James Strachey. In SE 10, 1–149.

Freud, Sigmund. 1910a. *Five Lectures on Psycho-Analysis*. Translated by James Strachey. In SE 11, 1–56.

Freud, Sigmund. 1910b. "A Special Type of Choice of Object Made by Men (Contributions to the Psychology of Love I)." Translated by Alan Tyson. In SE 11, 163–75.

Freud, Sigmund. 1910c. "The Psycho-Analytic View of Psychogenic Disturbance of Vision." Translated by Alix and James Strachey. In SE 11, 209–18.

Freud, Sigmund. 1912a. "Contributions to a Discussion on Masturbation." Translated by James Strachey. In SE 12, 239–54.

Freud, Sigmund. 1912b. "Recommendations to Physicians Practising Psycho-Analysis." Translated by Joan Riviere. In SE 12, 109–20.

Freud, Sigmund. 1912–1913. *Totem and Taboo*. Translated by James Strachey. In SE 13.

Freud, Sigmund. 1913a. "The Disposition to Obsessional Neurosis: A Contribution to the Problem of Choice of Neurosis." Translated by James Strachey. In SE 12, 311–20.

Freud, Sigmund. 1913b. "The Theme of the Three Caskets." Translated by C. J. M. Hubback. In SE 12, 289–301.

Freud, Sigmund. 1914. "On Narcissism: An Introduction." Translated by C. M. Baines. In SE 14, 67–102.

Freud, Sigmund. 1915a. "Instincts and Their Vicissitudes." Translated by C. M. Baines. In SE 14, 109–40.

Freud, Sigmund. 1915b. "Thoughts for the Times on War and Death." Translated by E. C. Mayne. In SE 14, 273–300.

Freud, Sigmund. 1915c. "On Transience." Translated by James Strachey. In SE 14, 303–7.

Freud, Sigmund. 1916. "Mourning and Melancholia." Translated by C. M. Baines. In SE 14, 237–58.

Freud, Sigmund. 1916–1917. *Introductory Lectures on Psycho-Analysis*. Translated by James Strachey. In SE 15–16.

Freud, Sigmund. 1917. "A Difficulty in the Path of Psycho-Analysis." Translated by James Strachey. In SE 17, 135–44.

Freud, Sigmund. 1918. "From the History of an Infantile Neurosis." Translated by Alix and James Strachey. In SE 17, 1–123.

Freud, Sigmund. 1919a. "'A Child Is being Beaten': A Contribution to the Study of the Origin of Sexual Perversions." Translated by Alix and James Strachey. In SE 17, 175–204.

Freud, Sigmund. 1919b. "Introduction to *Psycho-Analysis and the War Neuroses.*" Translated by James Strachey. In SE 17, 205–10.

Freud, Sigmund. 1920. *Beyond the Pleasure Principle.* Translated by James Strachey. In SE 18, 1–64.

Freud, Sigmund. 1921. *Group Psychology and Ego-Analysis.* Translated by James Strachey. In SE 18, 65–143.

Freud, Sigmund. 1923a. "Two Encyclopaedia Articles." Translated by James Strachey. In SE 18, 233–60.

Freud, Sigmund. 1923b. "The Ego and the Id." Translated by Joan Riviere. In SE 19, 1–66.

Freud, Sigmund. 1924a. "The Economic Problem of Masochism." Translated by Joan Riviere. In SE 19, 155–70.

Freud, Sigmund. 1924b. "The Loss of Reality in Neurosis and Psychosis." Translated by Joan Riviere. In SE 19, 183–87.

Freud, Sigmund. 1925a. "Negation." Translated by Joan Riviere. In SE 19, 233–39.

Freud, Sigmund. 1925b. "Some Psychical Consequences of the Anatomical Distinction Between the Sexes." Translated by Joan Riviere. In SE 19, 241–58.

Freud, Sigmund. 1926a. "Inhibitions, Symptoms and Anxiety." In SE 20, 75–175.

Freud, Sigmund. 1926b. "The Question of Lay Analysis." Translated by Alix Strachey. In SE 20, 177–258.

Freud, Sigmund. 1927a. "The Future of an Illusion." Translated by W. D. Robson-Scott. In SE 21, 3–56.

Freud, Sigmund. 1927b. "Humour." Translated by Joan Riviere. In SE 21, 159–66.

Freud, Sigmund. 1928. "Dostoevsky and Parricide." Translated by D. F. Tait. In SE 21, 173–96.

Freud, Sigmund. 1930. *Civilization and Its Discontents.* Translated by Joan Riviere. In SE 21, 57–145.

Freud, Sigmund. 1931. "Female Sexuality." Translated by Joan Riviere. In SE 21, 221–43.

Freud, Sigmund. 1932a. "The Acquisition and Control of Fire." Translated by Joan Riviere. In SE 22, 183–93.

Freud, Sigmund. 1932b. "Why War?" Translated by James Strachey. In SE 22, 22, 195–215.

Freud, Sigmund. 1933. *New Introductory Lectures on Psychoanalysis.* Translated by James Strachey. In SE 22, 1–182.

Freud, Sigmund. 1937. "Analysis Terminable and Interminable." Translated by Joan Riviere. In SE 23, 209–53.

Freud, Sigmund. 1938a. "Splitting of the Ego in the Process of Defence." Translated by Joan Riviere. In SE 23, 271–78.

Freud, Sigmund. 1938b. *An Outline of Psychoanalysis.* Translated by James Strachey. In SE 23, 139–207.

Freud, Sigmund. 1938c. "Findings, Ideas, Problems." In SE 23, 299–300.

Freud, Sigmund. 1939. *Moses and Monotheism.* Translated by James Strachey. In SE 23, 1–137.

Freud, Sigmund. 1942–1952 (= GW). *Gesammelte Werke: Chronologisch geordnet.* Edited by Anna Freud et al. London: Imago.

Freud, Sigmund. 1953–1974 (= SE). *The Standard Edition of the Complete Psychological Works of Sigmund Freud.* Edited by James Strachey et al. London: Hogarth.

Freud, Sigmund. 1954. *The Origins of Psychoanalysis: Letters to Wilhelm Fliess, Drafts and Notes: 1887–1902.* Edited by Marie Bonaparte, Anna Freud, and Ernst Kris. Translated by Eric Mosbacher and James Strachey. New York: Basic Books.

Friedrich, Jörg. (1984) 1994. *Die kalte Amnestie: NS-Täter in der Bundesrepublik.* Expanded and revised edition. Munich: Piper.

Frohn, Axel. 2008. "Klatsche für den Kanzler." *Spiegel Geschichte.* November 7, 2008. https://www.spiegel.de/geschichte/40-jahre-klarsfeld-skandal-a-948002.html

Gebirtig, Mordechai. 1936. "Es brent." Translated by Murray Citron. https://www.yiddishbookcenter.org/language-literature-culture/yiddish-translation/our-town-burning-and-beam-sunlight

Gillespie, W. H. 1971. "Aggression and Instinct Theory." *International Journal of Psychoanalysis* 52: 155–60.

Goethe, Johann Wolfgang. (1808/1832) 1994. Faust I & II. Edited and Translated by Stuart Atkins. In Goethe's Collected Works. Vol. 2. Princeton, NJ: Princeton University Press.

Greenson, Ralph R. 1967. *The Technique and Practice of Psychoanalysis.* Vol. 1. Madison, CT: International Universities Press.

Grimm, Jacob and Wilhelm. (1812) 1983. "Hans in Luck." In *Grimms' Tales for Young and Old: The Complete Stories.* Translated by Ralph Manheim, 287–91. New York: Doubleday Anchor.

Grodzicki, Wolf-Dietrich. 1967. "Einige Bemerkungen zur Struktur masochistischen Verhaltens im Zusammenhang mit Übertragungs- und Gegenübertragungsvorgängen." *Jahrbuch der Psychoanalyse* 4: 181–201.

Grubrich-Simitis, Ilse. 1976. "Extremtraumatisierung als kumulatives Trauma." *Psyche* 33, no. 11 (November): 991–1023.

Grubrich-Simitis, Ilse. 1984. "Vom Konkretismus zur Metaphorik: Gedanken zur psychoanalytischen Arbeit mit Nachkommen der Holocaust-Generation—anläßlich einer Neuerscheinung," *Psyche* 38, no. 1 (January): 1–28.

Grunert, Johannes, ed. 1981. *Leiden am Selbst: Zum Phänomen des Masochismus.* Munich: Kindler.

Gsell, Monika. 2016. "Was ist anders am 'anderen Ufer'? Zu Judith Le Soldats 'Grund zur Homosexualität.'" *Journal für Psychoanalyse* 57: 27–47.

Gsell, Monika, and Markus Zürcher. 2011. "Licht ins Dunkel der Bisexualität: Bisexualität, anatomische Geschlechtsdifferenz und die psychoanalytische Bedeutung von 'männlich' und 'weiblich,'" *Psyche* 65, no. 8 (August): 699–729.

Haas, Volkert. 1982. *Hethitische Berggötter und hurritische Steindämonen: Riten, Kulte und Mythen.* Mainz: Zabern.

Hartmann, Heinz. (1947) 1964. "On Rational and Irrational Action." In Hartmann 1964, 37–68.

Hartmann, Heinz. (1950) 1964. "Comments on the Psychoanalytic Theory of the Ego." In Hartmann 1964, 113–41.

Hartmann, Heinz. (1953) 1964. "Contribution to the Metapsychology of Schizophrenia." In Hartmann 1964, 182–206.

Hartmann, Heinz. (1955) 1964. "Notes on the Theory of Sublimation." In Hartmann 1964, 215–40.

Hartmann, Heinz. (1956) 1964. "Notes on the Reality Principle." In Hartmann 1964, 241–67.

Hartmann, Heinz. 1964. *Essays on Ego Psychology: Selected Problems in Psychoanalytic Theory*. New York: International Universities Press.
Hartmann, Heinz, Ernst Kris, and Rudolph M. Loewenstein. 1947. "Notes on the Theory of Aggression." *The Psychoanalytic Study of the Child* 3, no. 1 (1947): 9–36.
Hebbel, Christian Friedrich. (1844) 1914. *Maria Magdalena*. In *The German Classics of the Nineteenth and Twentieth centuries: Masterpieces of German Literature Translated into English*. Translated by Paul Bernard Thomas. Edited by Kuno Francke and William Guild Howard, 22–80. New York: German Publication Society.
Hermann, Imre. 1935. "Das Unbewußte und die Triebe vom Standpunkte einer Wirbeltheorie." *Imago* 21: 412–28.
Holder, Alex, and Christopher Dare. 1982. "Narzißmus, Selbstwertgefühl und Objektbeziehungen." Translated by Heidi Fehlhaber. *Psyche* 36, no. 9 (September): 788–812.
Horkheimer, Max. (1942) 1976. "Vernunft und Selbsterhaltung." In *Subjektivität und Selbsterhaltung: Beiträge zur Diagnose der Moderne*. Edited by Hans Ebeling, 41–75. Frankfurt: Suhrkamp.
Horkheimer, Max. (1955) 2004. "Schopenhauer and Society." Translated by Todd Cronan. *Qui Parle* 15, no. 1: 85–96.
Horkheimer, Max, and Theodor W. Adorno. (1944) 2002. *Dialectic of Enlightenment*. Translated by Edmund Jephcott. Edited by Gunzelin Schmid Noerr. Stanford, CA: Stanford University Press.
Horney, Karen. (1926) 1973. "The Flight from Womanhood: The Masculinity Complex in Women as Viewed by Men and Women." In Horney 1973, 54–70.
Horney, Karen. (1935) 1973. "The Problem of Feminine Masochism." In Horney 1973, 214–33.
Horney, Karen. 1936. "The Problem of the Negative Therapeutic Reaction." *Psychoanalytic Quarterly* 5, no. 1: 29–44.
Horney, Karen. 1973. *Feminine Psychology*. Edited by Harold Kelman. New York: Norton.
Jacobson, Edith. 1964. *The Self and the Object World*. New York: International Universities Press.
Jacoby, Russell. 1975. *Social Amnesia: A Critique of Contemporary Psychology from Adler to Laing*. Piscataway, NJ: Transaction.
Jaspers, Karl. 1966. *Wohin treibt die Bundesrepublik? Tatsachen, Gefahren, Chancen*. Munich: Piper.
Jaspers, Karl. (1966) 1967. *The Future of Germany*. Translated by E. B. Ashton. Chicago, IL: University of Chicago Press.
Jay, Martin. (1976) 1996. *The Dialectical Imagination: A History of the Frankfurt School and the Institute of Social Research 1923–1950*. Berkeley: University of California Press.
Khan, M. Masud R. 1979. *Alienation in Perversions*. New York: International Universities Press.
Kierkegaard, Søren. (1843) 1983. *Fear and Trembling*. Edited and translated by Howard V. Hong and Edna H. Hong. Vol. 6 of *Kierkegaard's Writings*. Princeton, NJ: Princeton University Press.
Kinder, Hermann, ed. (1966) 1980. *dtv-Atlas zur Weltgeschichte*. Munich: dtv.
Klaus, Georg, and Manfred Buhr, eds. (1964) 1972. *Marxistisch-leninistisches Wörterbuch der Philosophie*. Reinbek bei Hamburg: Rowohlt.
König, Marie E. P. 1973. *Am Anfang der Kultur: Die Zeichensprache des frühen Menschen*. Berlin: Mann.

Krafft-Ebing, Richard von. (1886) 2011. *Psychopathia Sexualis: The Case Histories*. Edited and translated by Domino Falls. Washington, DC: Solar Books in Association with Creation Books, 2011.

Kris, Ernst. (1950) 2000. "On Preconscious Mental Processes." In *Psychoanalytic Explorations in Art*. Edited by D. Rapaport, 303–18. New York: International Universities Press, 1952).

Kris, Ernst. 1951. "Some Comments and Observations on Early Autoerotic Activities." *The Psychoanalytic Study of the Child* 6, no. 1: 95–116.

Kristeva, Julia. (1980) 1982. *Powers of Horror: An Essay on Abjection*. Translated by Leon Roudiez. New York: Columbia University Press.

Krystal, Henry, ed. 1968. *Massive Psychic Trauma*. New York: International Universities Press.

Krystal, Henry, and William G. Niederland, eds. 1971. *Psychic Traumatization: Aftereffects in Individuals and Communities*. Boston: Little, Brown.

Kuhn, Thomas S. (1962) 2012. *The Structure of Scientific Revolutions*. Chicago: The University of Chicago Press.

Kurz, Thomas. 2020. "Otto Fenichel, Melanie Klein & Paula Heimann: Eine controversial discussion über Gegenübertragung und Übertragungsdeutung." Lecture at the Psychoanalytisches Seminar Bern, December 11, 2020.

La Boétie, Étienne de. (1574) 1980. *Von der freiwilligen Knechtschaft*. Edited and translated by Horst Günther. Frankfurt: Europäische Verlagsanstalt.

La Boétie, Étienne de. (1574) 2012. *Discourse on Voluntary Servitude*. Translated by James B. Atkinson and David Sices. Indianapolis, IN: Hackett.

Lacan, Jacques. (1959–1960) 1992. *The Ethics of Psychoanalysis 1959–1960: The Seminar of Jacques Lacan, Book VII*. Translated by Dennis Porter. Edited by Jacques-Alain Miller. New York: Norton.

Landauer, Gustav. (1907) 2010. "Revolution." In *Revolution and Other Writings: A Political Reader*. Edited and Translated by Gabriel Kuhn, 110–85. Oakland, CA: PM Press.

Laplanche, Jean, and Jean-Bertrand Pontalis. (1967) 1973. *The Language of Psycho-Analysis*. Translated by Donald Nicholson-Smith. London: Hogarth.

Le Soldat, Judith. 1983. "Freiwillige Knechte. Über Etienne de La Boétie: Von der freiwilligen Knechtschaft." *Der Alltag* 5: 41–45.

Le Soldat, Judith. 1985a. "Diskriminierende Toleranz. Zu einer Kritik an Fritz Morgenthalers Theorie der Homosexualität." *Journal Psychoanalytisches Seminar Zürich* 13: 30–32.

Le Soldat, Judith. 1985b. "Eine Parabel der Macht. Zu Ryszard Kapuscinski: König der Könige." *Neue Zürcher Zeitung*, no. 53: 37.

Le Soldat, Judith. 1986. "Sadismus, Masochismus und Todestrieb. Zum Problem von Sadismus und Masochismus." *Psyche* 40: 617–39.

Le Soldat, Judith. 1989. *Freiwillige Knechtschaft: Masochismus und Moral*. Frankfurt: Fischer.

Le Soldat, Judith. (1989) 2021. *Freiwillige Knechtschaft: Masochismus und Moral*. Edited by Monika Gsell. Stuttgart: Fromann-Holzboog.

Le Soldat, Judith. 1990. "Sozialer Masochismus." In *Schmerz*. Edited by Hans Jürgen Schultz, 248–60. Stuttgart: Kreuz-Verlag.

Le Soldat, Judith. 1993a. "Revenons à nos moutons! Irrungen im Übertragungskonflikt." In *Heilt die Psychoanalyse?* Edited by Brigitte Grossmann-Garger and Walter Parth, 63–71. Vienna: Orac.

Le Soldat, Judith. 1993b. "Kekulés Traum: Ergänzende Betrachtungen zum Benzolring." *Psyche* 47: 180–201.
Le Soldat, Judith. 1994. *Eine Theorie menschlichen Unglücks: Trieb, Schuld, Phantasie* Frankfurt: Fischer.
Le Soldat, Judith. (1994) 2020. *Raubmord und Verrat: Eine Analyse von Freuds Irma-Traum*. A critical edition of *Eine Theorie menschlichen Unglücks*. Edited by Monika Gsell. Judith Le Soldat Werkausgabe 3. Stuttgart: Frommann-Holzboog.
Le Soldat, Judith. 2000. "Der Strich des Apelles: Zwei homosexuelle Leidenschaften." *Psyche* 54: 742–67.
Le Soldat, Judith. 2001. "Kissing & Killing in Kyoto: Unordentliche Liebschaften im Triebwerk des Sadismus." In *Destruktivität: Wurzeln und Gesichter*. Edited by Michael Klöpper and Reinhard Lindner, 109–35. Göttingen: Vandenhoeck & Ruprecht.
Le Soldat, Judith. 2015. *Grund zur Homosexualität: Vorlesungen zu einer neuen psychoanalytischen Theorie der Homosexualität*. Edited by Monika Gsell. Judith Le Soldat Werkausgabe 1. Stuttgart: Fromann-Holzboog.
Le Soldat, Judith. 2018. *Land ohne Wiederkehr: Auf der Suche nach einer neuen psychoanalytischen Theorie der Homosexualität*. Edited by Monika Gsell. Judith Le Soldat Werkausgabe 2. Stuttgart: Fromann-Holzboog.
Le Soldat-Szatmary, Judit. 1973. *Vorstudie zu einem psychoanalytischen Konzept des Wohlbefindens: ein Regulationsmodell auf kybernetischer Grundlage*. Unpublished *Lizentiat* dissertation.
Le Soldat-Szatmary, Judit. 1978. *Wohlbefinden: Entwurf einer psychoanalytischen Theorie und Regulationsmodell*. Unpublished doctoral dissertation, University of Zurich.
Lenin, Vladimir Ilyich. (1902) 2006. "What Is to Be Done?," in *Lenin Rediscovered: What Is to Be Done? in Context*. Translated by Lars T. Lih, 673–840. Leiden: Brill.
Lichtenstein, David. 2019. "A Clinical Instance of the Death Drive in a Child Analysis." *Recherches en psychanalyse* 28, no. 2: 78a–82a.
Lincke, Harold. 1970. "Das Über-Ich – eine gefährliche Krankheit?" *Psyche* 24, no. 5 (May): 375–402.
Lohmann, Hans-Martin. 1983. "Wie harmlos dürfen Psychoanalytiker sein? Notizen zur verdrängten Thanatologie." In *Das Unbehagen in der Psychoanalyse: Eine Streitschrift*. Edited by Hans-Martin Lohmann, 50–59. Frankfurt: Qumran.
Lohmann, Hans-Martin, and Lutz Rosenkötter. 1982 "Psychoanalyse in Hitlerdeutschland: Wie war es wirklich?" *Psyche* 36, no. 11 (November): 961–88.
Löwenthal, Leo. (1945) 1990. "Individuum und Terror." In *Schriften*. Edited by Helmut Dubiel. Vol. 3, 163–74. Frankfurt: Suhrkamp.
Lowenthal, Leo. 1946. "Terror's Atomization of Man." *Commentary* (January): 1–8.
Lu, Xun. (1921) 2009. "The Real Story of Ah-Q." In *The Real Story of Ah-Q and Other Tales of China: The Complete Fiction of Lu Xun*. Translated by Julia Lovell, 79–123. New York: Penguin.
Lukács, Georg. (1922) 2016. Review of Freud 1921. Translated Ross Wolfe. https://thecharnelhouse.org/2016/06/12/early-marxist-criticisms-of-freudian-psychoanalysis-karl-korsch-and-georg-lukacs/
Lukács, Georg. (1923) 1968. *History and Class Consciousness: Studies in Marxist Dialectics*. Translated by Rodney Livingstone. Cambridge, MA: MIT Press.
Lukács, Georg. (1924) 2009. *Lenin: A Study on the Unity of His Thought*. Translated by Nicholas Jacobs. London: Verso.

Lukács, Georg. (1974) 2021. *The Destruction of Reason*. Translated by Peter Palmer. London: Verso.

Mahler, Margaret S., and Manuel Furer. 1968. *On Human Symbiosis and the Vicissitudes of Individuation: Infantile Psychosis*. New York: International Universities Press.

Mao, Tse-Tung. (1946) 1956. "Talk with the American Correspondent Anna Louise Strong." In *Selected Works*. Vol. 5: 1945–1949, 97–101. New York: International Publishers.

Marcuse, Herbert. (1955) 1956. *Eros and Civilization: A Philosophical Inquiry into Freud*. London: Routledge and Kegan Paul.

Marcuse, Herbert. (1956) 1970a. "Freedom and Freud's Theory of Instinct." In Marcuse 1970, 1–27.

Marcuse, Herbert. (1956) 1970b. "Progress and Freud's Theory of Instincts." In Marcuse 1970, 28–43.

Marcuse, Herbert. (1964) 2002. *One-dimensional Man: Studies in the Ideology of Advanced Industrial Society*. Abingdon: Routledge.

Marcuse, Herbert. 1965. "Repressive Tolerance." In *A Critique of Pure Tolerance*. By Robert Paul Wolff, Barrington Moore, and Herbert Marcuse, 81–117. Boston: Beacon Press.

Marcuse, Herbert. 1970. *Five Lectures: Psychoanalysis, Politics, and Utopia*. Translated by Jeremy J. Shapiro and Shierry M. Weber. London: Allen Lane.

Marx, Karl. (1845) 1970. "Theses on Feuerbach." In *The German Ideology*. Edited by C. J. Arthur, 121–23. London: Lawrence & Wishart.

Marx, Karl. (1867) 1990. *Capital: A Critical Analysis of Capitalist Production: London 1887*. In *Karl Marx Friedrich Engels Gesamtausgabe*. Div. 2, vol. 9. Translated by Samuel Moore and Edward Aveling. Edited by Waltraud Falk, Hanna Behrend, Marion Duparré, Hella Hahn, and Frank Zschaler. Berlin: Dietz.

Masserman, Jules H., ed. 1960. *Psychoanalysis and Human Values*, Science and Psychoanalysis 3. New York: Grune & Stratton.

Matteotti, Giacomo. 1924. Speech before the Chamber of Deputies, May 30, 1924. https://it.wikisource.org/wiki/Italia_-_30_maggio_1924,_Discorso_alla_Camera_dei_Deputati_di_denuncia_di_brogli_elettorali

Matz, Friedrich. 1956. *Kreta, Mykene, Troja: Die minoische und die homerische Welt*. Stuttgart: Cotta.

Mitscherlich, Alexander. (1963) 1969. *Society Without the Father: A Contribution to Social Psychology*. Translated by Eric Mosbacher. London: Tavistock.

Mitscherlich, Alexander. (1968) 1969. "Aggression—Spontaneität—Gehorsam." In *Bis hierher und nicht weiter: Ist die menschliche Aggression unbefriedbar?* Ders. (Hg.), 66–103. Munich: Piper.

Mitscherlich, Alexander, and Margarete Mitscherlich. (1967) 1975. *The Inability to Mourn: Principles of Collective Behavior*. Translated by Beverly R. Placzek. New York: Grove Press.

Modell, Arnold H. 1963. "Primitive Object Relationships and the Predisposition to Schizophrenia." *International Journal of Psycho-Analysis* 44, no. 3: 282–92.

Modena, Emilio (2002) 2017. *Mit den Mitteln der Psychoanalyse...* Gießen: Psychosozial-Verlag.

Mommsen, Hans. 2006. "Introduction." In *Eichmann in Jerusalem: Ein Bericht von der Banalität des Bösen*. By Hannah Arendt. Munich: Piper.

Monchy, René de. 1950. "Masochism as a Pathological and as a Normal Phenomenon in the Human Mind." *The International Journal of Psycho-Analysis* 31: 95–97.
Montagu, M. F. Ashley, ed. 1968. *Man and Aggression*. New York: Oxford University Press.
Morgenthaler, Fritz. 1969. "Aspekte der Anwendung der Psychoanalyse." *Jahrbuch der Psychoanalyse* 6: 9–18.
Morgenthaler, Fritz. 1974. "Die Stellung der Perversionen in Metapsychologie und Technik." *Psyche* 28, no. 12 (December): 1077–98.
Morgenthaler, Fritz. (1978) 2020. *On the Dialectics of Psychoanalytic Practice*. Translated by Nils F. Schott. Edited by Dagmar Herzog. London: Routledge.
Morgenthaler, Fritz (1984). *Homosexualität Heterosexualität Perversionen*. Frankfurt a.M.
Morgenthaler, Fritz. 1986. *Der Traum: Fragmente zur Theorie und Technik der Traumdeutung*. Edited by Paul Parin, Goldy Parin-Matthèy, Mario Erdheim, Ralf Binswanger, and Hans-Jürgen Heinrichs. Frankfurt: Campus.
Morgenthaler, Fritz. 2005. *Psychoanalyse, Traum, Ethnologie: Vermischte Schriften*. Edited by Judith Valk, Ralf Binswanger, and Christian Hauser. Gießen: Psychosozial-Verlag.
Moser, Ulrich. 1967. "Die Entwicklung der Objektbesetzung." *Psyche* 21, no. 1–3 (January–March): 97–124.
Moser, Ulrich, and Ilka von Zeppelin. 1973. "The Application of the Simulation Model of Neurotic Defence Mechanisms to the Psychoanalytic Theory of Psychosomatic Illness." Translated by J. Hull *The International Journal of Psychoanalysis* 54, no. 1: 79–84.
Mühsam, Erich. 1929. "Der revolutionäre Mensch Gustav Landauer." *Fanal* 3, no. 8 (May): 169–77.
Nacht, Sacha. 1938. "Le masochisme: Étude historique, clinique, psychogénétique, prophylactique et thérapeutique." *Revue française de psychanalyse* 10, no. 2: 171–291.
Nedelmann, Carl. "Apokalypseblindheit und Psychoanalyse." *Psyche* 36, no. 1 (January): 385–400.
Nietzsche, Friedrich Wilhelm. (1883–1885) 2006. *Thus Spoke Zarathustra: A Book for All and None*. Translated by Adrian del Caro. Edited by Adrian del Caro and Robert Pippin. Cambridge: Cambridge University Press.
Nitzschke, Bernd. 1989. "Marxismus und Psychoanalyse: Historische und aktuelle Aspekte der Marx-Freud-Debatte." *Luzifer–Amor: Zeitschrift zur Geschichte der Psychoanalyse* 2, no. 3: 108–138. Revised version: https://www.werkblatt.at/nitzschke/text/marx.htm
Olinick, Stanley L. 1954. "Some Considerations of the Use of Questioning as a Psychoanalytic Technique." *Journal of the American Psychoanalytic Association* 2, no. 1 (January): 57–66.
Oswald, Bernd. 2010. "Beate Klarsfeld über Filbinger: 'Wenn jemand stirbt, sind seine Verbrechen nicht ausgelöscht." *Süddeutsche Zeitung*. May 17, 2010.
Ottmann, Henning. 1977. *Individuum und Gemeinschaft bei Hegel: Hegel im Spiegel der Interpretationen*. New York: De Gruyter.
Otto, Hans-Uwe, Hans Thiersch, Rainer Treptow, and Holger Ziegler. 2022. *Handbuch Soziale Arbeit: Grundlagen der Sozialarbeit und Sozialpädagogik*. Munich: Reinhardt.
Parin, Paul. (1969) 1978. "Freiheit und Unabhängigkeit: Zur Psychoanalyse des politischen Engagements." In Parin 1978, 20–33.

Parin, Paul. (1973) 1978. "Triebschicksale der Aggression." In Parin 1978, 184–94.
Parin, Paul. 1975. "Is Psychoanalysis a Social Science?" *Annual of Psychoanalysis* 3: 371–93.
Parin, Paul. (1975) 1978. "Gesellschaftskritik im Deutungsprozess." In Parin 1978, 34–54.
Parin, Paul. (1977) 1978. "Das Ich und die Anpassungsmechanismen." In Parin 1978, 78–111.
Parin, Paul. 1977. "[Review of] Richter, Horst-Eberhard: Flüchten oder Standhalten." *Psyche* 31, no. 6 (June): 583–87.
Parin, Paul. 1978. *Der Widerspruch im Subjekt: Ethnopsychoanalytische Studien.* Frankfurt: Syndikat.
Parin, Paul. 1983. "Die therapeutische Aufgabe und die Verleugnung der Gefahr." *Psychosozial* 6, no. 19 (September): 17–30.
Parin, Paul. 2020. *Zurück aus Afrika. Die ethnopsychoanalytische Erweiterung der Psychoanalyse. Schriften 1957–1982.* Vienna: Mandelbaum.
Parin, Paul, Fritz Morgenthaler, and Goldy Parin-Matthèy. (1963) 1972. *Die Weissen denken zuviel: Psychoanalytische Untersuchungen in Westafrika.* Munich: Kindler.
Parin, Paul, Fritz Morgenthaler, and Goldy Parin-Matthey. (1977) 1980. *Fear Thy Neighbor as Thyself: Psychoanalysis and Society Among the Anyi of West Africa.* Translated by Patricia Klamerth. Chicago, IL: University of Chicago Press.
Passett, Peter, and Emilio Modena. 1983. *Krieg und Frieden aus psychoanalytischer Sicht.* Basel: Stroemfeld.
Reich, Wilhelm. (1932) 1938a. "The Masochistic Character." *The Psychoanalytic Review (1913–1957)* 25, no. 3: 218–19.
Reich, Wilhelm. (1932) 1938b. "Concluding Remarks on Bernfeld's Criticism." *The Psychoanalytic Review* 25, no. 3: 220.
Reich, Wilhelm. (1933) 1970. *The Mass Psychology of Fascism.* Translated by Vincent R. Carfagno. New York: Simon and Schuster.
Reiche, Reimut. 1995. "Von innen nach außen? Sackgassen im Diskurs über Psychoanalyse und Gesellschaft." *Psyche* 49, no. 3 (March): 227–58.
Reik, Theodor. (1940) 1941. *Masochism in Modern Man.* Translated by Margaret H. Beigel and Gertrud M. Kurth. New York: Farrar, Straus.
Reik, Theodor. (1948) 1949. *Listening with the Third Ear: The Inner Experience of a Psychoanalyst.* New York: Farrar, Straus, and Giroux.
Richter, Horst-Eberhard. 1976. *Flüchten oder Standhalten.* Reinbek bei Hamburg: Rowohlt.
Richter, Horst-Eberhard. 1983. "Frieden und Psychologie." *Psychosozial* 6, no. 19 (1983): 7–16.
Sacher-Masoch, Leopold von. (1869) 2006. *Venus in Furs.* Translated by Jean McNeil. In Masochism, 141–293. New York: Zone Books.
Sadger, Isidor. 1912. "Haut-, Schleimhaut- und Muskelerotik." *Jahrbuch für Psychoanalyse und psychopathologische Forschungen* 3: 525–56.
Salzman, Leon. 1960. "The Negative Therapeutic Reaction." In Masserman, ed., 1960, 303–13.
Sandkühler, Hans Jörg, ed. 1970. *Psychoanalyse und Marxismus: Dokumentation einer Kontroverse.* Frankfurt: Suhrkamp.
Sandler, Joseph. 1983. "Reflections on Some Relations between Psychoanalytic Concepts and Psychoanalytic Practice." *International Journal of Psycho-Analysis* 64: 35–44.

Sandler, Joseph, and W. G. Joffe. 1966. "On Skill and Sublimation." *Journal of the American Psychoanalytic Association* 14, no. 2: 335–55.

Sandler, Joseph, Christopher Dare, and Alex Holder. (1973) 2018. *The Patient and the Analyst: The Basis of the Psychoanalytic Process*. Revised by Joseph Sandler and rev. Anna Ursula Dreher. London: Routledge.

Schaeffer, Jacqueline. 2018. *The Universal Refusal: A Psychoanalytic Exploration of the Feminine Sphere and Its Repudiation*. London: Routledge.

Scheunert, Gerhart. 1976. "Das masochistische Phantasma als Abwehrmassnahme: Beobachtungen zur Beziehung zwischen psychischem Masochismus, Depression und masochistischer Perversion." *Jahrbuch der Psychoanalyse* 9: 161–73.

Schur, Max. 1966. *The Id and the Regulatory Principles of Mental Functioning*. New York: International Universities Press.

Specht, Ernst Konrad. 1972. "Der Traum des Sokrates." *Psyche* 26, no. 9 (September): 656–88.

Spitz, René A. 1957. *No and Yes: On the Genesis of Human Communication*. New York: International University Press.

Spitz, René A. 1962. "Autoerotism Re-Examined." *The Psychoanalytic Study of the Child* 17, no. 1 (January): 283–315.

Spitz, René A., and W. Godfrey Cobliner. 1965. *The First Year of Life: A Psychoanalytic Study of Normal and Deviant Development of Object Relations*. Madison, CT: International Universities Press.

Stekel, Wilhelm. (1925) 1968. *Sadism and Masochism: The Psychology of Hatred and Cruelty*. Translated by Louise Brink. New York: Washington Square Press.

Storck, Timo. 2020. "100 Jahre Rezeption des Todestriebkonzepts." *Psyche* 74, no. 11 (November): 831–67.

Tausk, Victor. 1951. "On Masturbation." *The Psychoanalytic Study of the Child* 6, no. 1 (January): 61–79.

Tolstoi, Leo N. 1910. *La Loi de l'Amour et la Loi de la Violence*. Paris: Dorbon aine (1 janvier 1910).

Torok, Maria. (1964) 1985. "The Significance of Penis Envy in Women." In Chasseguet-Smirgel, ed., 1985, 135–70.

Torok, Maria. 1968. "Maladie du deuil et fantasme du cadavre exquis." *Revue française de psychanalyse* 32, no. 4: 715–33.

Tsolas, Vaia, and Christine Anzieu-Premmereur, eds. 2023. *A Psychoanalytic Exploration of the Contemporary Search for Pleasure: The Turning of the Screw*. London: Routledge.

Weiss, Edoardo. 1935. *Todestrieb und Masochismus*. Imago 21, no. 4: 393–411.

Wheeler, William Morton. 1920. "On Instincts." *The Journal of Abnormal Psychology* 15, no. 5–6: 295–318.

Willard, Clara. 1939. "Hermann, Imre. The Unconscious and the Instincts from the Standpoint of a Vortex Theory." *Imago: Psychoanalytic Review* 26: 412.

Winnicott, Donald W. 1953. "Transitional Objects and Transitional Phenomena: A Study of the First Not-Me Possession." *International Journal of Psycho-Analysis* 34, no. 2: 89–97.

Index

Note: Page numbers followed by "n" denote endnotes.

Abraham, Karl 135
Adorno, Theodor W. 106, 107, 163
aggression/aggressiveness 71; alliance of 17; biological drive 71; defense against 110–11; destructive power of 68; early invasion of 181, 202–3; energies 13, 15; existence of free 212; explication of 19, 98; explicit theory 65–6; fission product 15; frustration 31, 67, 69, 177; genital 211–13, 242, 269; idealized 18; internalization of 54–5, 57, 168, 217, 238, 247, 251, 253, 261, 267, 281; liberated 75; and libido, relationship between 11–12, 17–18, 26, 177–8, 187, 201, 207, 252, 257, 281–4, 287n3; and morality 82; non-erotic 66; origin of 60, 193; pleasurable 32–3, 55, 121, 283; and power 71; problem of 19, 54, 217; psychoanalytic theory of 100; pulsional 7–8, 57, 63, 66, 71, 80, 87, 96, 98, 100, 101, 114, 122, 163, 188; reified 92; and sexuality, disentanglement of 57, 75, 87, 219–21, 285–6; social 63, 71, 73; superego's 260; tendency 34
aggression drive 7, 13, 28, 32–3, 37, 45n87; after oedipal internalization 259; causes and consequences 93; detour of superego 57; direct observation of 100; discovery of 53; genital excitation 269; goals of power 55; innate 72; internal agency 259; sovereignty of 111; success of 54
aggressive cathexes 16–17, 170n7, 178–80, 189, 206, 207, 210–12, 238, 241–2, 252, 283, 284

ambivalence 7, 143, 178, 203–4, 219–20, 251, 259, 262, 285–6; absence of 217, 225n10, 231, 275; conflict 208; of drives 56–7, 115, 169, 183, 225n10; emotional 132, 188; normal pulsional ambivalence 183; ordinary 187, 190n17; of repressed pulsional wishes 133, 134n10; of sadism 208; tension 187, 204, 208, 217–18, 231–2, 275
Amigorena, Horatio 162
amnesia 244, 272; collective 31, 61; infantile 41n26, 261; social 5, 30, 53, 58n3, 61, 82, 83n5, 156, 286–7
anger 131, 141, 170n8, 179, 185, 208, 234, 235, 242, 256, 263n11
anxiety 11; affects 136, 167, 185, 202, 274; with aggression 252; automatic 203; castration 11–13, 15, 116, 137, 141, 146, 167, 168, 170n7, 179, 192, 199n3, 205, 211–13, 214n8, 217, 231, 238, 240–2, 247, 248n3, 250–3, 259, 261, 262, 265–8, 271–5, 287; disavowal of 93; of ego 214n4, 224n6; genital 212, 275; and guilt 228, 232, 262; infantile 169, 274; neurotic 95n10; and pain 193; panic-like states 174; and pleasure 224n6; and power 100, 153; preoedipal 270, 272; pressure of 85; pulsional 43n45, 126n45, 147, 185–6, 213, 259, 261, 270; realistic 69, 88n4; and shame 208–9; as signal 88n4, 90, 93, 202–3, 224n6; signs of illness 136; unconscious 271, 277n9; unpleasure of 92–3, 155, 196, 209, 212; and wish 136, 141, 167
Arendt, Hannah 82

authoritarianism 86, 168
autocastration 141

Beradt, Charlotte 272
Beyond the Pleasure Principle (Freud) 38, 66, 117, 119, 193
border-crossing 22, 26, 42n39, 43n41, 43n50, 43n51
Borkenau, Franz 268
Bourke-White, Margaret 289
Busch, Günther 9

castration 144; anxieties 12, 13, 15, 116, 137, 141, 146, 167, 168, 170n7, 179, 192, 199n3, 205, 211–13, 214n8, 217, 231, 238, 240–2, 247, 248n3, 250–3, 259, 261, 262, 265–8, 271–5, 287; autocastration 141; endogenous 234; of the father 14–15; masturbatory self- 11, 14–16, 18, 206–7; pain as punishment 14, 141; phantasy 136, 164, 261, 266, 269, 270; revenge for 132–3; threat of 8, 12, 14, 167, 174, 205, 207, 234, 242, 248n3, 253, 258, 260–2, 267, 269, 277n16, 278n18, 279, 281, 284
cathexes: aggressive 16–17, 170n7, 178–80, 189, 206, 207, 210–12, 238, 241–2, 252, 283, 284; defense 174, 201; as defiance 188; displacement of 12, 61, 218–20, 224n4, 236, 238, 241, 243, 245, 247, 252, 277n9, 287n4, 288n6; of ego 189, 197; energy 185, 186, 231, 259, 284; of erogenous zones of body 208; of the father 12–13; of genitals 141, 170n7, 179, 182, 212–13; investment of 184; libidinous 16, 17, 183–4, 186, 211, 243, 259; of the mother 13; narcissistic 203; neurotic 14; object 13, 40n6, 175, 196, 201, 231, 232, 252, 259; psychical 90; pulsional 174, 182, 189, 224n6, 227, 259; quality of 141; sexual 207, 220; of tongue or teeth 212; of wishful phantasy 204; withdrawal 254
Civilization and Its Discontents (Freud) 65, 74, 96
collective amnesia 31, 61
collectively unconscious 29, 97
consciousness 7, 32, 53–5, 60–3, 90, 100, 130, 132, 160–1, 169, 172–3, 181–2, 201–2, 219, 221, 240, 241, 243, 250, 258, 260, 261, 272, 276, 280; class 73; false 121, 243; historical 70; subjective 56, 175; and unconscious 174, 204
countercathexis 41n26, 167, 175n4, 185, 211, 218, 228, 244, 254, 260, 261, 263n5, 282, 287n4

Dahmer, Helmut 27, 28, 30
death drive 28, 117–18, 120–1, 146–7; destruction drive 66, 104; Freud's concept of 39, 42n39, 65, 151, 172, 194; Le Soldat's conception 37–9; and Nirvana principle 119, 125n32; principle of 88n6, 89n6, 106, 191–223, 226, 230; the self 123
desire: to cause pain 114; for destruction 66; love object 135, 138n5, 172, 235, 251, 266; for pleasure 124; sexual 140, 228; tyrant 158
destruction (drive) 65–6, 100, 120, 123–4
disavowal 32–3, 58n4, 63, 64n3, 91–3, 94n2, 156, 259–60, 265, 272, 275; of anxiety 93; of danger 85, 100, 104; of death 205; of the dependence 281; of injustices committed 80; of objective 92; of pulsional source 60–1; socials 287; subjective 45n72, 146; techniques of 185; of threat of nuclear war 67
Discourse de le servitude volontaire (La Boétie) 158–62, 164, 287
drive binding and unbinding (disentangling) 14, 68, 204, 207, 219–20, 276, 286
drive discharge 197
Drives and Their Vicissitudes (Freud) 114
drive short-circuit 121–2
Dutschke, Rudi 289
dynamically unconscious 184–5, 260, 263n5

ego 13, 176–8; adult 167; auxiliary 18, 185; child's 260; defense structures in 183; erotic 38; functions in 100, 188–9, 203, 235, 258, 261; gravitation 196; hostility of 259; and id 24, 39, 119, 174, 194, 195, 197–8, 199n12, 202, 238; of "kitchen fairy" 257–8, 283; masochism of 122, 146, 188, 258, 259, 262; as narcissism 196; pleasure 186; sadistic 100, 122, 141; structure 156, 173, 193, 198,

201, 203, 213, 239n12; and superego 148, 166, 172, 175n4, 203, 258, 260, 266, 270
The Ego and the Id (Freud) 38, 117, 121, 166, 185, 193
Einstein, Albert 74, 92
Eissler, Kurt R. 18, 67
Engels, Friedrich 36
Erdheim, Mario 29, 31
erogenous zones 17, 183–6, 203–4, 208, 210, 212, 221, 240, 273, 282–3
excitation: of aggressive phantasies 186; erotic 284; genital 233–4, 269, 274, 283; infantile 266; of pain 120, 144; physical 186, 189n7, 213, 245, 265, 274; pleasant 227; pulsional 211; qualitative 184; quantity 201; sensorial 17, 109, 184, 283, 284; sexual 61, 116, 119, 120, 140–1, 171, 182, 192, 213, 234–6, 281; somatic 282, 284; violent 62; wished-for course 184, 222

fascism 34, 69, 86, 96, 98–9
Faust (Goethe) 227–9, 230
feminine masochism 22, 102n13, 116, 119–20, 250
Fenichel, Otto 33–5, 37–9, 67, 71, 96–9, 285
"fore-pleasure" 265, 276n1
Frankfurt School 27, 99
freedom 53, 74, 81, 92, 104, 159–60, 202, 245, 269, 275, 281, 286; vs. drive (unconscious pulsional strivings) 105, 284; love of 159
Freud, Anna 62, 93
Freud, Sigmund 7–8, 16, 18, 30–2, 53–4, 66, 68–70, 72–3, 86, 97, 99–101, 115–21, 124, 146–7, 149, 151, 172, 176–7, 198, 223, 226–7, 232; *Beyond the Pleasure Principle* 38, 66, 117, 119, 193; *Civilization and Its Discontents* 65, 74, 96; culture-critical writings 27, 75, 105; death drive hypothesis 38, 39, 194, 230; *Drives and Their Vicissitudes* 114; *The Ego and the Id* 38, 117, 121, 166, 185, 193; feminine masochism 119; *Group Psychology and the Analysis of the Ego* 74; "Instincts and Their Vicissitudes" 37; *The Interpretation of Dreams* 109–14, 120, 152; "non vixit" 58n4; posthumous writings 260–1; *premises* 123; self-destruction drive 65; theory of aggressiveness 65; *Thoughts for the Times on War and Death* 74; *Three Essays on the Theory of Sexuality* 113; *Why War?* 74
Friedrich, Jörg 80

genital aggression 211–13, 242, 269
Goethe, Johann Wolfgang 227
Group Psychology and the Analysis of the Ego (Freud) 74
guilt 30, 34; affect 75, 80, 85, 209, 212, 232, 258, 261, 270, 274; conflicts 227, 235, 244, 260, 274; defense against 134n8, 258; feelings of 8, 34, 44n68, 57, 62, 63, 88n5, 93, 99–100, 112, 141, 143–4, 153–4, 163, 173, 217, 236, 244, 257–8; and morality 55; parricide 270, 271; repression of 80–1; sadism 55; sense of 30, 55, 62, 98, 116–17, 119, 121–2, 136, 168, 169, 222, 244, 261–2, 269, 270, 272, 284, 287; unconscious sense of 62, 244

Hartmann, Heinz 176, 177
hatred 67, 85, 171, 178, 203–4, 218, 219, 240, 251–3, 255
Hebbel, Christian Friedrich 237
heterosexuality 251, 253, 273; becoming 19–22; love choice 135; object choice 241, 245; position of women 243; symptom formations 23
Hiroshima 86, 92, 118
homosexuality 4n4, 14, 23–4, 111, 113, 116, 137, 141, 192, 204, 253, 256, 273–4; aging 139; becoming 19–22; cure 8; discrimination of 37; female 241, 247n2, 249n9, 262n2; male 241, 243, 262n2, 283; and masochism 116; position of men 243; questions of 262n2; symptom formations 23
hypercathexes 195
hysteria 84, 151, 170n7, 235, 248n3, 248n5, 270

id: autoeroticism 275; centrifugal forces in 197, 226, 228; and ego 24, 39, 119, 174, 194, 195, 197–8, 199n12, 202, 238; energy reservoir in 194; gravitation 196–7, 226, 228; great reservoir of libido 218; pulsional forces 173, 183, 193–4, 197; and reality 223
idealized aggressiveness 18

identifications 155, 164, 171–2, 176, 180, 192; with the aggressor 7, 31, 60–4, 69, 86, 93, 94n6, 106, 147, 163, 168, 238, 244, 264n14; ego 236–8, 243, 275; object of 230–8; particularity of 144, 145n3; with victim of one's own hostility 147, 205
infantile amnesia 41n26, 261
infantile change of object 250
infantile depression 188, 191
infantile masochistic neurosis 188–9, 257
infantile masturbation 119, 182, 200, 201, 254, 285
infantile Oedipus complex 135, 281
infantile pulsional demands 266, 271
infantile sexuality 32, 132, 134n11
"intermediate realm," metaphor of: between individual and society 5, 27–9, 32–7, 44n57; between psychoanalysis and Marxism 28–9
internalized homophobia 37
The Interpretation of Dreams (Freud) 109–14, 120, 152
introjection 42n40, 56, 58n8, 70, 145n3, 147, 164, 168, 170n5, 195, 238, 242, 251, 253, 260

Jacoby, Russell 31, 70
Jaspers, Karl 82
Jensen, Wilhelm 114

La Boétie, Étienne de: *Discourse de le servitude volontaire* 158–62, 164, 287
Landauer, Gustav 153, 160
Le Soldat, Judith 2–3, 47; conception of death drive 37–9; fundamental positions 32–3; individual and society 27–8, 34–7; masochism concept 11–14; nuclei of later theory 14–27; psychoanalysis and Marxism, contradiction between 28–32; real problem of masochism 14; theory of "border crossing" 21–2, 25
liberated aggression 75
libido 284; and aggression 11–12, 17–18, 25–7, 40n6, 177–8, 187, 201, 207, 252, 257, 281–4, 287n3; cathexes 13, 16, 17, 183–4, 186, 211, 243, 259; and death drive 120–1, 123; energies 11–12, 15, 16, 173, 183, 201, 208, 220, 243; the "Eros" 194; and id 218; and masochism 123; pulsional qualities 17, 39n4, 56, 67, 112, 114, 217; sexual 7–8, 39, 68, 87, 118, 188, 194, 207, 221, 285–7
live drive *vs.* death drive (Nirvana) 118–19, 146–7, 199n9, 223; *see also* death drive
love: choice 135, 247; disappointment 13; early love for the mother 20, 42n36; forbidden 111, 235, 254; of freedom 159; frustrated 235; great 191; and hatred 203–4, 218–19, 253; homoerotic love for the father 42n28, 253; for mother 20, 180, 243, 248n3; object 12, 17, 19–20, 55, 58n8, 111, 121, 135, 138n5, 141, 153, 167, 172, 175n2, 180, 192, 205, 224n1, 231, 237, 239n11, 240–3, 246, 247, 247n2, 248n3, 251; oedipal love for the mother 12, 20; sexual 53, 117
Löwenthal, Leo 92, 160, 162, 164
Lukács, Georg 32, 33, 73

Marcuse, Herbert 86, 88
Marxism: defined 30; and psychoanalysis, relationship between 27–32
Marx, Karl 31
masochism 65–6; aggression, problem of 217; castration anxiety 242; and death drive 192–3, 223; defined 116; of ego 122; erogenous 120, 122, 284; feminine 119, 250; genuine 122; and homosexuality 116; individual-psychological 7; Le Soldat's theory 21–2; masturbation 282; masturbation, problem of 15; moral 117, 120–4; neurotic 9, 155, 192–3, 214n7, 285–6; Oedipus theory 15, 16, 224n1; passive counterpart 114; and pleasure principle 119; primary 114; problem of 14, 116–19, 125n39, 133, 188; psychosexual syndrome 5, 11–27; quantitative burden 212; and sadism 117, 120–1; secondary 114, 122; and sex 243, 285; social exploitation of 9, 152; symptom of social force 5, 27, 36; voluntary servitude 9, 101; and women 240, 245, 251
masochistic ego *vs.* sadism 258–9
masturbation 8, 11, 55, 233–6, 280–1; in adulthood 200; aggressive 213,

241; commanding dependence on 281; definitive prohibition on 204; drumming 137, 235; genital 237, 282; infantile 119, 182, 200, 201, 254, 285; masochistic development problem 14, 213, 240; obsessive 213; phantasies 136, 141, 180–2, 208, 240–1, 253, 262, 265, 281, 283; pleasurable 254, 256, 284; problem of 15, 19; taboo 11, 14, 15, 22, 281, 282; unsuccessful 237–8
Mitscherlich, Alexander 33, 67
moral masochism 117, 123; *see also* masochism
Morgenthaler, Fritz 232, 289

narcissism 115, 124n15, 196
Nazism 8, 44n68, 81–2, 86, 102n14, 272
need for punishment 117, 121, 123, 279–80
negation 138n4, 193, 198, 236, 278n18
negative oedipal outcome 42n29, 135, 243–4, 246, 249n7
negative therapeutic reaction 121
Newton, Isaac 92
Nietzsche, Friedrich Wilhelm 229n2
Nirvana principle 118–19, 125n32, 146–7, 199n9, 223
nuclear threat 8, 35, 84, 99

object cathexes 13, 40n6, 175, 196, 201, 231, 232, 252, 259
Oedipus complex: beginning of 15; central theorem of 19; characteristic of 14; demise of 13, 25; feminine change of object 22–3; girls' "common" change of object 22; infantile 135; masochistic 13–14; morality to 122
Oppenheimer, Robert 104
oppression 9, 28, 31–4, 71, 75, 87, 97, 101, 153, 159–61, 165, 276

pain 131; of death 274; excitation of 120; influence of 193; physical 14; as punishment for castration 14, 141; rituals 14; sadism 114; and suffering 100; unavoidable 279–87; unpleasure 284, 288n5
Parin, Paul 3, 9, 27, 33, 36, 67, 70, 100
perversion 149; active and passive forms 113; masochism 5, 32, 113, 116; sexual 60, 66, 102n13, 280, 285

pleasure: affect 81, 87n4, 184, 197, 224n6, 245; aggression as 32–3, 58n4, 85, 87n4, 283; and anxiety 170n7, 202, 224n6; attainment of 57; desire for 124; and duration 226–9; ego 186, 259; "end-pleasure" 276n1; "fore-pleasure" 265, 276n1; of functioning 188; gain 181, 183, 184, 186, 206–7, 209, 212–13, 217–19, 221–2, 237, 259, 281, 282, 284–5; masochistic 14, 119, 265, 280, 282; masturbation 254, 256, 284; pulsional 34, 56, 98, 100, 194, 213, 274; quality of 207, 223, 232, 236, 244, 276; sexual 67, 114, 137, 208, 240, 280; sources 182; and suffering 151
pleasure principle: *vs. Beyond the Pleasure Principle* 38, 42n39, 66, 117–19, 193; within individuals 107; and masochism 118; origin of aggression 60
preoedipal anxiety 270, 272
projections 8, 12, 13, 42n40, 58n8, 62, 81, 176, 182, 185, 259–60, 270, 275; of aggression 186, 242, 248n5, 252, 253; of childhood 63, 86; group 29, 97, 141; of shame 209; superego 145n3, 168
psyche *vs.* culture/socio-political forces 36
psychoeconomics 2, 63, 91, 107, 157n11, 194, 252, 257
pulsional cathexes 174, 182, 189, 224n6, 227, 259
pulsional defense 115, 144, 164, 174, 194, 271–2
punishment 171, 181–2, 208, 269, 276; dreams of 110, 112–13; fears of 141; need for 117, 121, 123, 279–80; pain as 14, 141, 284; self-punishment 114, 153, 257; threats of 55, 147, 253; unconscious expectations of 32, 62, 69, 111

rape 133, 137, 144, 270
reaction formation 147, 205, 254
reality principle 12, 36, 77n15, 118, 125n32, 167, 176, 194, 223, 243, 246–7, 250–2
recathexis 12–13, 40n6, 141, 209, 240–1, 243–7, 248n3, 250–4, 260, 263n3, 281
Reich, Wilhelm 37, 80, 96, 101

Reik, Theodor 68, 101, 276
repression 32, 60, 64n3, 91, 168, 174, 176, 185, 188, 196, 204, 207, 217–19, 236, 238, 241, 244–7, 250, 253–4, 260–2, 265, 281; and drive 83n3; of emotional isolation 13, 20; of guilt-affect 55, 80, 81; of pulsional forces 73; of sadism 120; of sexual phantasies (castration) 164; by superego 210

Sacher-Masoch, Leopold von 148
sadism 6, 28, 65–6, 68, 75, 85, 87; fights against 84, 111, 208; oral 238; originary 121, 139, 146, 267; pair of opposites 114; psychical 54; of superego 122, 258; transformation into masochism 114–15, 117, 120, 123; unsatisfied 55
satisfaction: aggressive 58n4, 71, 81, 87, 168, 182, 183, 185, 186, 190n9, 194, 213, 221, 228, 258, 262, 274, 286; bodily 17, 279; genital 170n7, 181, 184, 234, 236, 242, 266, 283; instinctual 73, 261; libidinous 123, 183, 228; physical 17, 147, 164, 184, 185, 196–7, 203, 208, 213, 219, 221–2, 224n7, 227, 282; pleasurable 9, 14, 42n8, 57n206, 124, 253; pulsional 17, 43n51, 55, 57, 60, 87n4, 96, 124, 188, 193, 196–7, 202, 209, 213, 218, 222–3, 227, 257, 259, 262, 264n16, 265, 271, 274–5, 285–7; sexual 124, 135, 140, 201, 221, 279, 284
Schmutzer, Ferdinand 289
secondary masochism 122
self-castration 11, 14–16, 18, 206–7
sexual cathexes 207, 220
sexual desire 140, 228
sexual difference 8, 12, 15–16, 41n27, 132, 167, 178, 181, 200, 212, 217, 241, 243, 248n5, 250, 256, 265, 267–8, 271, 273, 278n18, 281
sexuality 6; and aggression, disentanglement of 53–7, 75, 87, 219–21, 285–6; drumming 234; energy of 60; infantile 32; libidinous theory 99; masochistic 111; passive 17, 210; perversion 60, 66, 102n13, 280, 285; pulsional vicissitudes of 65, 124, 193
sexual libido 7–8, 39, 68, 87, 118, 188, 194, 207, 221, 285–7

sexual love 53, 117
sexual violence 140
shame 8, 57, 131, 136, 156, 165, 172, 179–80, 200, 208–10, 223, 234, 252, 272, 284
social amnesia 5, 30, 53, 58n3, 61, 82, 83n5, 156, 286–7
socially corrupted psyche/drive 176
social production of unconscious 5, 29, 64n3
somatization: excitation 282–4; instinctual source 37; psyche- 163, 279; pulsional source 61, 185, 196–8, 207, 210, 224n7; relaxation 282; theory of neuroses 279
Spitz, René A. 62
subjective factor 28–30, 36, 64, 99, 105, 154, 163–5, 287
superego 8, 82, 86, 88n5, 141, 171–2, 195–6, 210–11, 250; agency of conscience 57; of child 83n6, 90, 167; defense process 173, 181, 185; and ego 148, 172, 175n4, 203, 258, 260, 266, 270; establishment of 13, 168, 254, 263n5; feeling of guilt 63, 117; function of 166, 170n1; identification 243; influence of 204; masochistic 172, 204, 218, 253, 254, 259; motivation 113; preautonomous 178; problem 147; prohibitions 221, 256, 279; to protect consciousness 55; psychical agency 54; pulsional forces 188–9; and reality 221; sadistic 32, 121–2, 146, 237; threats of 169; two-fold mechanism 168; tyrannical agency 162; see also ego

Thoughts for the Times on War and Death (Freud) 74
Three Essays on the Theory of Sexuality (Freud) 113
totalitarianism 162

the uncanny 85, 227
unconscious 45n74; aggressive 81–2, 110, 117, 130, 169; anxiety 271, 277n9; collectively 29, 97; conflicts 71–2, 130, 136, 280; and consciousness 204; dynamically 184–5, 260, 263n5; expectations of punishment 32, 69; impulse experiences 245–6; of individuals 8, 61, 97, 154, 220; phantasies 8, 57, 117, 130, 169, 199n3,

201, 204, 269, 271, 273, 277n6; pleasure-seeking 60; powerless conflicts 71, 72; primary activity of 109; psychical processes 30, 69, 246, 250; rescue 132; sense of guilt 62, 144, 163, 217, 244; social production of 5, 29, 64n3; states of affairs 105; *see also* consciousness

Vignar, Marcel 162
violence 54–5, 75, 81, 87, 91, 97, 98, 100, 246, 268, 270, 276; collaborators of 160; in ego 147; external 161; internalizing 287; in masochism 19; open 162; of originary sadism 267; physical 33, 63, 71, 272; psychical 33, 71, 132; sexual 140; social 275; threats of 154; victim of 132
voluntary servitude 243, 245; collaborators of violence 160; on double internal mechanism 100; *vs.* freedom 158–60; habit 160; oppression 159–60; political dominion 158; psychological causes of 160; question of 34, 99; sociological theory of 7, 8; subjective factor 287; as symptom of oppression 9; and violence 161; *see also* masochism

Why War? (Freud) 74
wish(es): and anxiety 136, 141, 167; cathexes of phantasy 204; excitation 184, 222; fulfillment 57, 60, 68, 75, 90, 110, 112, 131, 171, 184, 192, 195, 203, 208, 210, 222, 227, 232, 236, 259, 267, 274, 282, 285–6; genital 11, 15, 16, 18, 135–7, 141, 180, 182, 211, 262; incestuous 13, 133, 167, 231, 232, 240, 242, 244, 246–7, 251, 253–4, 260–2, 269–70, 274–5, 281; oedipal 122, 132, 136, 153, 169, 232, 244, 259, 274; pulsional 8–9, 16–17, 19, 21, 32, 35, 67, 69, 80, 87, 93, 98, 105, 114–17, 119, 123, 133, 134n10, 164, 166–8, 173–4, 177, 183–5, 195, 196, 200, 202, 207, 211, 220, 222, 231, 236, 241, 242, 252, 260, 262, 279, 287; sexual 13, 57, 116, 135–6, 140–1, 169, 181, 186, 207, 209, 220, 250, 261, 265–6, 269–71, 274, 276, 283
World Wars 32, 75, 255

Made in the USA
Columbia, SC
20 December 2024

c7d7d598-27e8-45fa-8b29-67f526715575R01